Williams
OBSTETRICS
STUDY GUIDE

NOTICE

Medicine is an ever-changing science. As new research and clinical experience broaden our knowledge, changes in treatment and drug therapy are required. The authors and the publisher of this work have checked with sources believed to be reliable in their efforts to provide information that is complete and generally in accord with the standards accepted at the time of publication. However, in view of the possibility of human error or changes in medical sciences, neither the authors nor the publisher nor any other party who has been involved in the preparation or publication of this work warrants that the information contained herein is in every respect accurate or complete, and they disclaim all responsibility for any errors or omissions or for the results obtained from use of the information contained in this work. Readers are encouraged to confirm the information contained herein with other sources. For example and in particular, readers are advised to check the product information sheet included in the package of each drug they plan to administer to be certain that the information contained in this work is accurate and that changes have not been made in the recommended dose or in the contraindications for administration. This recommendation is of particular importance in connection with new or infrequently used drugs.

Williams
OBSTETRICS
STUDY GUIDE
24th Edition

Robyn Horsager, MD
Holder, Luis Leib, MD Professorship in Obstetrics and Gynecology
Chief, Obstetrics and Gynecology
University Hospital St. Paul
Professor
Department of Obstetrics and Gynecology
University of Texas Southwestern Medical Center at Dallas

Scott W. Roberts, MD
Medical Director, High-Risk Obstetrical Unit
Parkland Hospital
Professor
Department of Obstetrics and Gynecology
University of Texas Southwestern Medical Center at Dallas

Vanessa L. Rogers, MD
Director, Obstetrics and Gynecology Residency Program
Associate Professor
Department of Obstetrics and Gynecology
University of Texas Southwestern Medical Center at Dallas

Patricia C. Santiago-Muñoz, MD
Associate Professor
Department of Obstetrics and Gynecology
University of Texas Southwestern Medical Center at Dallas

Kevin C. Worley, MD
Associate Director, Obstetrics and Gynecology Residency Program
Assistant Professor
Department of Obstetrics and Gynecology
University of Texas Southwestern Medical Center at Dallas

Barbara L. Hoffman, MD
Associate Professor
Department of Obstetrics and Gynecology
University of Texas Southwestern Medical Center at Dallas

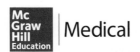

New York   Athens   Chicago   San Francisco   London   Madrid   Mexico City
Milan   New Delhi   Singapore   Sydney   Toronto

Williams Obstetrics Study Guide, 24th edition

Copyright © 2015 by McGraw-Hill Education. All rights reserved.
Printed in China. Except as permitted under the United States
Copyright Act of 1976, no part of this publication may be reproduced or distributed in any form or by any means, or stored in a
data base or retrieval system, without the prior written permission of
the publisher.

1 2 3 4 5 6 7 8 9 0 CTP/CTP 19 18 17 16 15 14

ISBN 978-0-07-179327-8
MHID 0-07-179327-5

This book was set in Adobe Garamond Pro by Aptara, Inc.
The editors were Alyssa Fried and Cindy Yoo.
The production supervisor was Richard Ruzycka.
Project management was provided by Amit Kashyap.
The cover designer was Thomas De Pierro.
China Translation and Printing Services, Ltd., was printer and
binder.

This book is printed on acid-free paper.

McGraw-Hill Education books are available at special quantity
discounts to use as premiums and sales promotions or for use in
corporate training programs. To contact a representative, please visit
the Contact Us pages at www.mhprofessional.com.

International Edition ISBN 978-1-259-25556-4; MHID 1-259-25556-5.
Copyright © 2015. Exclusive rights by McGraw-Hill Education for
manufacture and export. This book cannot be re-exported from the
country to which it is consigned by McGraw-Hill Education. The
International Edition is not available in North America.

DEDICATION

During our training and careers, we have had the privilege to learn from many of the great physicians in the fields of obstetrics and reproductive medicine. These giants taught us the importance of basing clinical care on good scientific evidence—decades before the phrases "evidence-based medicine" and "best practices" became part of the medical lexicon. They inspired us to be logical, meticulous, curious, and courageous. With great admiration and appreciation, we dedicate this edition of our *Williams Obstetrics Study Guide* to our heroes: Jack Pritchard, Paul McDonald, Peggy Whalley, Norman Gant, Ken Leveno, and Gary Cunningham.

Robyn Horsager
Scott W. Roberts
Vanessa L. Rogers
Patricia C. Santiago-Muñoz
Kevin C. Worley
Barbara L. Hoffman

CONTENTS

SECTION 4

PRECONCEPTIONAL AND PRENATAL CARE

SECTION 5

THE FETAL PATIENT

SECTION 6

EARLY PREGNANCY COMPLICATIONS

SECTION 7

LABOR

SECTION 8

DELIVERY

SECTION 9

THE NEWBORN

SECTION 10

THE PUERPERIUM

SECTION 11

OBSTETRICAL COMPLICATIONS

SECTION 12

MEDICAL AND SURGICAL COMPLICATIONS

PREFACE

The *Williams Obstetrics 24th Edition Study Guide* is designed to assess comprehension and retention of information presented in *Williams Obstetrics*, 24th edition. The questions for each section have been selected to emphasize the key points from each chapter. In total, nearly 2100 questions have been created from the 65 chapters. Questions are in a multiple-choice format, and one single best answer should be chosen for each. With this edition, we have also included more than 250 full-color images as question material. In addition, clinical case questions have been added to test implementation of content learned. At the end of each chapter, answers are found, and a page guide directs readers to the section of text that contains the answer. We hope that our clinical approach to this guide translates into a more accurate test of important clinical knowledge.

Robyn Horsager
Scott W. Roberts
Vanessa L. Rogers
Patricia C. Santiago-Muñoz
Kevin C. Worley
Barbara L. Hoffman

OVERVIEW

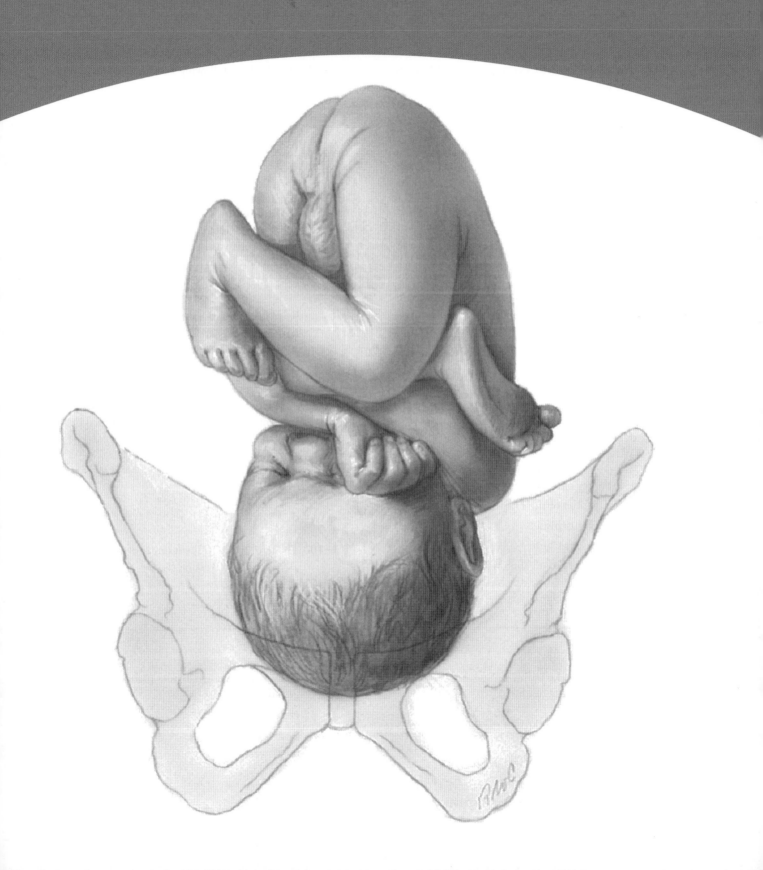

CHAPTER 1

Overview of Obstetrics

1–1. The field of obstetrics encompasses all **EXCEPT** which of the following?

  a. Prenatal care

  b. Management of labor

  c. Infertility treatments

  d. Immediate newborn care

1–2. Registration of live births is currently assigned to which national agency?

  a. Bureau of the Census

  b. National Institutes of Health

  c. National Center for Health Statistics

  d. Department of Health and Human Services

1–3. How does the National Vital Statistics System, using data from the National Center for Health Statistics, define fetal death for its reports?

  a. Fetal weight > 350 g

  b. Fetal weight > 500 g

  c. Gestational age > 20 weeks

  d. Gestational age > 24 weeks

1–4. The perinatal period starts after delivery at 20 weeks' gestation or older. When does it end?

  a. 7 days after birth

  b. 1 year after birth

  c. 28 days after birth

  d. 1 calendar month after birth

1–5. Which of the following is synonymous with fetal death rate?

  a. Stillbirth rate

  b. Perinatal death rate

  c. Spontaneous abortion rate

  d. Early neonatal death rate

1–6. At the state level, which of the following is used to define fetal death?

  a. Fetal death > 20 weeks' gestation

  b. Fetal death with a birthweight of ≥ 500 g

  c. Any fetal death regardless of gestational age

  d. Each has been used

1–7. Which of the following is defined as the sum of stillbirths and neonatal deaths per 1000 total births?

  a. Fetal death rate

  b. Neonatal mortality rate

  c. Perinatal mortality rate

  d. None of the above

1–8. A patient presents at 22 weeks' gestation with spontaneous rupture of membranes and delivers a 489-g male infant who dies at 4 hours of life. Her last menstrual period and early sonographic evaluation confirm her gestational dating. All **EXCEPT** which of the following definitions accurately apply to this delivery?

  a. Abortus

  b. Preterm neonate

  c. Early neonatal death

  d. Extremely low birthweight

1–9. A death of a newborn at 5 days of life due to congenital heart disease would be counted in which of the following rates?

  a. Infant mortality rate

  b. Perinatal mortality rate

  c. Early neonatal death rate

  d. All of the above

1–10. The fertility rate is the number of live births per 1000 females of what age?

  a. 9–39 years

  b. 11–55 years

  c. 15–44 years

  d. 18–49 years

1–11. Delivery at what age divides preterm from term gestations?

  a. 34 weeks

  b. 36 weeks

  c. 37 weeks

  d. 38 weeks

1–12. Which of the following is an example of an indirect maternal death?

   a. Septic shock following an abortion

   b. Aspiration following an eclamptic seizure

   c. Hemorrhage following a ruptured ectopic pregnancy

   d. Aortic rupture at 36 weeks' gestation in a patient with Marfan syndrome

1–13. A patient with no prenatal care presents to Labor and Delivery with abdominal pain. Her fundal height is 21 cm. She spontaneous delivers a 475-g female fetus with no heart rate. According to the Centers for Disease Control, which of the following terminology correctly describes the death?

   a. Abortus

   b. Fetal death

   c. Neonatal death

   d. None of the above

1–14. A patient presents with severe preeclampsia at 25 weeks' gestation. Labor is induced and she spontaneously delivers a 692-g neonate. In the recovery room she complains of a severe headache and suddenly collapses. She is unable to be resuscitated. An autopsy reveals the following finding. How would her death be classified?

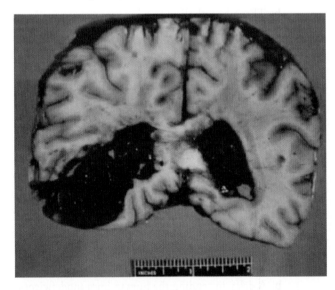

Reproduced with permission from Cunningham FG, Leveno KJ, Bloom SL, et al (eds): Hypertensive disorders. In Williams Obstetrics, 24th ed. New York, McGraw-Hill, 2014, Figure 40-11.

   a. Perinatal death

   b. Nonmaternal death

   c. Direct maternal death

   d. Indirect maternal death

1–15. The death of the patient in Question 1–14 should also be classified as which of the following?

   a. Maternal death

   b. Pregnancy-related death

   c. Pregnancy-associated death

   d. All of the above

1–16. Which of the following definitions most specifically applies to the neonate in the previous clinical scenario?

   a. Low birthweight

   b. Growth restricted

   c. Very low birthweight

   d. Extremely low birthweight

1–17. A 30-year-old multigravida presents with ruptured membranes at term but without labor. Following induction with misoprostol, her labor progresses rapidly, and she spontaneously delivers a liveborn 3300-g neonate. Immediately after delivery, she complains of dyspnea. She becomes apneic and pulseless and is unable to be resuscitated. Photomicrographs from her autopsy reveal fetal squames (*arrows*) within the pulmonary vasculature. How would her death be classified?

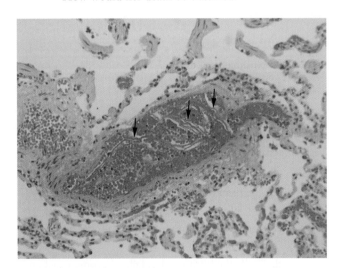

   a. Perinatal death

   b. Nonmaternal death

   c. Direct maternal death

   d. Indirect maternal death

1–18. A 24-year-old primigravida with no prior prenatal care presents with active preterm labor at 33 weeks' gestation. Following admission to Labor and Delivery, she complains of dyspnea, suddenly collapses, and is unable to be resuscitated. Her fetus dies during attempted maternal resuscitation. Autopsy of the mother reveals marked right ventricular hypertrophy, and her peripheral pulmonary arteries microscopically show marked hypertrophy of the tunica media. How would her death be classified? RV = right ventricle; LV = left ventricle.

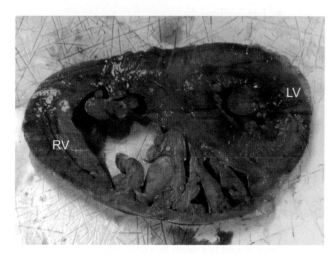

Used with permission from Dr. David Nelson.

a. Perinatal death

b. Nonmaternal death

c. Direct maternal death

d. Indirect maternal death

1–19. Which of the following is an accurate statement regarding the birth rate in the United States?

a. It is at an all-time low.

b. The teenage birth rate has slowly increased in the past 20 years.

c. The greatest decrease in birth rate has been seen in women older than 30 years.

d. While the birth rate has fallen in some racial and ethnic groups, it has increased in other groups.

1–20. Which of the following makes the largest contribution to infant death in the United States?

a. Home births

b. Multifetal gestations

c. Congenital fetal anomalies

d. Preterm birth < 32 weeks' gestation

1–21. What percentage of all pregnancies in the United States end in a live birth?

a. 30%

b. 50%

c. 65%

d. 90%

1–22. Which of the following is an accurate reflection of fetal death rates between 20 and 28 weeks' gestation?

a. They have fallen significantly since 1990.

b. They have remained relatively stable since 1990.

c. The fetal mortality rate at 20–27 weeks' gestation approximates that at > 28 weeks' gestation.

d. None of the above

1–23. Which of the following is the largest contributor to the perinatal mortality rate?

a. Fetal deaths

b. Neonatal deaths

c. Spontaneous abortions < 16 weeks' gestation

d. None of the above

1–24. Which of the following obstetrical complications contributes the least to the pregnancy-related death rate in the United States?

a. Hemorrhage

b. Thromboembolism

c. Ectopic pregnancy

d. Anesthetic complications

1–25. What is the most recent estimate of maternal mortality in the United States?

a. 4/10,000 live births

b. 14/10,000 live births

c. 14/100,000 live births

d. 41/100,000 live births

1–26. All **EXCEPT** which of the following is an example of a "near miss?"

a. A postpartum patient who falls in shower without injury

b. A delay in sending the human immunodeficiency virus (HIV) screening test of a laboring patient who ultimately has a negative test result

c. Failure to give Rh immunoglobulin to an Rh-negative postpartum patient who ultimately has no change in antibody screen

d. High spinal anesthesia resulting in intubation, admission to the intensive-care unit, and a ventilator-associated pneumonia

1–27. Which of the following is an accurate statement regarding current health care for women in the United States?

    a. Uninsured women with breast cancer have a 50% higher mortality rate than insured women.

    b. The United States is ranked in the top 10 countries with the lowest neonatal mortality rates.

    c. The Affordable Care Act mandates expanded Medicaid coverage for poor women, improving availability to prenatal services.

    d. The availability of Medicaid coverage for prenatal care has eliminated disparities in perinatal outcomes between insured and uninsured women.

1–28. How are programs supported by Title V Maternal and Child Health Services Block Grants funded?

    a. States match federally provided funds.

    b. States generate revenue through property taxes.

    c. Private contributions support individual state initiatives.

    d. A percentage of Social Security revenue is apportioned for Title V and Title X.

1–29. All **EXCEPT** which of the following contribute to the increasing cesarean delivery rate?

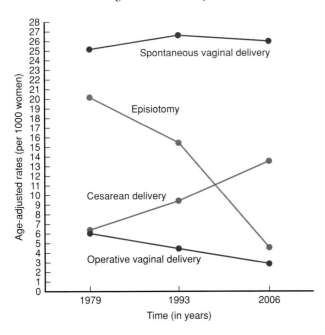

Reproduced with permission from Cunningham FG, Leveno KJ, Bloom SL, et al (eds): Overview of obstetrics. In Williams Obstetrics, 24th ed. New York, McGraw-Hill, 2014, Figure 1-8.

    a. Increasing rates of labor dystocia

    b. Increasing rates of labor induction

    c. Increasing rates of breech presentation

    d. Decreasing rates of vaginal birth after cesarean section

1–30. For which of the following purposes would fetal chromosomal microarray analysis be potentially beneficial?

    a. Evaluating a stillborn fetus

    b. Screening the fetus of an advanced-age mother

    c. Evaluating the fetus with trisomy 21 and a double-outlet right ventricle

    d. Screening the fetus at 12 weeks' gestation whose mother personally carries a balanced translocation

1–31. Which of the following are reported physician responses to the current liability environment in the United States?

    a. Higher cesarean delivery rates

    b. Reduction in number of obstetric patients accepted for care

    c. Refusal to care for women whose pregnancies are considered high-risk

    d. All of the above

1–32. Which of the following is accurate regarding home births in the United States?

    a. Certified nurse midwives attend most home births.

    b. They have a higher associated perinatal mortality rate than births occurring in medical facilities.

    c. Randomized trials suggest their outcomes are equivalent to those of births occurring in medical facilities.

    d. None of the above

CHAPTER 1 ANSWER KEY

Question number	Letter answer	Page cited	Header cited
1–1	c	p. 2	Introduction
1–2	c	p. 2	Vital Statistics
1–3	c	p. 3	Definitions
1–4	c	p. 3	Definitions
1–5	a	p. 3	Definitions
1–6	d	p. 3	Definitions
1–7	c	p. 3	Definitions
1–8	a	p. 3	Definitions
1–9	d	p. 3	Definitions
1–10	c	p. 3	Definitions
1–11	c	p. 3	Definitions
1–12	d	p. 3	Definitions
1–13	a	p. 3	Definitions
1–14	c	p. 3	Definitions
1–15	d	p. 3	Definitions
1–16	d	p. 3	Definitions
1–17	c	p. 3	Definitions
1–18	d	p. 3	Definitions
1–19	a	p. 4	Pregnancy Rates
1–20	d	p. 4	Infant Deaths
1–21	c	p. 4	Table 1-2
1–22	b	p. 5	Figure 1-3
1–23	a	p. 4	Perinatal Mortality
1–24	d	p. 6	Table 1-3
1–25	c	p. 5	Maternal Mortality
1–26	d	p. 6	Severe Maternal Morbidity
1–27	a	p. 7	Health Care for Women and Their Infants
1–28	a	p. 7	Health Care for Women and Their Infants
1–29	c	p. 9	Rising Cesarean Delivery Rate
1–30	a	p. 9	Genomic Technology
1–31	d	p. 10	Medical Liability
1–32	b	p. 11	Home Births

MATERNAL ANATOMY AND PHYSIOLOGY

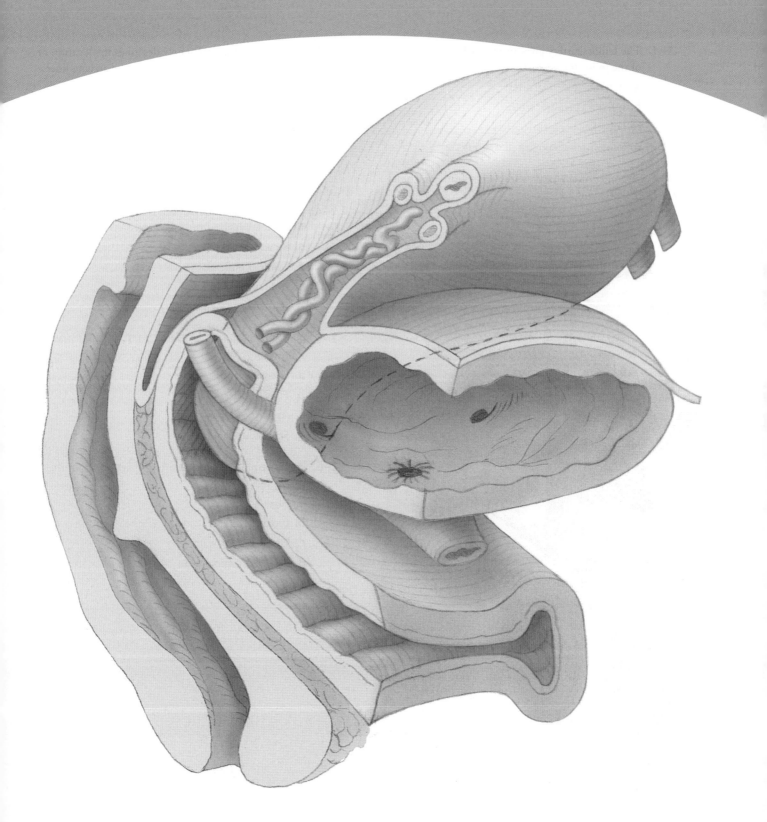

CHAPTER 2

Maternal Anatomy

2–1. The femoral artery gives rise to all **EXCEPT** which of the following vessels?

   a. External pudendal artery

   b. Inferior epigastric artery

   c. Superficial epigastric artery

   d. Superficial circumflex iliac artery

2–2. The inferior epigastric artery arises from which of the following?

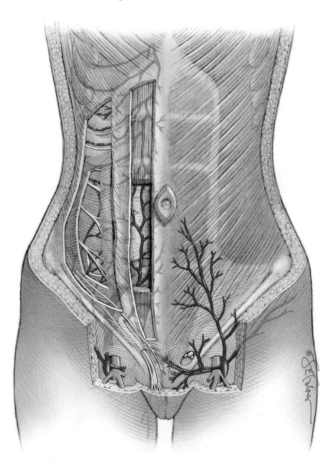

   a. Aorta

   b. Femoral artery

   c. Hypogastric artery

   d. External iliac artery

2–3. Which statement accurately describes the location of the inferior epigastric artery above the arcuate line?

   a. Ventral to the anterior rectus sheath

   b. Dorsal to the posterior rectus sheath

   c. Ventral to the external oblique muscle aponeurosis

   d. Ventral to the transversus abdominis muscle aponeurosis

2–4. The anterior abdominal wall is innervated by all **EXCEPT** which of the following?

   a. Subcostal nerve

   b. Internal pudendal nerve

   c. Intercostal nerves (T_7–T_{11})

   d. Iliohypogastric nerve (L_1)

2–5. The labia minora lack all **EXCEPT** which of the following?

   a. Eccrine glands

   b. Hair follicles

   c. Apocrine glands

   d. Sebaceous glands

2–6. The internal pudendal artery supplies which of the following?

   a. Bladder trigone

   b. Proximal vagina

   c. Distal vaginal walls

   d. Posterior vaginal wall

2–7. The vagina and its investing musculature are supplied by all **EXCEPT** which of the following arteries?

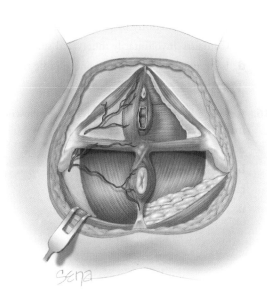

Reproduced with permission from Cunningham FG, Leveno KJ, Bloom SL, et al (eds): Maternal anatomy. In Williams Obstetrics, 23rd ed. New York, McGraw-Hill, 2010, Figure 2-5.

a. Perineal artery
b. Pudendal artery
c. Inferior rectal artery
d. Posterior labial artery

2–8. Which of the following is true concerning the anal sphincters?
a. The external anal sphincter measures 3 to 4 cm in length.
b. The external sphincter remains in a state of constant relaxation.
c. The internal anal sphincter contributes the bulk of anal canal resting pressure.
d. The external anal sphincter receives blood supply from the superior rectal artery.

2–9. The perineal body is formed partly by which of the following muscles?
a. Levator ani muscle
b. Gluteus maximus muscle
c. Bulbocavernosus muscle
d. Ischiocavernosus muscle

2–10. The vestibule is an almond shaped area bound by which of the following?
a. Laterally by the Hart line
b. Anteriorly by the fourchette
c. Laterally by the labia minora
d. Laterally by the external surface of hymen

2–11. The cervix contains little of which of the follow components?
a. Elastin
b. Collagen
c. Smooth muscle
d. Proteoglycans

2–12. Concerning the endometrium, which of the following is true?

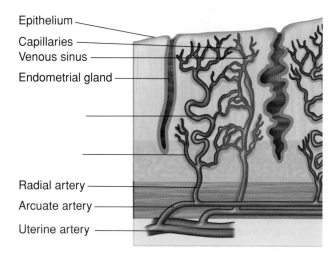

Reproduced with permission from Hoffman BL: Abnormal uterine bleeding. In Hoffman BL, Schorge JO, Schaffer JI, et al (eds): Williams Gynecology, 2nd ed. New York, McGraw-Hill, 2012, Figure 8-3.

a. The basal artery comes directly from the arcuate artery.
b. Spiral arteries extend directly from radial arteries.
c. The spiral arteries extend directly from the arcuate artery.
d. Functionalis layer contains spiral arteries and radial arteries.

2–13. During postpartum tubal sterilization, which of the following correct anatomical information may assist you?
a. The round ligament lies anterior to the fallopian tube.
b. The fallopian tube lies anterior to the round ligament.
c. The uteroovarian ligament lies anterior to the round ligament.
d. The fallopian tube lies posterior to the uteroovarian ligament.

2–14. Which of the following arteries is marked by the arrow?

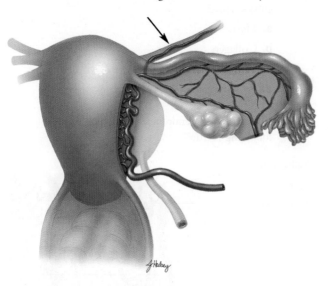

Reproduced with permission from Cunningham FG, Leveno KJ, Bloom SL, et al (eds): Maternal anatomy. In Williams Obstetrics, 23rd ed. New York, McGraw-Hill, 2010, Figure 2-15.

a. Sampson artery

b. Uterine artery

c. Obturator artery

d. Internal iliac artery

2–15. Which of the following is true regarding the external anal sphincter?

a. Is bound anteriorly by the perineal body

b. Is bound anteriorly by the posterior vagina

c. Contains involuntarily innervated smooth muscle

d. Is supplied by the superior and middle rectal arteries

2–16. Referring to the drawing, which of the following is marked by the letter A?

a Ureter

b. Uterine artery

c. Uteroovarian ligament

d. Infundibulopelvic ligament

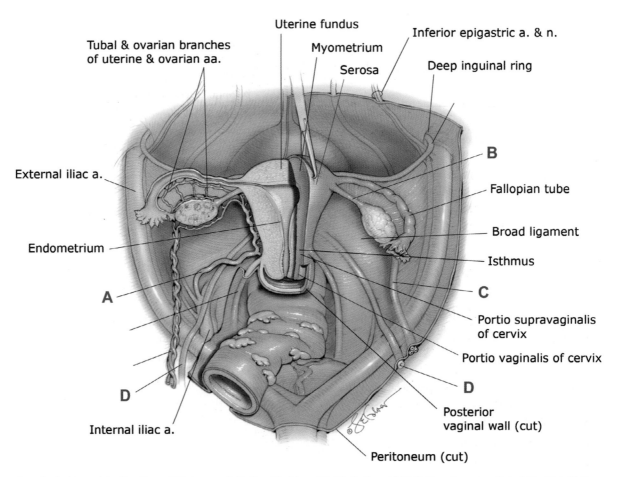

Reproduced with permission from Corton MM: Anatomy. In Hoffman BL, Schorge JO, Schaffer JI, et al (eds): Williams Gynecology, 2nd ed. New York, McGraw-Hill, 2012, Figure 38-14.

2–17. Referring to the drawing in Question 2–16, which of the following is marked by the letter B?

   a. Ureter

   b. Uterine artery

   c. Uteroovarian ligament

   d. Infundibulopelvic ligament

2–18. Referring to the drawing in Question 2–16, which of the following is marked by the letter C?

   a. Ureter

   b. Uterine artery

   c. Uteroovarian ligament

   d. Infundibulopelvic ligament

2–19. Referring to the drawing in Question 2–16, which of the following is marked by the letter D?

   a. Ureter

   b. Uterine artery

   c. Uteroovarian ligament

   d. Infundibulopelvic ligament

2–20. The common iliac artery arises directly from which of the following?

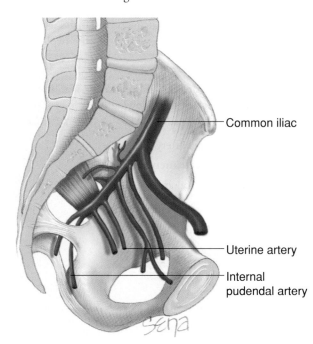

Reproduced with permission from Cunningham FG, Leveno KJ, Bloom SL, et al (eds): Maternal anatomy. In Williams Obstetrics, 23rd ed. New York, McGraw-Hill, 2010, Figure 2-16.

   a. Aorta

   b. External iliac artery

   c. Internal iliac artery

   d. None of the above

2–21. The uterine artery is a main branch of which of the following vessels?

   a. Iliolumbar artery

   b. Common iliac artery

   c. External iliac artery

   d. Internal iliac artery

2–22. From proximal (uterus) to distal (fimbriae), the correct progression of fallopian tube anatomy is which of the following?

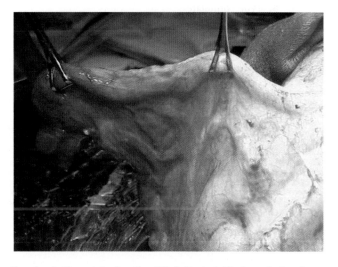

Reproduced with permission from Hnat MD: Parkland tubal ligation at the time of cesarean section (update). In Cunningham FG, Leveno KL, Bloom SL, et al (eds): Williams Obstetrics, 22nd ed. Online. New York, McGraw-Hill, 2006, http://www.accessmedicine.com. Figure 1.

   a. Isthmus, infundibulum, ampulla

   b. Isthmus, ampulla, infundibulum

   c. Infundibulum, ampulla, isthmus

   d. Ampulla, infundibulum, isthmus

2–23. The pelvis is formed by which of the following bone(s)?

   a. Sacrum

   b. Coccyx

   c. Innominate

   d. All of the above

2–24. Which of the following is true regarding relaxation of the pelvic joints at term in pregnancy?

   a. Is permanent and not accentuated in subsequent pregnancies

   b. Allows for an increase in the transverse diameter of the midpelvis

   c. Results in marked mobility of the pelvis at term because of a downward gliding movement of the sacroiliac (SI) joint

   d. Displacement of the SI joint increases outlet diameters by 1.5 to 2.0 cm in dorsal lithotomy position

2–25. Which of the following statements best describes the origin of the internal branch of the common iliac artery?

    a. Proximal to the iliolumbar artery

    b. Distal to the lateral sacral artery

    c. Distal to the superior rectal artery

    d. Proximal to where the ureters cross the pelvic brim

2–26. The clinical evaluation of the pelvic inlet requires manual measurement of which diameter?

    a. True conjugate

    b. Diagonal conjugate

    c. Obstetric conjugate

    d. Pelvic inlet transverse diameter

2–27. Engagement occurs when the biparietal diameter of the fetal head descends below the level of which of the following?

    a. Midpelvis

    b. Pelvic inlet

    c. Pelvic floor

    d. Ischial tuberosities

2–28. In this diagram, which of the following is demonstrated?

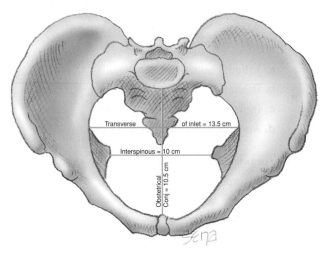

Reproduced with permission from Cunningham FG, Leveno KJ, Bloom SL, et al. Williams Obstetrics. 23rd ed. New York: McGraw-Hill Professional, 2010.

    a. Ischial tuberosities

    b. Midpelvis ischial spines

    c. Important pelvic outlet diameters

    d. An inadequate obstetrical conjugate

2–29. The lower uterine segment incised at the time of cesarean delivery is formed by which of the following?

    a. Cornu

    b. Cervix

    c. Isthmus

    d. Uterine corpus

2–30. Hegar sign refers to which of the following?

    a. Cervical softening

    b. Bluish tint to ectocervix

    c. Replacement of collagen by smooth muscle in the cervix

    d. Replacement of ectocervix by endocervix commonly seen during pregnancy

2–31. Which of the following statements best describes the pelvic outlet?

    a. The base of the posterior triangle is the coccyx.

    b. The angle of the pubic arch is usually < 90 degrees.

    c. The lateral boundaries of the posterior triangle are the descending inferior rami of the pubic bones.

    d. The common base of the two triangles is formed by a line drawn between the two ischial tuberosities.

2–32. The posterior division of the internal iliac artery contains which of the following?

    a. Iliolumbar artery

    b. Middle rectal artery

    c. Superior rectal artery

    d. Superior vesical artery

CHAPTER 2 ANSWER KEY

Question number	Letter answer	Page cited	Header cited
2–1	b	p. 16	Blood Supply
2–2	d	p. 17	Blood Supply; Figure 2-1
2–3	d	p. 18	Skin, Subcutaneous layer, and Fascia; Figure 2-2
2–4	b	p. 17	Innervation; Figure 2-1
2–5	d	p. 18	Mons Pubis, Labia, and Clitoris
2–6	c	p. 20	Vagina and Hymen
2–7	c	p. 20	Vagina and Hymen; Figure 2-8
2–8	c	p. 24	Anal Sphincter Complex
2–9	c	p. 21	Perineum
2–10	a	p. 20	Vestibule
2–11	c	p. 26	Cervix
2–12	b	p. 28	Blood Supply
2–13	a	p. 27	Ligaments
2–14	a	p. 27	Ligaments
2–15	a	p. 24	Anal Sphincter Complex; Figure 2-4
2–16	b	p. 26	Figure 2-10
2–17	c	p. 26	Figure 2-10
2–18	d	p. 26	Figure 2-10
2–19	a	p. 26	Figure 2-10
2–20	a	p. 28	Blood Supply
2–21	d	p. 28	Blood Supply
2–22	b	p. 30	Fallopian Tube
2–23	d	p. 31	Pelvic Bones
2–24	d	p. 32	Pelvic Joints
2–25	a	p. 29	Figure 2-13
2–26	b	p. 32	Pelvic Inlet
2–27	b	p. 32	Pelvic Inlet
2–28	b	p. 33	Midpelvis and Pelvic Outlet
2–29	c	p. 25	Uterus
2–30	a	p. 26	Cervix
2–31	d	p. 33	Midpelvis and Pelvic Outlet
2–32	a	p. 29	Figure 2-13

CHAPTER 3

Congenital Genitourinary Abnormalities

3–1. Which of the following is not derived from the müllerian ducts?

a. Ovary

b. Uterus

c. Proximal vagina

d. All derive from the müllerian ducts

3–2. In females, what does the metanephros ultimately form?

a. Uterus

b. Kidney

c. Embryonic remnants

d. None of the above

3–3. The urogenital sinus gives rise to which of the following?

a. Bladder

b. Urethra

c. Distal vagina

d. All of the above

3–4. In this image, which of the following ultimately develops into the uterus?

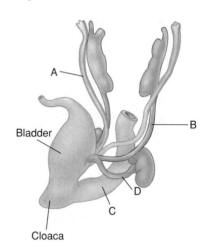

Modified with permission from Bradshaw KB: Anatomic disorders. In Schorge JO, Schaffer JI, Halvorson LM, et al (eds): Williams Gynecology. New York, McGraw-Hill, 2008, Figure 18-1C.

a. A

b. B

c. C

d. D

3–5. Compared with the general population, women with müllerian anomalies are at increased risk for which of the following?

a. Urinary tract anomalies

b. Premature ovarian failure

c. Gastrointestinal anomalies

d. All of the above

3–6. If a müllerian anomaly is identified during pregnancy, which of the following modalities may be preferred to initially search for an associated renal anomaly?

   a. Renal sonography

   b. Computed tomography

   c. Intravenous pyelography

   d. Magnetic resonance imaging

3–7. Your patient presents with vaginal spotting in the first trimester. During transvaginal 2-dimensional (2-D) sonographic evaluation, a live singleton fetus is seen, and a uterine müllerian anomaly is suspected. Three-dimensional (3-D) sonography is performed at the same visit and shows this banana-shaped uterus containing a gestational sac. What is the next clinically prudent step during this pregnancy?

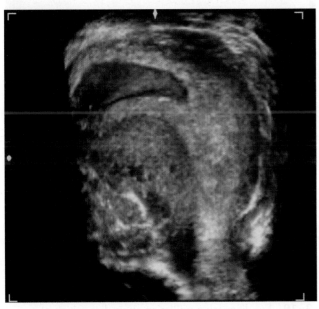

Reproduced with permission from Moschos E, Twickler DM: Techniques used for imaging in gynecology. In Hoffman BL, Schorge JO, Schaffer JI, et al (eds): Williams Gynecology, 2nd ed. New York, McGraw-Hill, 2012, Figure 2-23.

   a. Schedule renal sonographic examination

   b. Schedule computed tomography with contrast

   c. Perform prophylactic cervical cerclage at 14 weeks' gestation

   d. Recommend pregnancy termination due to the high rate of uterine horn rupture

3–8. Mesonephric duct remnants may lead to which of the following?

   a. Skene gland cyst

   b. Gartner duct cyst

   c. Urethral diverticulum

   d. Bartholin gland duct cyst

3–9. Cloacal exstrophy, bladder exstrophy, and epispadias all originate from premature embryological rupture of which of the following?

   a. Yolk sac

   b. Sinovaginal bulb

   c. Cloacal membrane

   d. Hymeneal membrane

3–10. In this sagittal image of the early fetal pelvis, incomplete resorption at the point marked (*) leads to which anomaly?

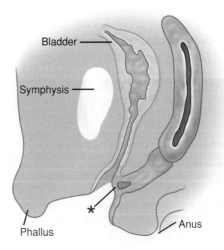

Modified with permission from Bradshaw KD: Anatomic disorders. In Schorge JO, Schaffer JI, Halvorson LM, et al (eds): Williams Gynecology. New York, McGraw-Hill, 2008, Figure 18-4B.

   a. Vaginal adenosis

   b. Gartner duct cyst

   c. Imperforate hymen

   d. Ambiguous genitalia

3–11. Imperforate hymen typically first presents in which age group and with which symptoms?

   a. Perimenarche with amenorrhea

   b. Fetal period with polyhydramnios

   c. Neonatal period with urinary retention

   d. Reproductive age with primary infertility

3–12. Classically, the pathogenesis of a müllerian defect involves which of the following?

   a. Agenesis of one mesonephric duct

   b. Duplication of one paramesonephric duct

   c. Faulty fusion of the two mesonephric ducts

   d. None of the above

3–13. Mayer-Rokitansky-Küster-Hauser (MRKH) syndrome is characterized by upper vaginal agenesis that is typically associated with uterine hypoplasia or agenesis. Other systems that may also be affected include all **EXCEPT** which of the following?

   a. Renal

   b. Skeletal

   c. Auditory

   d. Gastrointestinal

3–14. A 19-year-old presents at 14 weeks' gestation with this vaginal anomaly, which extends the full vaginal length. Additional evaluation reveals no associated uterine defect. You counsel her that this anomaly is typically associated with a greater risk for which of the following peripartum complications?

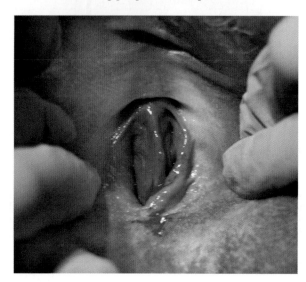

Used with permission from Dr. Alison Brooks.

   a. Urinary retention

   b. Face presentation

   c. Breech presentation

   d. None of the above

3–15. During labor, a transverse vaginal septum may be managed appropriately with all **EXCEPT** which of the following strategies?

   a. Permit normal labor

   b. Avoid labor augmentation

   c. Perform cesarean delivery

   d. Cruciate incision of the septum once cervical dilatation is complete

3–16. Which of the following is the more common uterine müllerian anomaly?

   a. Uterine agenesis

   b. Bicornuate uterus

   c. Uterine didelphys

   d. Unicornuate uterus

3–17. For diagnosing müllerian anomalies, which of the following tools is the most accurate?

   a. Hysterosalpingography

   b. Saline infusion sonography

   c. Magnetic resonance imaging

   d. Two-dimensional transvaginal sonography

3–18. This hysterosalpingogram depicts a unicornuate uterus. For diagnosing müllerian anomalies in nonpregnant women, which of the following are disadvantages of hysterosalpingography?

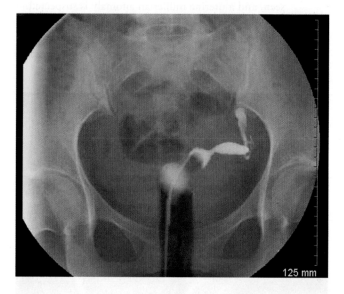

   a. Dye will not fill noncavitary horns.

   b. No outer uterine fundal contour is seen.

   c. Dye will not fill noncommunicating horns.

   d. All of the above

3–19. For diagnosing müllerian anomalies, which of the following are advantages to 3-dimensional sonography?

   a. Displays the contour of the endometrium

   b. Less expensive than magnetic resonance imaging

   c. Displays the contour of the outer uterine fundus

   d. All of the above

3–20. With magnetic resonance imaging, a septate uterus is displayed here. For diagnosing müllerian anomalies, which of the following are advantages to this modality?

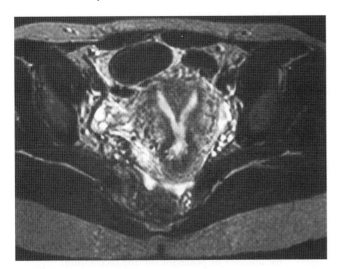

Reproduced with permission from Moschos E, Twickler DM: Techniques used for imaging in gynecology. In Schorge JO, Schaffer JI, Halvorson LM et al (eds): Williams Gynecology. New York, McGraw-Hill, 2008, Figure 2-27.

    a. Is nearly 100-percent accurate

    b. Displays fundal, myometrial, and endometrial contours

    c. Permits identification of concurrent skeletal or renal anomalies

    d. All of the above

3–21. The pathogenesis of poor pregnancy outcomes with a unicornuate uterus is thought to be related to all **EXCEPT** which of the following primary factors?

    a. Cervical incompetence

    b. Reduced uterine capacity

    c. Poor implantation into endometrium

    d. Anomalous distribution of the uterine artery

3–22. Rates for all **EXCEPT** which of the following obstetrical complications are increased in women with uterine müllerian anomalies?

    a. Twinning

    b. Miscarriage

    c. Malpresentation

    d. Preterm delivery

3–23. Which category of unicornuate uterus poses the greatest risk for ectopic pregnancy?

    a. Agenesis of one horn

    b. Communicating noncavitary rudimentary horn

    c. Noncommunicating cavitary rudimentary horn

    d. Noncommunicating noncavitary rudimentary horn

3–24. A longitudinal vaginal septum is **LEAST** commonly seen with which of the following müllerian anomalies?

    a. Septate uterus

    b. Unicornuate uterus

    c. Bicornuate uterus

    d. Uterine didelphys

3–25. Which uterine müllerian anomaly is seen in this hysterosalpingogram?

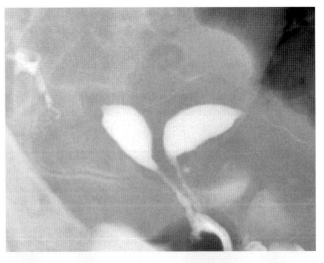

Reproduced with permission from Halvorson LM: Evaluation of the infertile couple. In Schorge JO, Schaffer JI, Halvorson LM, et al (eds): Williams Gynecology. New York, McGraw-Hill, 2008, Figure 19-7C.

    a. Arcuate uterus

    b. Septate uterus

    c. Uterine didelphys

    d. Bicornuate uterus

3–26. With magnetic resonance imaging, a bicornuate uterus is most reliably differentiated from a septate uterus by which of the following characteristics?

    a. Intrafundal cleft < 1 cm deep

    b. Intrafundal cleft > 1 cm deep

    c. Two distinct endometrial cavities

    d. Partition running the full uterine cavity length

3–27. Reparative excision is most feasible and easiest for which of the following uterine müllerian anomalies?

    a. Septate uterus

    b. Uterine didelphys

    c. Bicornuate uterus

    d. Unicornuate uterus with a communicating cavitary rudimentary horn

3–28. The highest miscarriage rate is associated with which of the following uterine müllerian anomalies?

    a. Septate uterus

    b. Bicornuate uterus

    c. Uterine didelphys

    d. Unicornuate uterus with a noncommunicating noncavitary rudimentary horn

3–29. A 22-year-old G1P0 presents to your office as a new patient for prenatal care. During transvaginal 2-dimensional (2-D) sonographic evaluation, a live singleton fetus is seen, but a müllerian anomaly is suspected. Three-dimensional (3-D) sonography is subsequently performed, and this image shows an arcuate uterus containing a gestational sac. The outer uterine contour rounds slightly outward. The endometrial contour indents only slightly inward. Which of the following untoward outcomes has been consistently associated with this particular finding?

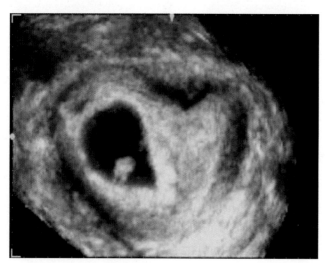

    a. Miscarriage

    b. Preterm delivery

    c. Incompetent cervix

    d. None of the above

3–30. For which of the following müllerian anomalies should prophylactic cervical cerclage be recommended in most cases?

    a. Bicornuate uterus

    b. Uterine didelphys

    c. Unicornuate uterus

    d. None of the above

3–31. All **EXCEPT** which of the following are common symptoms associated with a retroflexed incarcerated uterus?

    a. Abdominal pain

    b. Pelvic pressure

    c. Vaginal bleeding

    d. Urinary retention

3–32. Which of the following is the most common complication encountered during cesarean delivery for anterior or posterior uterine sacculation?

    a. Placenta previa

    b. Placenta accreta

    c. Urinary retention

    d. Distorted anatomy

CHAPTER 3 ANSWER KEY

Question number	Letter answer	Page cited	Header cited
3–1	a	p. 36	Embryology of the Urinary System
3–2	b	p. 36	Embryology of the Urinary System
3–3	d	p. 36	Embryology of the Urinary System
3–4	a	p. 37	Embryology of the Genital Tract
3–5	a	p. 37	Embryology of the Genital Tract
3–6	a	p. 37	Embryology of the Genital Tract
3–7	a	p. 37	Embryology of the Genital Tract
3–8	b	p. 37	Mesonephric Remnants
3–9	c	p. 38	Bladder and Perineal Anomalies
3–10	c	p. 38	Defects of the Hymen
3–11	a	p. 38	Defects of the Hymen
3–12	d	p. 38	Müllerian Abnormalities
3–13	d	p. 39	Vaginal Abnormalities
3–14	d	p. 39	Vaginal Abnormalities
3–15	b	p. 39	Vaginal Abnormalities
3–16	b	p. 40	Uterine Abnormalities
3–17	c	p. 40	Uterine Abnormalities
3–18	d	p. 40	Uterine Abnormalities
3–19	d	p. 40	Uterine Abnormalities
3–20	d	p. 40	Uterine Abnormalities
3–21	c	p. 40	Unicornuate Uterus (Class II)
3–22	a	p. 40	Unicornuate Uterus (Class II)
3–23	c	p. 40	Unicornuate Uterus (Class II)
3–24	b	p. 41	Uterine Didelphys (Class III); Bicornuate Uterus (Class IV); Septate Uterus (Class V)
3–25	c	p. 41	Uterine Didelphys (Class III)
3–26	b	p. 41	Bicornuate Uterus (Class IV)
3–27	a	p. 42	Septate Uterus (Class V)
3–28	a	p. 42	Septate Uterus (Class V)
3–29	d	p. 42	Arcuate Uterus (Class VI)
3–30	d	p. 42	Treatment with Cerclage
3–31	c	p. 42	Retroflexion
3–32	d	p. 43	Sacculation

CHAPTER 4

Maternal Physiology

4-1. Changes in maternal blood volume and cardiac output in pregnancy may mimic which following disease states?

    a. Hypertension

    b. Thyrotoxicosis

    c. Diabetes insipidus

    d. Chronic renal disease

4-2. Regarding Braxton Hicks contractions, which of the following is true?

    a. Their intensity varies between 20 and 40 mm Hg.

    b. They occur early in pregnancy and may be palpated in the second trimester.

    c. Late in pregnancy, these contractions become more regular and may cause discomfort.

    d. B and C

4-3. Uterine blood flow near term most closely approximates which of the following?

    a. 150 mL/min

    b. 350 mL/min

    c. 550 mL/min

    d. 850 mL/min

4-4. In this photograph, cervical eversion is demonstrated. As shown, what kind of epithelium makes up most of the visible portion of the cervix?

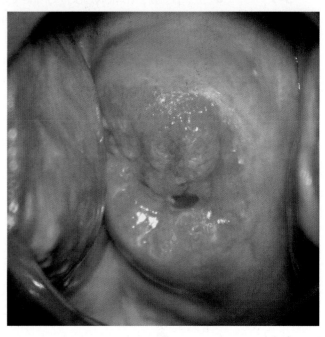

Reproduced with permission from Cunningham FG, Leveno KJ, Bloom SL, et al (eds): Maternal physiology. In Williams Obstetrics, 24th ed. New York, McGraw-Hill, 2014, Figure 4-1.

    a. Serous

    b. Columnar

    c. Squamous

    d. Transitional

4–5. This pattern of cervical mucus is typically seen in which of the following clinical settings?

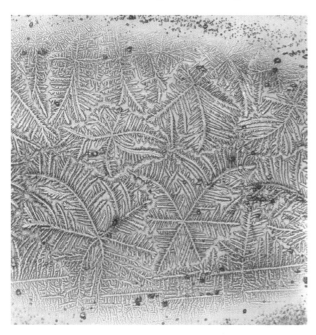

Reproduced with permission from Cunningham FG, Leveno KJ, Bloom SL, et al (eds): Maternal physiology. In Williams Obstetrics, 24th ed. New York, McGraw-Hill, 2014, Figure 4-2.

a. Ovulation

b. Uncomplicated pregnancy

c. Pregnancy with amnionic fluid leakage

d. A and C

4–6. Your pregnant patient in her second trimester presents with breasts that have enlarged during the past few months. This photograph illustrates which of the following?

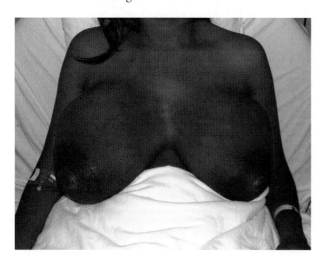

Used with permission from Dr. Mary Jane Pearson.

a. Gigantomastia

b. Inflammatory breast carcinoma

c. Pathologic enlargement that may ultimately require surgery.

d. A and C

4–7. The graphic below illustrates which of the following pregnancy-related concepts? LMP = last menstrual period; MP = menstrual period.

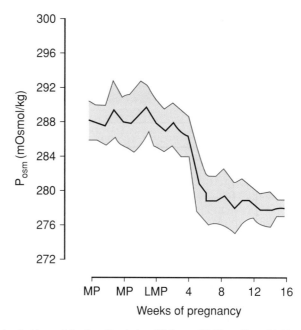

Reproduced with permission from Cunningham FG, Leveno KJ, Bloom SL, et al (eds): Maternal physiology. In Williams Obstetrics, 24th ed. New York, McGraw-Hill, 2014, Figure 4-4.

a. Maternal plasma osmolality decreases early in pregnancy.

b. Maternal plasma osmolality increases throughout pregnancy.

c. Maternal plasma osmolality does not change during pregnancy.

d. Maternal plasma osmolality is affected most by increases in sodium.

4–8. This graphic concerning insulin and glucose levels during pregnancy suggests which of the following?

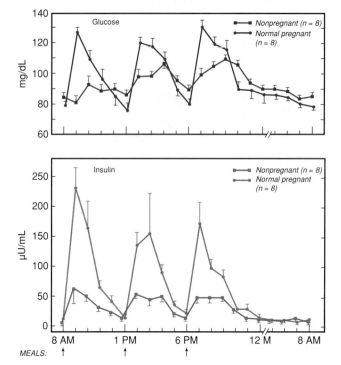

Reproduced with permission from Cunningham FG, Leveno KJ, Bloom SL, et al (eds): Maternal physiology. In Williams Obstetrics, 24th ed. New York, McGraw-Hill, 2014, Figure 4-5.

a. Hypoinsulinemia
b. Hyperinsulinemia
c. Postprandial hypoglycemia
d. Mild fasting hyperglycemia

4–9. The total increase in protein during pregnancy approximates which of following?
a. 500 g
b. 1000 g
c. 500 g for contractile protein in the uterus
d. B and C

4–10. Related to calcium metabolism, which of the following occurs during pregnancy?
a. Serum magnesium levels increase.
b. Total serum calcium levels decline.
c. The fetal skeleton accrues 70 g of calcium by term.
d. Maximums of 500 mEq of sodium and 200 mEq of potassium are retained.

4–11. As illustrated by this graphic, which of the following occurs during pregnancy?

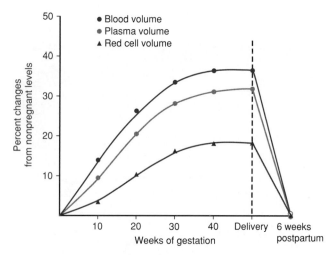

Reproduced with permission from Cunningham FG, Leveno KJ, Bloom SL, et al (eds): Maternal physiology. In Williams Obstetrics, 24th ed. New York, McGraw-Hill, 2014, Figure 4-6.

a. The hematocrit increases.
b. Total blood volume increases 40% by term.
c. Red cell volume does not increase until 20 weeks.
d. The hematocrit increases due to an increased red cell volume relative to plasma volume.

4–12. This graphic suggests which of the following?

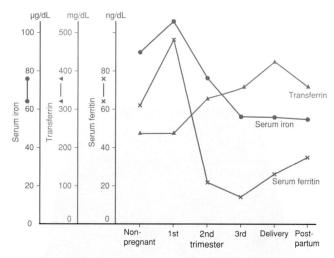

Reproduced with permission from Cunningham FG, Leveno KJ, Bloom SL, et al (eds): Maternal physiology. In Williams Obstetrics, 23rd ed. New York, McGraw-Hill, 2014, Figure 5-6.

a. Serum iron is decreased in the first trimester.
b. Serum ferritin is increased in the second trimester.
c. Serum ferritin is increased by the end of pregnancy.
d. Serum transferrin is increased by the end of pregnancy.

4–13. Average blood loss for a vaginal delivery is which the following?

    a. 500 mL

    b. 1000 mL

    c. Half of that lost during cesarean delivery of twins

    d. A and C

4–14. Regarding immunological function during pregnancy, which of the following statements is true?

    a. Th1 response is suppressed.

    b. Th2 cells are downregulated.

    c. There is up regulation of T-cytotoxic cells.

    d. All of the above

4–15. Regarding the coagulation system in pregnancy, which of the following statements is true?

    a. Mean platelet count is 250,000/μL.

    b. Fibrinolytic activity is usually reduced.

    c. Fibrinogen levels are increased to a median of 250 mg/dL.

    d. Decreases in platelet concentration are solely due to hemodilution.

4–16. The graphic below demonstrates which of the following points?

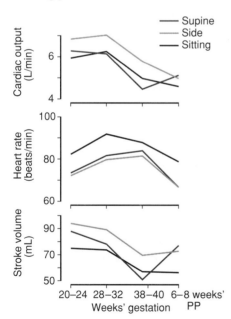

Reproduced with permission from Cunningham FG, Leveno KJ, Bloom SL, et al (eds): Maternal physiology. In Williams Obstetrics, 24th ed. New York, McGraw-Hill, 2014, Figure 4-7.

    a. Cardiac output increases between 20 and 40 weeks' gestation.

    b. Heart rate increases when pregnant women are sitting compared with lying supine.

    c. Cardiac output increases when postpartum women are sitting compared with lying supine.

    d. Stroke volume increases when pregnant women are supine compared with lying on their sides.

4–17. During pregnancy, the venous pressure does which of the following?

    a. Decreases when the woman is lying in the lateral position

    b. Declines from 24 mm Hg to 8 mm Hg at term in the lower extremities

    c. Is responsible for dependent edema in the lower extremities

    d. A and C

4–18. Which of the following are true regarding infused angiotensin II and its vascular effects during pregnancy?

    a. Hypertensive patients become and then remain refractory.

    b. The vascular response is believed to be progesterone related.

    c. Normotensive nulliparas near term are responsive to the effects of angiotensin II.

    d. Increased vessel refractoriness to angiotensin II results primarily from altered renin-angiotensin secretion.

4–19. Concerning acid-base equilibrium during pregnancy, which of the following statement is true?

    a. Plasma bicarbonate concentration decreases from 26 to approximately 22 mmol/L.

    b. The maternal oxygen-disassociation curve is shifted to the right.

    c. Physiological dyspnea results from slightly decreased tidal volume that lowers CO_2 levels.

    d. Estrogen acts centrally, where it lowers the threshold and increases the sensitivity of the chemoreflex response to CO_2.

4–20. Regarding lung volumes during pregnancy, which of the following is true?

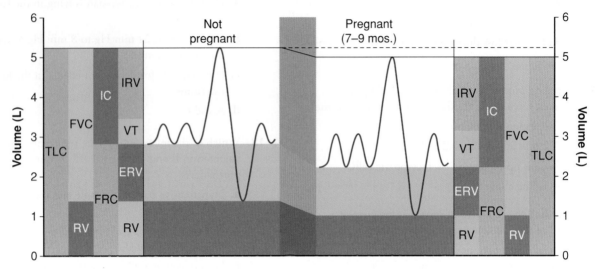

Expiratory reserve volume (ERV); Functional residual capacity (FRC); Forced vital capacity (FVC); Inspiratory capacity (IC); Inspiratory reserve volume (IRV); Residual volume (RV); Tidal volume (VT); Total lung capacity (TLC). Reproduced with permission from Cunningham FG, Leveno KJ, Bloom SL, et al (eds): Maternal physiology. In Williams Obstetrics, 24th ed. New York, McGraw-Hill, 2014, Figure 4-13.

    a. Tidal volume is increased.

    b. Reserve volume is increased.

    c. Total lung capacity increases by approximately 5% by term.

    d. A and C

4–21. The maternal arteriovenous oxygen difference decreases during pregnancy because of which of the following?

    a. Increased tidal volume

    b. Increased cardiac output

    c. Increased hemoglobin mass

    d. All of the above

4–22. Regarding the bladder during pregnancy, which of the following is true?

    a. There is increased bladder capacity.

    b. Absolute and functional urethral length increases.

    c. Bladder pressure decreases from 15 to 8 cm H_2O by term.

    d. Approximately three fourths of all pregnant women experience incontinence during pregnancy.

4–23. Regarding the gastrointestinal tract during pregnancy, which of the following is true?

    a. Gastric emptying time is shortened during labor.

    b. Gastric emptying time is lengthened in each trimester.

    c. Pyrosis is caused by reflux of acidic secretions into the lower esophagus.

    d. Epulis gravidarum is a highly vascular swelling that may affect any mucosal membrane.

4–24. Which of the following is true regarding the gallbladder during pregnancy?

    a. It empties more completely.

    b. It has reduced contractility caused by progesterone.

    c. Stasis leads to formation of pyruvate-containing stones.

    d. Cholestasis is linked to high circulating levels of progesterone.

4–25. Regarding the pituitary gland during pregnancy, which of the following is true?

    a. Growth of microadenomas is likely.

    b. Serum prolactin levels remain unchanged throughout pregnancy.

    c. It enlarges due to estrogen-stimulated hypertrophy and hyperplasia of the lactotrophs.

    d. A and C

4–26. Regarding the thyroid gland during pregnancy, which of the following is true?

Mother

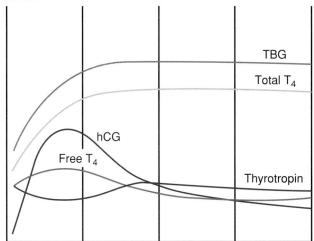

Fetus

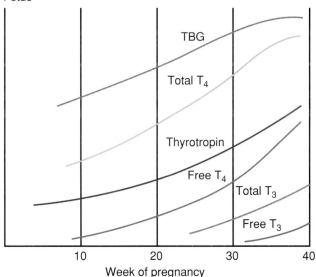

Reproduced with permission from Cunningham FG, Leveno KJ, Bloom SL, et al (eds): Maternal physiology. In Williams Obstetrics, 24th ed. New York, McGraw-Hill, 2014, Figure 4-17.

    a. It undergoes enlargement through hypertrophy.

    b. Total T_4 concentration increases during pregnancy.

    c. Free T_4 concentration increases its mean value by term.

    d. Human chorionic gonadotropin (hCG), which mimics thyroid-stimulating hormone, has declining levels beginning at approximately 20 weeks.

4–27. Regarding iodine during pregnancy, which of the following is true?

    a. Maternal requirements remain the same during normal pregnancy.

    b. Fetal neurodevelopment is dependent on adequate thyroid hormone exposure.

    c. Iodine deficiency is the most preventable cause of fetal neurological deficiency.

    d. In women with low or marginal intake, deficiency may manifest as decreased thyroid-stimulating hormone (TSH) levels.

4–28. Regarding fetal skeletal mineralization, which of the following is true?

    a. The calcium required by the fetus represents only 3% of maternal stores.

    b. A total of 3 g of calcium is required, primarily during the third trimester.

    c. Calcium absorption reaches approximately 100 mg/day in the third trimester.

    d. A and B

4–29. This graphic illustrates which of the following?

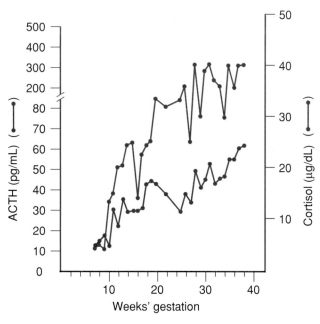

Reproduced with permission from Cunningham FG, Leveno KJ, Bloom SL, et al (eds): Maternal physiology. In Williams Obstetrics, 24th ed. New York, McGraw-Hill, 2014, Figure 4-19.

    a. Maximum secretion of cortisol is reached by 20 weeks.

    b. Serum cortisol secretion decreases throughout pregnancy.

    c. Serum adrenocorticotropic hormone (ACTH) secretion increases across pregnancy.

    d. None of the above

4–30. Regarding aldosterone during pregnancy, which of the following is true?

   a. It is the principal mineralocorticoid.

   b. Secretion is decreased by sodium restriction.

   c. Increased aldosterone levels protect against the antinatriuretic effect of progesterone and atrial natriuretic peptide.

   d. A and B

4–31. Regarding the central nervous system during pregnancy, which of the following is true?

   a. Memory decline is typically limited to the third trimester.

   b. Pregnancy significantly alters cerebrovascular autoregulation.

   c. Attention and memory are typically decreased in women receiving magnesium sulfate.

   d. Mean blood flow in the middle cerebral artery (MCA) and posterior cerebral artery (PCA) increases in the third trimester.

CHAPTER 4 ANSWER KEY

Question number	Letter answer	Page cited	Header cited
4–1	b	p. 46	Introduction
4–2	d	p. 47	Uterine Contractility
4–3	c	p. 47	Uteroplacental Blood Flow
4–4	b	p. 48	Cervix
4–5	d	p. 48	Cervix
4–6	d	p. 50	Breasts
4–7	a	p. 51	Water Metabolism
4–8	b	p. 53	Carbohydrate Metabolism
4–9	d	p. 53	Protein Metabolism
4–10	b	p. 54	Electrolyte and Mineral Metabolism
4–11	b	p. 55	Blood Volume
4–12	d	p. 55	Iron Metabolism
4–13	a	p. 56	The Puerperium
4–14	a	p. 56	Immunological Functions
4–15	b	p. 57	Coagulation and Fibrinolysis
4–16	b	p. 58	Cardiovascular System
4–17	d	p. 60	Circulation and Blood Pressure
4–18	b	p. 61	Renin, Angiotensin II, and Plasma Volume
4–19	a	p. 63	Acid–Base Equilibrium
4–20	a	p. 62	Pulmonary Function
4–21	d	p. 63	Oxygen Delivery
4–22	b	p. 66	Bladder
4–23	c	p. 66	Gastrointestinal Tract
4–24	b	p. 67	Gallbladder
4–25	c	p. 67	Pituitary Gland
4–26	b	p. 68	Thyroid Gland
4–27	b	p. 69	Iodine Status
4–28	a	p. 70	Parathyroid Hormone
4–29	c	p. 70	Adrenal Gland
4–30	a	p. 70	Aldosterone
4–31	a	p. 72	Memory

PLACENTATION, EMBRYOGENESIS, AND FETAL DEVELOPMENT

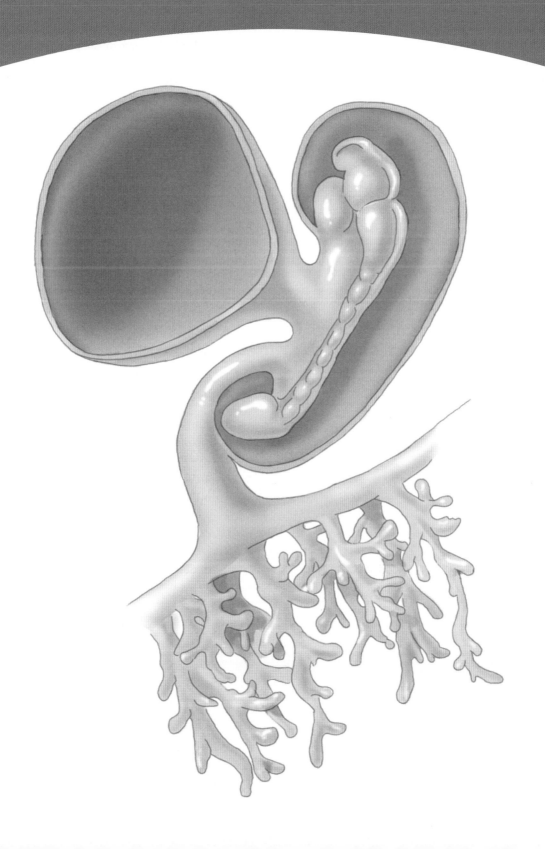

Implantation and Placental Development

5–1. What is the average duration of a normal menstrual cycle?

   a. 14–28 days

   b. 25–32 days

   c. 28–55 days

   d. 40–50 days

5–2. Of 2 million oocytes in the human ovary present at birth, how many are present at the onset of puberty?

   a. 200,000

   b. 300,000

   c. 400,000

   d. 500,000

5–3. Which hormone is required for the late-stage development of antral follicles?

   a. Estradiol

   b. Androstenedione

   c. Luteinizing hormone

   d. Follicle-stimulating hormone

5–4. Which cells of the dominant follicle are responsible for estrogen production during the follicular phase of the menstrual cycle?

   a. Theca

   b. Decidual

   c. Granulosa

   d. Endometrial

5–5. What name is given to the process through which the corpus luteum develops from the remains of the Graafian follicle?

   a. Luteinization

   b. Thecalization

   c. Decidualization

   d. Graafian transformation

5–6. What is the approximate peak production of ovarian progesterone during midluteal phase?

   a. 10–20 mg/day

   b. 25–50 mg/day

   c. 60–80 mg/day

   d. 75–100 mg/day

5–7. Which of the following is the most biologically potent naturally occurring estrogen?

   a. Estriol

   b. Estrone

   c. Estetrol

   d. 17β-Estradiol

5–8. Which of the following is the endometrial layer that is shed with every menstrual cycle?

   a. Basalis layer

   b. Decidual layer

   c. Luteinized layer

   d. Functionalis layer

5–9. Within the glandular epithelium of the endometrium, what is the first histological sign of ovulation?

   a. Cessation of glandular cell mitosis

   b. Vacuoles at the apical portion of the secretory nonciliated cells

   c. Secretory nonciliated cells devoid of glycoprotein and mucopolysaccharide

   d. Subnuclear vacuoles and pseudostratification in the basal portion of the glandular epithelium

5–10. In the following image, which letter identifies the spiral arteries?

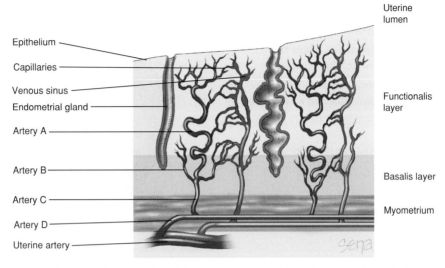

Modified with permission from Cunningham FG, Leveno KJ, Bloom SL, et al (eds): Implantation and placental development. In Williams Obstetrics, 24th ed. New York, McGraw-Hill, 2014, Figure 5-4.

a. A

b. B

c. C

d. D

5–11. Which prostaglandin plays a role in vasoconstriction of the spiral arteries, leading to menstruation?

a. Prostaglandin E_1

b. Prostaglandin E_2

c. Prostaglandin D_2

d. Prostaglandin $F_{2\alpha}$

5–12. In sequence from letters A to C, please identify the three types of deciduas in the figure:

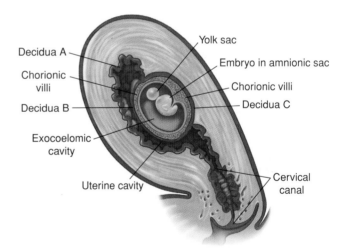

Modified with permission from Cunningham FG, Leveno KJ, Bloom SL, et al (eds): Implantation and placental development. In Williams Obstetrics, 24th ed. New York, McGraw-Hill, 2014, Figure 5-6.

a. Basalis, capsularis, parietalis

b. Capsularis, basalis, parietalis

c. Parietalis, basalis, capsularis

d. Parietalis, capsularis, basalis

5–13. What is the Nitabuch layer?

    a. A layer of the decidua made of large, distended glands

    b. An area of the decidua with large, closely packed epithelioid, polygonal cells

    c. A zone of fibrinoid degeneration where the invading trophoblast and decidua meet

    d. An area of superficial fibrin deposition at the bottom of the intervillous space and surrounding the anchoring villi

5–14. Which of the following functions does the placenta not perform for the fetus?

    a. Renal

    b. Hepatic

    c. Adrenal

    d. Pulmonary

5–15. At 5 days postfertilization, the blastocyst is released and hatched from which surrounding structure?

    a. Morula

    b. Chorion laeve

    c. Trophectoderm

    d. Zona pellucida

5–16. Which of the following gives rise to the chorionic structures that transport oxygen and nutrients between fetus and mother?

    a. Villous trophoblast

    b. Interstitial trophoblast

    c. Extravillous trophoblast

    d. Endovascular trophoblast

5–17. In this drawing of implantation, which of the following labeled structures will eventually become the fetus?

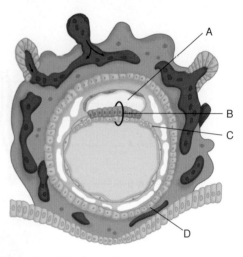

Modified with permission from Cunningham FG, Leveno KJ, Bloom SL, et al (eds): Implantation and placental development. In Williams Obstetrics, 24th ed. New York, McGraw-Hill, 2014, Figure 5-9B.

    a. A

    b. B

    c. C

    d. D

5–18. Which of the following statements is accurate regarding the chorion frondosum?

    a. It is the same as the chorion laeve.

    b. It is the maternal component of the placenta.

    c. It is the area of villi in contact with the decidua basalis.

    d. It is the avascular area that abuts the decidua parietalis.

5–19. Maternal regulation of trophoblast invasion and vascular growth is mainly controlled by which of the following?

    a. CD4 T cells

    b. Progesterone

    c. Cellular adhesion molecules

    d. Decidual natural killer (DNK) cells

5–20. Remodeling of maternal spiral arteries by invading trophoblasts is completed by which week(s) of pregnancy?

    a. 8th week

    b. 12th week

    c. 12–16 weeks

    d. 16–18 weeks

5–21. End-diastolic blood flow can be identified in the fetal umbilical artery by the end of which week of pregnancy?

   a. 10th week

   b. 14th week

   c. 18th week

   d. 22nd week

5–22. Regarding the orientation of spiral blood vessels in relationship to the uterus, which of the following is true?

   a. Both arteries and veins are parallel to the uterine wall.

   b. Both arteries and veins are perpendicular to the uterine wall.

   c. Arteries are perpendicular and veins are parallel to the uterine wall.

   d. Veins are perpendicular and arteries are parallel to the uterine wall.

5–23. What is the name given to the phenomenon that describes how fetal cells can become engrafted in the mother during pregnancy and then be identified decades later?

   a. Microchimerism

   b. Histocompatibility

   c. Hemochorial invasion

   d. Immunological neutrality

5–24. Which of the following is a component of the amnion?

   a. Nerves

   b. Lymphatics

   c. Blood vessels

   d. Acellular zona spongiosa

5–25. Which of the following is accurate regarding a Meckel diverticulum?

   a. It is an allantoic duct remnant.

   b. It is a failure of the right umbilical vein to involute.

   c. It is a portion of one umbilical artery that remains patent postnatally.

   d. It is a failure of the intraabdominal portion of the umbilical vesicle to atrophy.

5–26. As shown in this figure, blood coming from the placenta to the fetus travels first from the umbilical vein into which of the following structures?

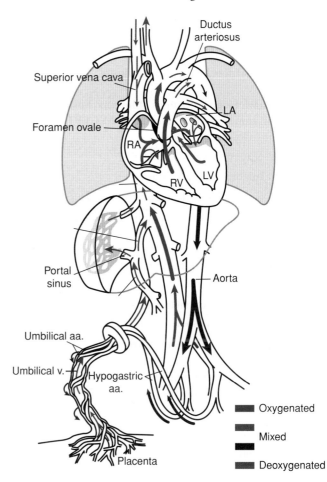

Modified with permission from Cunningham FG, Leveno KJ, Bloom SL, et al (eds): Embryogenesis and fetal morphological development. In Williams Obstetrics, 24th ed. New York, McGraw-Hill, 2014, Figure 7-8.

   a. The portal vein

   b. The hepatic vein

   c. The ductus venosus

   d. The inferior vena cava

5–27. The amino acid sequence of the α-subunit of human chorionic gonadotropin (hCG) is identical in all **EXCEPT** which of the following?

   a. Luteinizing hormone

   b. Thyroid-stimulating hormone

   c. Follicle-stimulating hormone

   d. Corticotropin-releasing hormone

5–28. Abnormally low levels of human chorionic gonado-tropin (hCG) may be found most typically with which of the following?

   a. Down syndrome

   b. Ectopic pregnancy

   c. Erythroblastosis fetalis

   d. Gestational trophoblastic disease

5–29. Known biological actions of human chorionic gonadotropin (hCG) include all **EXCEPT** which of the following?

   a. Maternal thyroid stimulation

   b. Inhibition of relaxin secretion

   c. Sexual differentiation of the male fetus

   d. Rescue and maintenance of the corpus luteum

5–30. Which of the following has the greatest production rate of any known human hormone?

   a. Progesterone

   b. Human placental lactogen

   c. Human chorionic gonadotropin

   d. Chorionic adrenocorticotropin

5–31. Among placental peptide hormones, which has shown a correlation with birthweight?

   a. Leptin

   b. Activin

   c. Inhibin

   d. Neuropeptide Y

5–32. Which of the following is true of bilateral oophorectomy at 9 weeks' gestation?

   a. It will cause a miscarriage.

   b. It will cause a significant drop in progesterone.

   c. It will not alter the maternal excretion of urinary pregnanediol.

   d. None of the above

5–33. Ichthyosis, an X-linked disorder that affects male fetuses, is associated with which of the following?

   a. Fetal adrenal hypoplasia

   b. Fetal adrenal hyperplasia

   c. Fetal placental sulfatase deficiency

   d. Fetal placental aromatase deficiency

5–34. Which of the following conditions is associated with increased estrogen levels in pregnancy?

   a. Fetal demise

   b. Down syndrome

   c. Fetal anencephaly

   d. Erythroblastosis fetalis

CHAPTER 5 ANSWER KEY

Question number	Letter answer	Page cited	Header cited
5–1	b	p. 80	The Ovarian Endometrial Cycle
5–2	c	p. 80	Follicular and Preovulatory Ovarian Phase
5–3	d	p. 80	Follicular and Preovulatory Ovarian Phase
5–4	c	p. 80	Follicular and Preovulatory Ovarian Phase
5–5	a	p. 82	Luteal or Postovulatory Ovarian Phase
5–6	b	p. 82	Luteal or Postovulatory Ovarian Phase
5–7	d	p. 83	Estrogen and Progesterone Action
5–8	d	p. 84	The Endometrial Cycle; Proliferative and Preovulatory Endometrial Phase
5–9	d	p. 85	Secretory or Postovulatory Endometrial Phase
5–10	a	p. 86	Figure 5-4
5–11	d	p. 86	Prostaglandins and Menstruation
5–12	d	p. 87	Decidual Structure; Figure 5-6
5–13	c	p. 88	Decidual Histology
5–14	c	p. 89	Implantation and Early Trophoblast Invasion
5–15	d	p. 90	The Blastocyst
5–16	a	p. 90	Trophoblast Differentiation
5–17	b	p. 92	Early Trophoblast Invasion; Figure 5-9
5–18	c	p. 93	Chorion and Decidua Development
5–19	d	p. 93	Maternal Regulation of Trophoblast Invasion and Vascular Growth
5–20	c	p. 93	Invasion of Spiral Arteries
5–21	a	p. 95	Fetal Circulation
5–22	c	p. 96	Maternal Circulation
5–23	a	p. 97	Breaks in the Placental "Barrier"
5–24	d	p. 98	The Amnion
5–25	d	p. 100	Cord Development
5–26	c	p. 101	Cord Function
5–27	d	p. 101	hCG; Chemical Characteristics
5–28	b	p. 103	Abnormally High or Low hCG Levels
5–29	b	p. 103	Biological Functions of hCG
5–30	b	p. 103	Human Placental Lactogen; Chemical Characteristics
5–31	a	p. 106	Leptin
5–32	c	p. 106	Placental Progesterone Production
5–33	c	p. 110	Fetal Placental Sulfatase Deficiency
5–34	d	p. 109	Fetal Conditions That Affect Estrogen Production

Placental Abnormalities

6-1. For which situation is pathological examination of the placenta considered most informative and cost effective?

   a. Multifetal gestation

   b. Cholestasis of pregnancy

   c. Maternal seizure disorder

   d. All obstetrical deliveries

6-2. At term, which of the following most closely approximates typical placental disk measurements?

   a. 200 g weight, 10 cm diameter, 15 mm thickness

   b. 500 g weight, 20 cm diameter, 25 mm thickness

   c. 1000 g weight, 15 cm diameter, 35 mm thickness

   d. 1500 g weight, 25 cm diameter, 45 mm thickness

6-3. Which of the following terms describes this surface of the placenta?

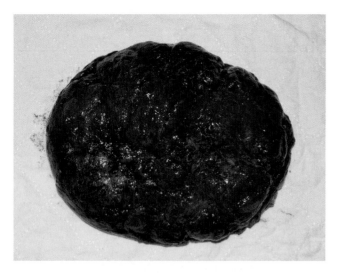

   a. Basal plate

   b. Amniochorion

   c. Placental bed

   d. Chorionic plate

6-4. This is which type of placental variant?

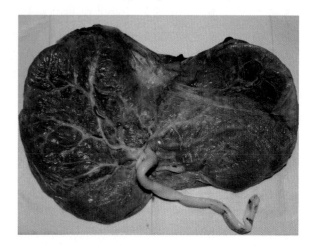

Used with permission from Dr. Jaya George.

   a. Bilobate placenta

   b. Succenturiate lobe

   c. Placenta fenestrata

   d. Circumvallate placenta

6-5. Which placental variant is marked by arrowheads in this image?

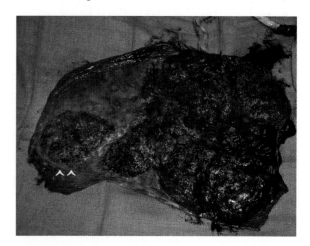

Used with permission from Dr. Heather Lytle.

   a. Bilobate placenta

   b. Succenturiate lobe

   c. Placenta fenestrata

   d. Circumvallate placenta

6–6. Compared with a normally shaped placenta, which complication of third-stage labor is more common with an undiagnosed succenturiate lobe?

a. Cord avulsion

b. Chorioamnionitis

c. Uterine inversion

d. Retained cotyledon

6–7. The placenta in this image meets sonographic criteria for placentomegaly. Common causes of an increased placental thickness include all **EXCEPT** which of the following?

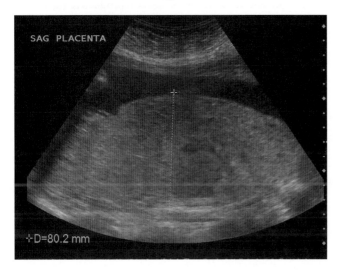

Reproduced with permission from Hoffman BL, Ziadie MS, Dashe JS, et al: Placental Chorioangioma (update). In Cunningham FG, Leveno KL, Bloom SL, et al (eds): Williams Obstetrics, 23rd ed. Online. Accessmedicine.com. New York, McGraw-Hill, 2009, Figure 15.

a. Syphilis

b. Diabetes mellitus

c. Fatty liver of pregnancy

d. Gestational trophoblastic neoplasia

6–8. Extrachorial placentation describes which of the following structural abnormalities?

a. Amnion rupture

b. Total chorion surface area significantly exceeds that of the amnion

c. Excessive folds of amnion are present at the cord insertion site

d. Placental basal plate surface area significantly exceeds that of the chorionic plate

6–9. Pregnancies with this type of extrachorial placentation are at increased risk for which of the following complications?

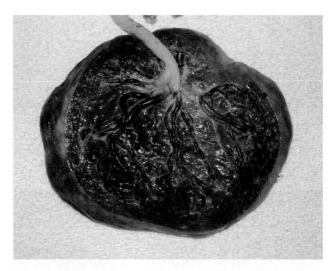

a. Stillbirth

b. Placental abruption

c. Intrapartum fetal acidosis

d. None of the above

6–10. Which term best describes the small opaque plaque (*arrow*) seen on the fetal surface of this placenta?

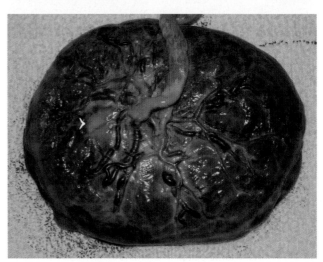

a. Subamnionic hematoma

b. Maternal floor infarction

c. Fetal thrombotic vasculopathy

d. Subchorionic fibrin deposition

6–11. Which of the following is most consistently associated with poor fetal outcomes such as miscarriage, growth restriction, preterm birth, and stillbirth?

a. Subamnionic hematoma

b. Maternal floor infarction

c. Perivillous fibrin deposition

d. Subchorionic fibrin deposition

6–12. Which of the following is most consistently associated with placental abruption?

    a. Subamnionic hematoma

    b. Subchorial thrombosis

    c. Retroplacental hematoma

    d. Perivillous fibrin deposition

6–13. The following placental tumor was found during routine fetal anatomic survey. The differential diagnosis includes chorioangioma, placental hematoma, partial hydatidiform mole, teratoma, tumor metastasis, and leiomyoma. What is most commonly first employed to help distinguish among these?

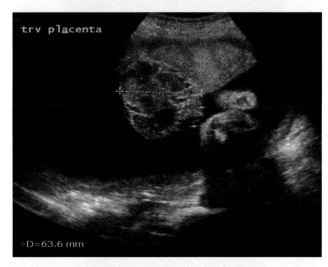

Reproduced with permission from Hoffman BL, Dashe JS: Placental chorioangioma (update). In Cunningham FG, Leveno KL, Bloom SL, et al (eds): Williams Obstetrics, 22nd ed. Online. Accessmedicine.com. New York, McGraw-Hill, 2009, Figure 9.

    a. Color Doppler imaging

    b. Chorionic villus sampling

    c. Magnetic resonance imaging

    d. Three-dimensional sonography

6–14. Which of the following is true regarding calcium deposits within the placenta?

    a. These most commonly form just beneath the chorionic plate.

    b. Increasing calcium deposits should prompt delivery at 39 weeks' gestation.

    c. Deposits are associated with advancing gestation, nulliparity, and smoking.

    d. Grannum grade 3 lesions are consistently linked with intrapartum fetal acidosis and low Apgar scores.

6–15. Which of the following is most consistently associated with large chorioangiomas?

    a. Fetal hydrops

    b. Pulmonary embolism

    c. Severe preeclampsia

    d. Gestational diabetes

6–16. Which of the following cancers most frequently metastasizes to the placenta?

    a. Colon

    b. Gastric

    c. Ovarian

    d. Melanoma

6–17. Which route of bacterial inoculation causes most cases of chorioamnionitis?

    a. Hematogenous spread from maternal blood

    b. Direct spread through the fallopian tubes

    c. Ascension from the lower reproductive tract

    d. Needle inoculation during intraamnionic procedures

6–18. Which of the following risk factors is most commonly associated with chorioamnionitis?

    a. Maternal drug abuse

    b. Poor maternal hygiene

    c. Prior cesarean delivery

    d. Prolonged rupture of membranes

6–19. With chorioamnionitis, fetal contact with bacteria through which of the following routes may lead to fetal infection?

    a. Aspiration

    b. Swallowing

    c. Hematogenous

    d. All of the above

6–20. The multiple, small, raised lesions of amnion nodosum are most commonly associated with which of the following?

    a. Oligohydramnios

    b. Chorioamnionitis

    c. Meconium staining

    d. Placental abruption

6–21. Sonographically, an amnionic sheet or band may reflect several different clinical conditions. Which of the following poses the greatest fetal risk?

    a. Amnionic band

    b. Amniochorion of a vanishing twin

    c. Amniochorion of a circumvallate placenta

    d. Amniochorion of a pregnancy in one horn of a partial bicornuate uterus

6–22. A short umbilical cord may be associated with which of the following perinatal outcomes?

    a. Intrapartum distress

    b. Fetal-growth restriction

    c. Congenital malformations

    d. All of the above

6–23. A long umbilical cord may be more commonly associated with which of the following?

　　a. Cord prolapse

　　b. Cord false knots

　　c. Cord pseudocysts

　　d. Velamentous insertion

6–24. The number of complete coils per centimeter of cord length has been termed the umbilical coiling index. Which of the following is true of cord coiling?

　　a. A normal coiling index in a postpartum cord approximates 1.2.

　　b. Hypocoiling has not been associated with adverse fetal outcomes.

　　c. Hypercoiling has been associated with greater rates of intrapartum fetal acidosis.

　　d. All of the above

6–25. A transverse-plane sonographic image of the lower abdomen from a 17-week fetus is shown here. What is the most reasonable next step?

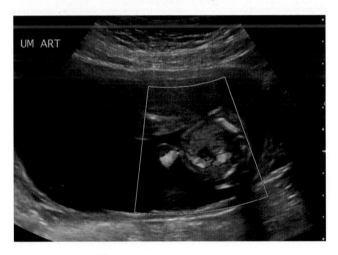

　　a. Fetal karyotyping

　　b. Continued routine prenatal care only

　　c. Detailed sonographic anatomic survey

　　d. Radiofrequency ablation of this anomaly

6–26. Sectioning of a term umbilical cord after delivery may reveal embryonic remnants. Which of the following would not be possibly found?

　　a. Wolffian duct

　　b. Vitelline duct

　　c. Allantoic duct

　　d. Second umbilical vein

6–27. A single umbilical cord cyst is found during a first-trimester scan performed for vaginal bleeding. What is the most reasonable next step?

　　a. Chorionic villus sampling

　　b. Ultrasound-guided percutaneous cyst drainage

　　c. Repeated sonographic evaluation in the second trimester

　　d. Counsel regarding pregnancy termination of this anomalous pregnancy

6–28. This cord insertion variant is most commonly associated with a higher rate of which of the following?

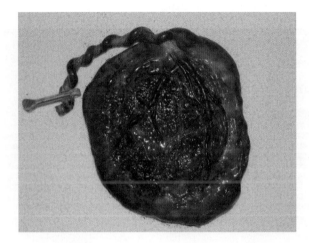

　　a. Cord avulsion

　　b. Fetal anomalies

　　c. Uterine inversion

　　d. Single umbilical artery

6–29. In which of the following clinical settings is the cord insertion variant seen here most likely to develop?

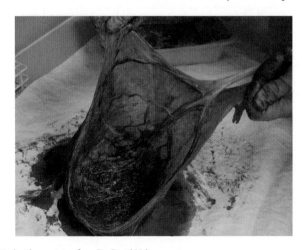

Used with permission from Dr. David Nelson.

　　a. Multifetal gestation

　　b. Fetus with trisomy 21

　　c. Concurrent cocaine substance abuse

　　d. Poorly controlled chronic hypertension prior to conception

6–30. The cord insertion abnormality seen in Question 6-28 may more commonly be associated with which of the following complications?

    a. Funisitis

    b. Vasa previa

    c. Placenta percreta

    d. Maternal floor infarction

6–31. At 28 weeks' gestation, this finding is noted during subsequent sonographic evaluation of a placenta previa that was identified earlier at 18 weeks. The patient is asymptomatic. What is the most reasonable next step?

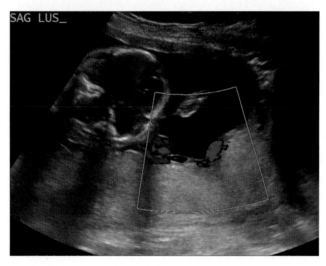

Used with permission from Dr. Jodi Dashe.

    a. Immediate cesarean delivery

    b. Cesarean delivery at 39 weeks' gestation

    c. Cesarean delivery at 34 to 35 weeks' gestation

    d. Administer corticosteroids to promote lung maturation and perform cesarean delivery 24 hours later

6–32. A true knot in the umbilical cord is associated with an increased risk of which of the following fetal complications?

    a. Stillbirth

    b. Cerebral palsy

    c. Chromosomal anomalies

    d. Amnionic band sequence

6–33. This umbilical cord finding is more commonly associated with which of the following fetal complications?

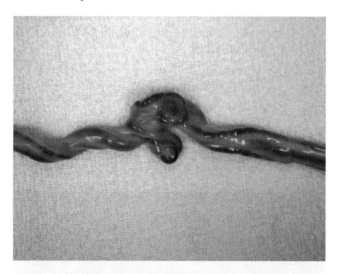

    a. Stillbirth

    b. Trisomy 13

    c. Cardiac anomalies

    d. None of the above

CHAPTER 6   ANSWER KEY

Question number	Letter answer	Page cited	Header cited
6–1	a	p. 117	Table 6-1
6–2	b	p. 116	Normal Placenta
6–3	a	p. 116	Normal Placenta
6–4	a	p. 117	Shape and Size
6–5	b	p. 117	Shape and Size
6–6	d	p. 117	Shape and Size
6–7	c	p. 117	Shape and Size
6–8	d	p. 118	Extrachorial Placentation
6–9	d	p. 118	Extrachorial Placentation
6–10	d	p. 119	Subchorionic Fibrin Deposition
6–11	b	p. 119	Maternal Floor Infarction
6–12	c	p. 119	Hematoma
6–13	a	p. 120	Subamnionic Hematoma
6–14	c	p. 120	Placental Calcification
6–15	a	p. 120	Chorioangioma
6–16	d	p. 121	Tumors Metastatic to the Placenta
6–17	c	p. 121	Chorioamnionitis
6–18	d	p. 121	Chorioamnionitis
6–19	d	p. 121	Chorioamnionitis
6–20	a	p. 121	Other Membrane Abnormalities
6–21	a	p. 121	Other Membrane Abnormalities
6–22	d	p. 121	Length
6–23	a	p. 121	Length
6–24	c	p. 121	Coiling
6–25	c	p. 122	Vessel Number
6–26	a	p. 122	Remnants and Cysts
6–27	c	p. 122	Remnants and Cysts
6–28	a	p. 122	Insertion
6–29	a	p. 122	Insertion
6–30	b	p. 122	Insertion
6–31	c	p. 123	Vasa Previa
6–32	a	p. 123	Knots, Strictures, and Loops
6–33	d	p. 123	Knots, Strictures, and Loops

CHAPTER 7

Embryogenesis and Fetal Morphological Development

7–1. A patient reports that the first day of her last menstrual period was September 19th. Based on Naegele rule, her due date is which of the following?

    a. July 10th

    b. June 14th

    c. June 26th

    d. December 12th

7–2. Pregnancy can be divided into three units or trimesters each lasting how many weeks?

    a. 12

    b. 13

    c. 15

    d. 16

7–3. At the beginning of which week following fertilization is a conceptus termed an embryo?

    a. 1st week

    b. 2nd week

    c. 3rd week

    d. 4th week

7–4. How many weeks does the embryonic period last?

    a. 4

    b. 8

    c. 10

    d. 12

7–5. During which week of development is the primitive heart partitioned?

    a. 4th week

    b. 6th week

    c. 8th week

    d. 10th week

7–6. At 10 weeks' gestation based on the last menstrual period, all **EXCEPT** which of the following are true?

    a. Arms bend at the elbows.

    b. Crown-rump length is 7 cm.

    c. The upper lip is complete.

    d. Heart is completely formed.

7–7. Corresponding with midbrain maturation, when do eye movements begin?

    a. 10–12 weeks

    b. 12–14 weeks

    c. 14–16 weeks

    d. 16–18 weeks

7–8. At 28 weeks' gestation, what is the chance of survival without physical or neurological impairment?

    a. 10%

    b. 25%

    c. 50%

    d. 90%

7–9. All **EXCEPT** which of the following pass through placental tissue by simple diffusion?

    a. IgG

    b. Water

    c. Oxygen

    d. Anesthetic gases

7–10. What is the average oxygen saturation of intervillous space blood?

    a. 10–20%

    b. 30–35%

    c. 65–75%

    d. 90–95%

7–11. Which of the following statements regarding the transfer of carbon dioxide across the placenta is true?

    a. Carbon dioxide traverses the chorionic villus more slowly than oxygen.

    b. Fetal blood has more affinity for carbon dioxide than maternal blood.

    c. The partial pressure of carbon dioxide in the umbilical arteries averages 50 mm Hg.

    d. Mild maternal hypoventilation results in a fall in P_{CO_2} levels, favoring a transfer of carbon dioxide from the fetal compartment to maternal blood.

7-12. Which of the following is found in higher concentrations in the mother than the fetus?

a. Iron

b. Zinc

c. Ascorbic acid

d. Human placental lactogen

7-13. Which of the following maternal immunoglobulins (Ig) reach the fetus?

a. Only IgA

b. Only IgG

c. Only IgM

d. IgA and IgG

7-14. How is iodide transported across the placenta?

a. Endocytosis

b. Simple diffusion

c. Carrier-mediated process

d. Iodide does not cross the placenta

7-15. In early pregnancy, amnionic fluid is composed of which of the following?

a. Fetal urine

b. Fetal pulmonary fluid

c. Ultrafiltrate of maternal plasma

d. Extracellular fluid that diffuses through fetal skin

7-16. Amnionic fluid volume peaks at what gestational age?

a. 24 weeks

b. 28 weeks

c. 34 weeks

d. 38 weeks

7-17. Which of the following statements regarding the fetal cardiovascular system is true?

a. Fetal heart chambers work in series.

b. The portal sinus is the major branch of the umbilical vein.

c. Oxygen is delivered from the placenta by the umbilical artery.

d. The ductus venosus traverses the liver to enter the inferior vena cava directly.

7-18. After birth, the intraabdominal remnants of the umbilical vein form which of the following?

a. Ligamentum teres

b. Ligamentum venosum

c. Ligament of Treitz

d. Umbilical ligaments

7-19. The order in which hemopoiesis is seen in the embryo/fetus from earliest to latest is which of the following?

a. Liver, yolk sac, bone marrow

b. Yolk sac, liver, bone marrow

c. Bone marrow, liver, yolk sac

d. Yolk sac, bone marrow, liver

7-20. Which of the following has the lowest erythrocyte mean cell volume (MCV)?

a. Embryo

b. Term fetus

c. Aneuploid fetus

d. The MCV remains the same throughout gestation

7-21. A fetus weighs 3000 g at term. What is the expected fetoplacental blood volume?

a. 125 mL

b. 250 mL

c. 375 mL

d. 500 mL

7-22. Where is fetal hemoglobin F produced?

a. Liver

b. Yolk sac

c. Bone marrow

d. Yolk sac and liver

7-23. Infants attain adult levels of IgM at what age?

a. 3 months

b. 6 months

c. 9 months

d. 12 months

7–24. Which of the following sequences correctly identifies the bones labeled in the image?

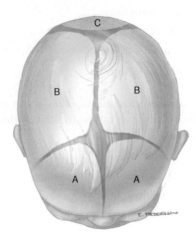

Modified with permission from Cunningham FG, Leveno KJ, Bloom SL, et al (eds): Embryogenesis and Fetal Morphological Development. In Williams Obstetrics, 24th ed. New York, McGraw-Hill, 2014, Figure 7-11.

a. A is the frontal bone, B is the parietal bone, C is the occipital bone.

b. A is the parietal bone, B is the occipital bone, C is the frontal bone.

c. A is the temporal bone, B is the frontal bone, C is the occipital bone.

d. A is the frontal bone, B is the temporal bone, C is the parietal bone.

7–25. In the figure of Question 7-24, the suture bordered by the bones labeled A and B is which of the following?

a. Coronal suture

b. Lambdoid suture

c. Frontal suture

d. Sagittal suture

7–26. Which of the following sequences correctly identifies the dimensions labeled in this image?

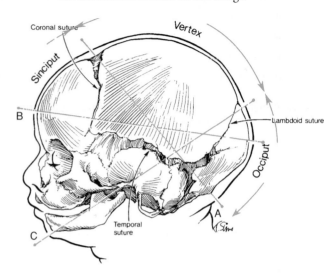

Modified with permission from Cunningham FG, Leveno KJ, Bloom SL, et al (eds): Fetal Growth and Development. In Williams Obstetrics, 22nd ed. New York, McGraw-Hill, 2005, Figure 4-9.

a. A is suboccipitobregmatic, B is occipitofrontal, C is occipitomental.

b. A is occipitofrontal, B is suboccipitobregmatic, C is occipitomental.

c. A is occipitomental, B is occipitofrontal, C is suboccipitobregmatic.

d. A is occipitofrontal, B is occipitomental, C is suboccipitobregmatic.

7–27. Which of the statements regarding fetal swallowing is true?

a. Swallowing begins at 20 weeks' gestation.

b. Term fetuses swallow between 200 and 760 mL per day.

c. If swallowing is inhibited in late pregnancy, oligohydramnios will occur.

d. Swallowing greatly affects amnionic fluid volume, particularly in early pregnancy.

7–28. The limits of fetal viability are determined by which of the following processes?

a. Pulmonary growth

b. Kidney formation

c. Hepatic development

d. Fetal immunocompetence

7–29. A 25-year-old G1P0 presents with rupture of membranes at 19 weeks. She subsequently delivers. On histological evaluation of the lungs of the nonviable fetus, you would expect which of the following?

    a. Mature alveoli

    b. No cartilage development

    c. Presence of terminal sacs

    d. Normal bronchial branching

7–30. You deliver an infant with ambiguous genitalia. During examination, you note a small phallus that you suspect is clitoral hypertrophy. A photograph is provided below. You counsel the mother and order karyotyping. The karyotype is 46,XY. The most likely diagnosis is which of the following?

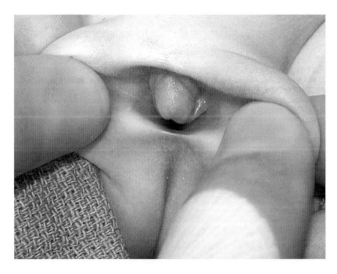

Reproduced with permission from Cunningham FG, Leveno KJ, Bloom SL, et al (eds): Fetal growth and development. In Williams Obstetrics, 23rd ed. New York, McGraw-Hill, Figure 4-20.

    a. True hermaphroditism

    b. Fetal aromatase deficiency

    c. Male pseudohermaphroditism

    d. Congenital adrenal hyperplasia

7–31. The child below has a webbed neck, streak gonads, and genital infantilism. Her mother reports that when pregnant with her, her ultrasound was abnormal, with fluid collecting on the back of the child's neck. The most likely diagnosis is which of the following?

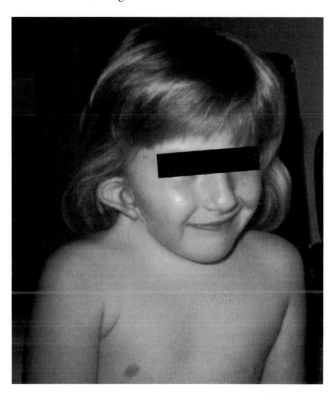

Reproduced with permission from Fuster V, Walsh RA, Harrington RA (eds): Hurst's The Heart, 13th ed. New York, McGraw-Hill, 2011, Figure 14-14.

    a. Gonadal dysgenesis

    b. True hermaphroditism

    c. Reifenstein syndrome

    d. Androgen insensitivity syndrome

7–32. A woman presents to labor and delivery after having a vaginal birth at home. She has had no prenatal care. After attending to her, you examine the newborn. A photograph is provided. You note a hemiscrotum among other things. The likely diagnosis is which of the following?

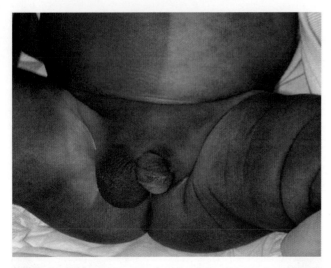

Reproduced with permission from Cunningham FG, Leveno KJ, Bloom SL, et al (eds): Fetal growth and development. In Williams Obstetrics, 23rd ed. New York, McGraw-Hill, Figure 4-21B.

a. True hermaphroditism

b. Fetal aromatase deficiency

c. Male pseudohermaphroditism

d. Congenital adrenal hyperplasia

CHAPTER 7 ANSWER KEY

Question number	Letter answer	Page cited	Header cited
7–1	c	p. 127	Gestational Age Variously Defined
7–2	b	p. 127	Gestational Age Variously Defined
7–3	c	p. 128	Embryonic Period
7–4	c	p. 128	Embryonic Period
7–5	a	p. 128	Embryonic Period
7–6	b	p. 128	Embryonic Period
7–7	d	p. 129	16 Gestational Weeks
7–8	d	p. 129	28 Gestational Weeks
7–9	a	p. 132	Mechanisms of Transfer
7–10	c	p. 132	Transfer of Oxygen and Carbon Dioxide
7–11	c	p. 132	Transfer of Oxygen and Carbon Dioxide
7–12	d	p. 133	Glucose and Fetal Growth
7–13	b	p. 134	Proteins
7–14	c	p. 134	Ions and Trace Metals
7–15	c	p. 135	Amnionic Fluid Formation
7–16	c	p. 135	Amnionic Fluid Formation
7–17	d	p. 135	Cardiovascular System
7–18	a	p. 137	Circulatory Changes at Birth
7–19	b	p. 137	Hemopoiesis
7–20	b	p. 137	Hemopoiesis
7–21	c	p. 137	Fetoplacental Blood Volume
7–22	a	p. 137	Fetal Hemoglobin
7–23	c	p. 139	Immunoglobulin M and A
7–24	a	p. 139	Skull
7–25	a	p. 139	Skull
7–26	a	p. 139	Skull
7–27	b	p. 140	Gastrointestinal System
7–28	a	p. 142	Anatomical Maturation
7–29	d	p. 142	Anatomical Maturation
7–30	c	p. 148	Genital Ambiguity of the Newborn
7–31	a	p. 148	Genital Ambiguity of the Newborn
7–32	a	p. 148	Genital Ambiguity of the Newborn

SECTION 4

PRECONCEPTIONAL AND PRENATAL CARE

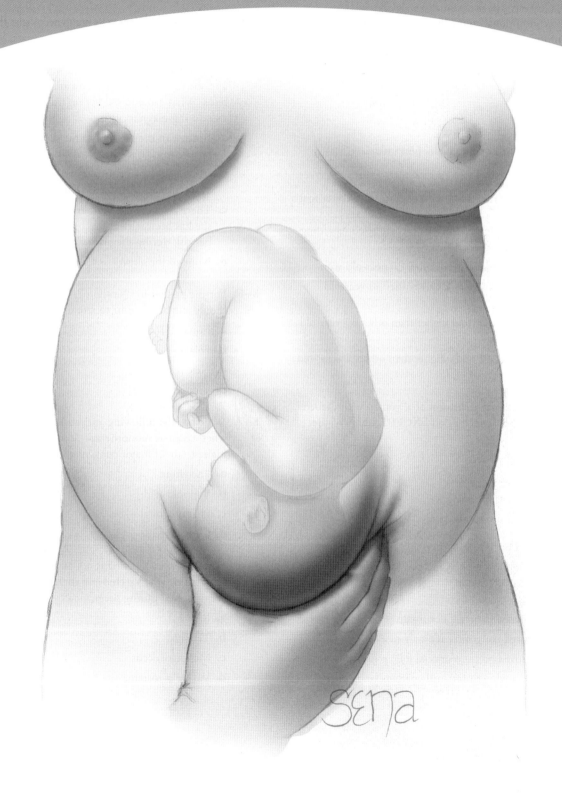

CHAPTER 8

Preconceptional Counseling

8-1. Preconceptional counseling involves collection of information regarding previous pregnancy outcomes, medical conditions, and family history. What is the optimal method of collecting this information?

 a. Nurse visit

 b. Paper intake form

 c. Online questionnaire

 d. Combined questionnaire plus interview

8-2. A 30-year-old woman with no known medical conditions is noted to have 3+ glucosuria at her first prenatal visit. A fasting blood glucose level is 144 mg/dL. How should she be counseled regarding her risk for fetal anomalies?

 a. Her risk is the same as other 30-year-old women.

 b. Her risk is twice as high as other 30-year-old women.

 c. Her risk is fourfold higher than other 30-year-old women.

 d. Her risk is 10 times higher than other 30-year-old women.

8-3. Preconceptional evaluation of a woman with diabetes mellitus should include all **EXCEPT** which of the following?

 a. Hemoglobin A_{1c}

 b. Retinal examination

 c. Bone density testing

 d. 24-hour urine collection

8-4. All **EXCEPT** which of the following can be expected following preconceptional counseling and its implementation in women with pregestational diabetes?

 a. Decreased perinatal death rate

 b. Reduced congenital anomaly rate

 c. Improved preconceptional folic acid use

 d. Decreased need for antihypertensive therapy

8-5. A 23-year-old patient tells her gynecologist that she wants to have a child in the next few years. She is concerned as she has a seizure disorder and takes valproic acid. It has been 1 year since her last seizure, and she has heard that seizures are dangerous for the fetus. What can you tell her regarding her seizure risk during pregnancy?

 a. Because of the length of time she has been seizure-free, it is reduced 50%.

 b. If she delays pregnancy for an additional 12 months, her risk will be reduced by 50%.

 c. There is an inverse relationship between the time she has been seizure-free before pregnancy and her risk during pregnancy.

 d. None of the above

8-6. For the patient in Question 8-5, what supplement should she begin prior to attempting conception?

 a. Iron

 b. Folate

 c. Niacin

 d. Vitamin D

8-7. Which of the following antiseizure medications, when taken as monotherapy, is associated with the highest rate of major congenital malformations?

 a. Phenytoin

 b. Valproic acid

 c. Phenobarbital

 d. Carbamazepine

8-8. Which of the following is not an example of a killed bacterial or viral vaccine and therefore should not be administered during pregnancy?

 a. Rabies

 b. Tetanus

 c. Meningococcus

 d. Varicella-zoster

8–9. A woman presents for a screening sonographic evaluation at 21 weeks' gestation. A fetal leg is imaged below. She and her partner ask about the frequency of birth defects in the general population. What is the correct response to their question?

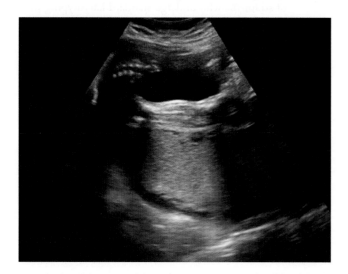

a. 0.1%

b. 1%

c. 3%

d. 11%

8–10. Birth defects are responsible for what percentage of infant mortality?

a. 2%

b. 5%

c. 10%

d. 20%

8–11. What is the significance of the individual identified by the arrow in the following image?

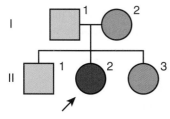

Reproduced with permission from Cunningham FG, Leveno KJ, Bloom SL, et al (eds): Preconceptional counseling. In Williams Obstetrics, 24th ed. New York, McGraw-Hill, 2014, Fig. 8-2.

a. She is one of a triplet gestation.

b. She is affected by the condition in question.

c. She is being evaluated for a suspected condition.

d. She is the only one in her family unaffected by the condition in question.

8–12. The incidence of fetal cardiac abnormalities is increased in all **EXCEPT** which of the following maternal conditions?

a. Lead exposure

b. Phenylketonuria

c. Diabetes mellitus

d. Methylene tetrahydrofolate reductase mutation carrier

8–13. What percent of fetuses with the following condition are born to women at low risk for the anomaly?

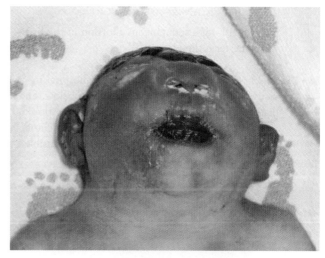

Used with permission from Dr. Tiffany Woodus.

a. 10%

b. 50%

c. 75%

d. 90%

8–14. Preconception supplementation and fortification of some food products with folate has had what impact on pregnancy outcomes?

a. Reduced the rate of preeclampsia

b. Reduced the incidence of childhood seizures

c. Reduced the incidence of neural-tube defects

d. Reduced the incidence of spontaneous abortions

8–15. A woman with phenylketonuria presents to her primary care physician's office 1 week after her missed menses. A home urine pregnancy test was positive. The pregnancy was unplanned, and her blood phenylalanine level is 1012 µmol/L, which is essentially unchanged from her baseline levels over the past several months. How should she be counseled regarding about her pregnancy outcomes?

   a. Her risk for congenital anomalies is not increased.

   b. There is a 50% chance for neurological impairment in her fetus.

   c. The risk for congenital cardiac abnormalities in her fetus is 12%.

   d. Her risk for a spontaneous abortion in the first trimester is doubled.

8–16. A 23-year-old woman presents to the hospital in active labor and delivers the infant seen below. She had received no prenatal care and upon questioning admits she has some medical problems. Which of the following conditions is most likely responsible for the infant's condition?

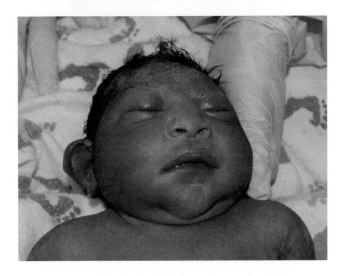

   a. Gaucher disease

   b. Phenylketonuria

   c. Diabetes mellitus

   d. None of the above

8–17. What are the most common single-gene disorders worldwide?

   a. Hemophilias

   b. Thalassemias

   c. Cystic fibrosis mutations

   d. Glycogen storage diseases

8–18. A 33-year-old multipara presents to Labor and Delivery complaining of decreased fetal movement for 2 days at 33 weeks' gestation. Sonographic evaluation confirms the diagnosis of fetal demise. No other abnormalities are noted. What percentage of stillbirths who undergo standard karyotyping will have a chromosomal abnormality detected?

   a. 0.1%

   b. 1%

   c. 13%

   d. 21%

8–19. What benefit does chromosomal microarray analysis have over standard karyotyping in the evaluation of stillbirth?

   a. Can be performed on maternal blood

   b. Can be performed on nonviable tissue

   c. Detects lower levels of tissue mosaicism

   d. None of the above

8–20. All **EXCEPT** which of the following obstetrical complications is increased in adolescent pregnancies compared with women aged 20 to 35 years?

   a. Anemia

   b. Preeclampsia

   c. Preterm labor

   d. Postpartum hemorrhage

8–21. For women older than 40 years, pregnancy-related mortality rates are increase by what magnitude compared with women in their twenties?

   a. Twofold

   b. Fivefold

   c. Eightfold

   d. Tenfold

8–22. Which of the following is the most common pregnancy complication in women older than 35 years?

   a. Diabetes

   b. Hypertension

   c. Preterm birth

   d. Low birthweight

8–23. In 2005, what percentage of all multifetal gestations were due to assisted reproductive technologies?

a. 20%

b. 30%

c. 40%

d. 50%

8–24. Which of the following assisted reproductive technologies is associated with a higher rate of congenital abnormalities in the fetus?

a. Cryopreservation

b. Ovulation induction

c. In vitro fertilization

d. Intracytoplasmic sperm injection

8–25. An infant with achondroplasia is born to a 41-year-old diabetic woman and her 51-year-old husband who uses testosterone supplementation. Which of the factors in their backgrounds is most likely related to the infant's condition?

a. Maternal age

b. Paternal age

c. Maternal diabetes

d. Paternal sex steroid use

8–26. Which of the following obstetrical complications is not increased in obese patients?

a. Hypertension

b. Fetal anomalies

c. Cesarean delivery

d. Group B streptococcal carrier frequency

8–27. A 23-year-old primigravida who is seeking pregnancy presents for her annual examination, and you ascertain that she smokes approximately one pack of cigarettes daily. She is considering pregnancy and is concerned about the effect of tobacco use on pregnancy outcomes. Which of the following is an accurate statement?

a. Her risk of preterm delivery continues to fall during the first 6 months she abstains from cigarette use.

b. Her risk for pulmonary edema complicating preeclampsia remains higher than that of the nonsmoking population.

c. The risk of fetal-growth restriction should be no higher that the general population if she quits before she conceives.

d. None of the above

8–28. What percent of women giving birth in the United States are smokers?

a. 2%

b. 6%

c. 14%

d. 24%

8–29. Pregnant women should limit their weekly dietary intake of canned tuna to 12 ounces and should eliminate consumption of certain kinds of fish such as mackerel and swordfish to minimize exposure to which fetal neurotoxin?

a. Cadmium

b. Methyl mercury

c. Organic phosphate

d. Algae-related toxin

8–30. A 19-year-old G3P2 at 28 weeks' gestation is embarrassed to admit she has been craving and eating ice and dirt. She thinks she must be "going crazy." What test is likely to be abnormal?

a. Toxicology screen

b. Liver function tests

c. Complete blood count

d. Electroencephalogram

8–31. What diagnostic test should be performed either prior to pregnancy or early in prenatal care to assess the risk to the fetus and the pregnancy from the disease that is typified by the blood smear shown in this image?

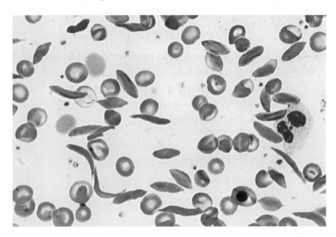

Reproduced with permission from Longo DL: Atlas of hematology and analysis of peripheral blood smears. In Longo DL, Fauci AS, Kasper DL, et al (eds): Harrison's Principles of Internal Medicine, 18th ed. New York, McGraw-Hill, 2012, Figure e17-12.

a. Serum ferritin

b. Antiglobulin test

c. Indirect Coombs test

d. Hemoglobin electrophoresis

8–32. Ashkenazi Jewish individuals should be offered preconceptional screening for all **EXCEPT** which of the following?

a. Canavan disease

b. Cystic fibrosis

c. Beta thalassemia

d. Tay-Sachs disease

8–33. You have recently taken the practice from a retiring obstetrician and are meeting a patient for her first prenatal appointment. In reviewing her old chart, you see the following photo and notes that state her husband was responsible. Why are you concerned for this patient?

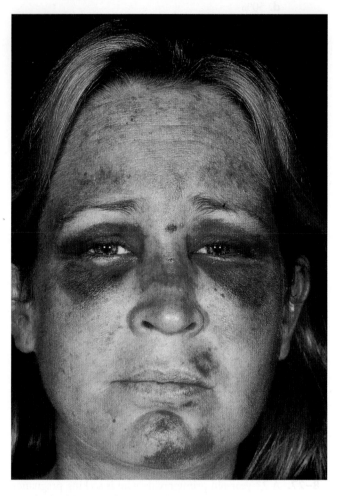

Reproduced with permission from Knoop KJ, Stack LB, Storrow AB, et al (eds): The Atlas of Emergency Medicine, 3rd ed. New York, McGraw-Hill, 2010, Figure 1-3.

a. Rate of successful breastfeeding is reduced.

b. Risk for violence against your patient is higher during pregnancy.

c. There is reduced bonding between the father and infant in the setting of domestic violence.

d. None of the above

CHAPTER 8 ANSWER KEY

Question number	Letter answer	Page cited	Header cited
8–1	d	p. 156	Counseling Session
8–2	c	p. 157	Diabetes Mellitus
8–3	c	p. 163	Table 8-4
8–4	d	p. 157	Diabetes Mellitus
8–5	a	p. 158	Epilepsy
8–6	b	p. 158	Epilepsy
8–7	b	p. 158	Table 8-2
8–8	d	p. 158	Immunizations
8–9	c	p. 159	Genetic Disease
8–10	d	p. 159	Genetic Diseases
8–11	b	p. 160	Figure 8-2
8–12	a	p. 159	Neural-Tube Defects
8–13	d	p. 159	Neural-Tube Defects
8–14	c	p. 159	Neural-Tube Defects
8–15	a	p. 159	Table 8-3
8–16	b	p. 159	Table 8-3
8–17	b	p. 160	Thalassemias
8–18	c	p. 161	Reproductive History
8–19	b	p. 161	Reproductive History
8–20	d	p. 161	Maternal Age
8–21	b	p. 161	Maternal Age
8–22	a	p. 161	Figure 8-3
8–23	c	p. 161	Assisted Reproductive Technologies
8–24	d	p. 161	Assisted Reproductive Technologies
8–25	b	p. 162	Paternal Age
8–26	d	p. 162	Diet
8–27	c	p. 162	Recreational Drugs and Smoking
8–28	c	p. 162	Recreational Drugs and Smoking
8–29	b	p. 163	Table 8-4
8–30	c	p. 162	Diet
8–31	d	p. 163	Table 8-4
8–32	c	p. 161	Individuals of Eastern European Jewish Descent
8–33	b	p. 163	Intimate Partner Violence

CHAPTER 9

Prenatal Care

9–1. Which of the following statements accurately describes racial differences in prenatal care usage?

  a. Hispanic women are least likely to obtain care.

  b. Ten percent of African American women receive no prenatal care.

  c. Minority women now access prenatal care as readily as nonminority women.

  d. Minority women have made the largest gains in timely access to prenatal care during the past 2 decades.

9–2. Common reasons cited by women as barriers to enrolling in prenatal care include which of the following?

  a. Lack of funding

  b. Late identification of pregnancy

  c. Inability to obtain an appointment

  d. All of the above

9–3. Fetal movements are typically first perceived by the mother at approximately what gestational age?

  a. 8 weeks

  b. 14 weeks

  c. 16 weeks

  d. 22 weeks

9–4. A false-positive human chorionic gonadotropin (hCG) test result due to circulating heterophilic antibodies is most likely to occur in which individuals?

  a. Women carrying a twin gestation

  b. Women with a history of a molar pregnancy

  c. Women who have worked closely with animals

  d. Women with autoimmune conditions such as systemic lupus erythematosus

9–5. A 29-year-old primigravida with an unknown last menstrual period presents complaining of vaginal spotting and cramping. Transvaginal sonographic examination is performed as part of her evaluation. One image is shown here. This finding would represent a pregnancy of approximately what gestational age?

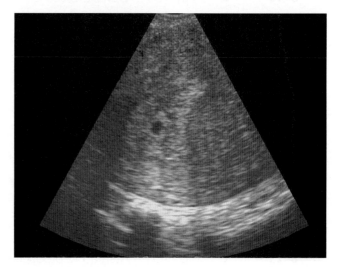

Used with permission from Dr. Elysia Moschos.

  a. 3 weeks

  b. 5 weeks

  c. 7 weeks

  d. 9 weeks

9–6. Referring to the patient and image described in Question 9-5, which of the following increases the certainty that this finding represents an intrauterine pregnancy?

  a. An echogenic rim along one side of the decidua

  b. Two concentric echogenic rings surrounding the sac

  c. A sac positioned eccentrically within the endometrium

  d. All of the above

9–7. Referring to the patient described in Question 9-5, an examination was performed and identified a closed cervical os and no bleeding. Bimanual examination was benign. What is the most appropriate management plan?

a. Dilation and curettage

b. Methotrexate administration

c. Obtain serial serum β-hCG levels

d. Repeat sonographic examination in 48 hours

9–8. Provided it occurs in the first trimester, all **EXCEPT** which of the following are typically performed or obtained at the initial prenatal care evaluation?

a. Urine culture

b. Neural-tube defect screening

c. Complete physical examination

d. Blood type and antibody screen

9–9. Which of the following women could be classified as a *nulligravida*?

a. A 30-year-old who has never been pregnant before

b. A 23-year-old who is pregnant for the first time at 22 weeks' gestation

c. A 25-year-old who is 6 weeks postpartum after her first term delivery

d. A 34-year-old who has two previous pregnancies that ended in miscarriages at 8 weeks' gestation

9–10. How should a woman who has had 4 pregnancies delivered at term, one of which was a twin pregnancy, be designated?

a. Gravida 5 para 4

b. Gravida 4 para 5

c. Gravida 4 para 4

d. Gravida 5 para 5

9–11. Adding 7 days to the first day of the last menstrual period and counting back 3 months to estimate the day of delivery is termed what?

a. Hegar rule

b. Naegele rule

c. Kessner rule

d. Chadwick rule

9–12. Approximately how often will delivery dates be estimated incorrectly using the device shown in the image below?

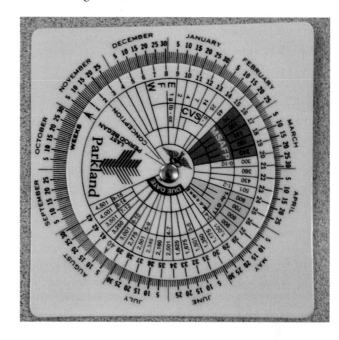

a. 10%

b. 30%

c. 50%

d. 70%

9–13. The accuracy of gestational age dating using the last menstrual period is affected by which of the following?

a. Anovulatory bleeding

b. Menstrual cycle length

c. Oral contraceptive use

d. All of the above

9–14. Which groups of women should receive psychosocial screening as a part of their prenatal care?

a. All women

b. Women who use illicit substances

c. Women at risk for domestic violence

d. Women of minority race or ethnicity

9–15. All **EXCEPT** which of the following adverse outcomes have been linked to smoking in pregnancy?

a. Preeclampsia

b. Preterm birth

c. Placental abruption

d. Sudden infant death syndrome

9–16. According to the Centers for Disease Control and Prevention, which of the following are characteristics of women who are most likely to use alcohol in pregnancy?

    a. Teenagers

    b. Unemployed

    c. College educated

    d. African American race

9–17. Intimate partner violence has been associated with all **EXCEPT** which of the following untoward pregnancy outcomes?

    a. Perinatal death

    b. Preterm delivery

    c. Gestational hypertension

    d. Fetal-growth restriction

9–18. As demonstrated in the image below, fundal height measurements in centimeters correlate closely with gestational age between 20 and 34 weeks. All **EXCEPT** which of the following can introduce error into this measurement?

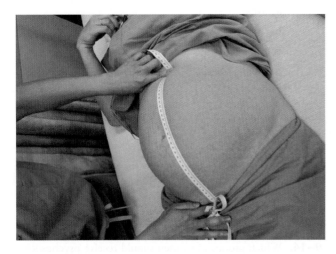

Used with permission from Dr. Heather Lytle.

    a. Obesity

    b. An empty bladder

    c. Uterine leiomyomas

    d. Multifetal gestation

9–19. Which of the following statements is true regarding the current recommendations for weight gain by the Institute of Medicine?

    a. Recommended weight gain differs by ethnicity.

    b. Adolescents should gain slightly more weight than adults.

    c. Women of normal weight should gain between 15 to 25 pounds.

    d. Recommendations are stratified based on prepregnancy body mass index.

9–20. At least how much elemental iron should be given daily as a supplement to pregnant women?

    a. 15 mg

    b. 27 mg

    c. 42 mg

    d. 60 mg

9–21. Which of the following strategies may decrease side effects from iron supplementation?

    a. Ingestion at bedtime

    b. Taking it on an empty stomach

    c. Avoiding it in the first trimester

    d. All of the above

9–22. Which women who are planning a pregnancy should receive 0.4–0.8 mg of supplemental folate?

    a. All women

    b. Those with proven folate deficiency

    c. Those with a previous child affected by a neural-tube defect

    d. Those who do not receive adequate dietary intake of grains

9–23. A 29-year-old G1P1 was just delivered of a newborn with a large posterior encephalocele as demonstrated in the image. Assuming she takes the appropriate dose of folate in the periconceptional period of her next pregnancy, the risk for recurrence is decreased by approximately what percentage?

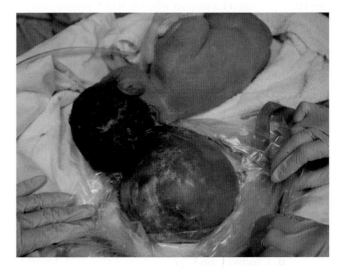

Used with permission from Dr. Heather Lytle.

    a. 20%

    b. 40%

    c. 70%

    d. 90%

9–24. Doses of vitamin A in excess of what amount have been associated with congenital malformations?

    a. > 1,000 IU per day

    b. > 10,000 IU per day

    c. > 100,000 IU per day

    d. > 1,000,000 IU per day

9–25. Which of the following vitamins, when combined with the antihistamine doxylamine, has been found to be helpful in cases of nausea and vomiting?

    a. Vitamin C

    b. Vitamin D

    c. Vitamin B_6

    d. Vitamin B_{12}

9–26. Maternal deficiency of vitamin D has been associated with which of the following complications in the offspring?

    a. Anemia

    b. Jaundice

    c. Seizures

    d. Congenital rickets

9–27. Which of the following conditions would be considered absolute contraindications to exercise in pregnancy?

    a. Mild hypertension

    b. Restrictive lung disease

    c. Placenta previa at 16 weeks' gestation

    d. All of the above

9–28. Which of the following types of fish should be avoided in pregnancy due to potentially high methylmercury levels?

    a. Tuna

    b. Salmon

    c. Flounder

    d. Swordfish

9–29. Which of the following is a blood lead concentration threshold, above which would indicate lead poisoning that requires treatment?

    a. > 5 µg/dL

    b. > 20 µg/dL

    c. > 45 µg/dL

    d. > 75 µg/dL

9–30. Air travel in pregnancy is not recommended after what gestational age?

    a. 12 weeks

    b. 22 weeks

    c. 30 weeks

    d. 36 weeks

9–31. Which of the following statements regarding vaccinations in pregnancy is true?

    a. Tdap should be given to all pregnant women between 16 and 20 weeks.

    b. All pregnant women should be offered influenza vaccine during the appropriate season.

    c. Varicella vaccine should be offered to all women who have a chicken pox exposure in pregnancy.

    d. Measles-mumps-rubella (MMR) vaccine should be given to all pregnant women who are rubella nonimmune.

9–32. The condition shown in the image is a common complaint in pregnancy that results from increased pelvic venous pressure. Treatment of this condition is typically conservative, but surgery can be required in what situation?

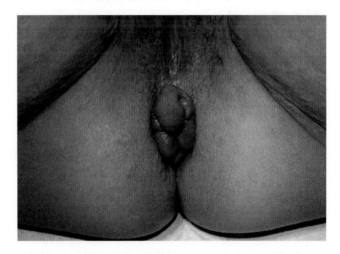

    a. If they are multiple

    b. If they are thrombosed

    c. If they are associated with vulvar varicosities

    d. None of the above

CHAPTER 9 ANSWER KEY

Question number	Letter answer	Page cited	Header cited
9–1	d	p. 167	Prenatal Care in the United States
9–2	d	p. 167	Assessing Prenatal Care Adequacy
9–3	c	p. 169	Fetal Movement
9–4	c	p. 169	Measurement of hCG
9–5	b	p. 170	Sonographic Recognition of Pregnancy
9–6	d	p. 170	Sonographic Recognition of Pregnancy
9–7	c	p. 170	Sonographic Recognition of Pregnancy
9–8	b	p. 171	Table 9-2
9–9	a	p. 170	Definitions
9–10	c	p. 170	Definitions
9–11	b	p. 172	Normal Pregnancy Duration
9–12	c	p. 172	Normal Pregnancy Duration
9–13	d	p. 172	Previous and Current Health Status
9–14	a	p. 172	Psychosocial Screening
9–15	a	p. 172	Cigarette Smoking
9–16	c	p. 173	Alcohol
9–17	c	p. 174	Intimate Partner Violence
9–18	b	p. 176	Fundal Height
9–19	d	p. 177	Weight Gain Recommendations; Table 9-5
9–20	b	p. 179	Iron
9–21	d	p. 179	Iron
9–22	a	p. 181	Folic Acid
9–23	c	p. 181	Folic Acid
9–24	b	p. 181	Vitamin A
9–25	c	p. 181	Vitamin B_6—Pyridoxine
9–26	d	p. 181	Vitamin D
9–27	b	p. 182	Table 9-7
9–28	d	p. 183	Seafood Consumption
9–29	c	p. 183	Lead Screening
9–30	d	p. 183	Automobile and Air Travel
9–31	b	p. 184	Immunization and Table 9-9
9–32	b	p. 188	Varicosities and Hemorrhoids

THE FETAL PATIENT

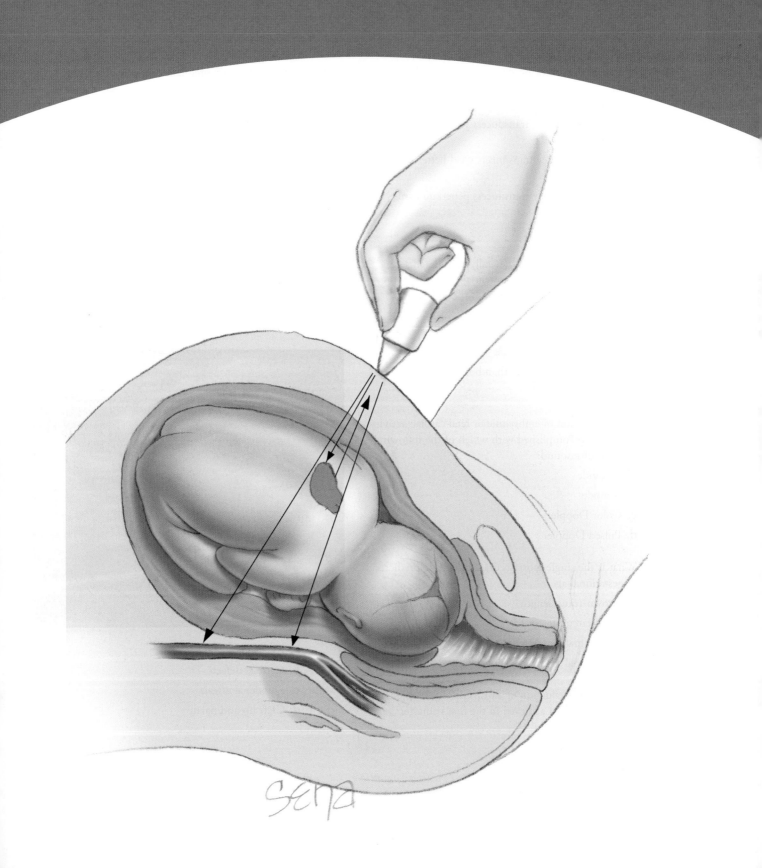

CHAPTER 10

Fetal Imaging

10–1. Which of the following statements accurately describes the relationship between tissue penetration and image resolution in ultrasound?

    a. Higher-frequency transducers yield better image resolution.

    b. Lower-frequency transducers yield better image resolution.

    c. Higher-frequency transducers penetrate tissue more effectively.

    d. None of the above

10–2. Although sonography is generally considered safe in human pregnancy, the potential for temperature elevation is increased in which of the following situations?

    a. Third trimester

    b. Longer examination time

    c. Near soft tissue rather than bone

    d. All of the above

10–3. Documentation of embryonic or fetal cardiac activity should be accomplished with which of the following types of ultrasound?

    a. M-mode

    b. L-mode

    c. Color Doppler

    d. Pulsed Doppler

10–4. What is the single most accurate biometric predictor of gestational age?

    a. Crown-rump length

    b. Head circumference

    c. Abdominal circumference

    d. Gestational sac mean diameter

10–5. Sonographic evaluation of all **EXCEPT** which of the following are best achieved in the first trimester?

    a. Adnexa

    b. Cervical length

    c. Ectopic pregnancy

    d. Chorionicity of twins

10–6. An anembryonic pregnancy may be accurately diagnosed at what mean gestational sac diameter when using transvaginal ultrasound?

    a. 5 mm

    b. 10 mm

    c. 15 mm

    d. 20 mm

10–7. A 41-year-old G3P2 presents at 12 weeks' gestation for a first-trimester sonographic evaluation. The nuchal translucency is measured as shown in the image and is noted to be increased at 4.6 mm. She subsequently undergoes chorionic villus sampling, and the fetal karyotype is 46,XY. Her fetus still needs to be evaluated in the second trimester for which of the following?

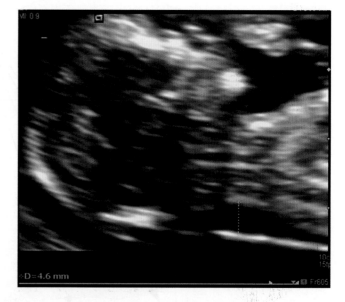

    a. Aneuploidy

    b. Cardiac defects

    c. Duodenal atresia

    d. Cleft lip and palate

10–8. The fetal head circumference should be measured in which of the following views?

    a. Transatrial view

    b. Transthalamic view

    c. Transcerebellar view

    d. Any of the above are acceptable

10–9. Which of the biometric parameters measured in the second trimester has the greatest variation for gestational age estimation?

    a. Femur length

    b. Head circumference

    c. Biparietal diameter

    d. Abdominal circumference

10–10. A 39-year-old multipara with chronic hypertension is noted to have lagging fundal growth at 29 weeks' gestation. Sonographic evaluation is completed, and the fetal weight estimate is less than the 3rd percentile for this gestational age. According to recommendations from the American Institute of Ultrasound in Medicine, when would it be appropriate to repeat sonographic evaluation of interval fetal growth?

    a. 2 days

    b. 1 week

    c. 3 weeks

    d. 5 weeks

10–11. The following sonographic image is taken from a pregnancy in which polyhydramnios is suspected. The distance between the two calipers must exceed what value to confirm this diagnosis?

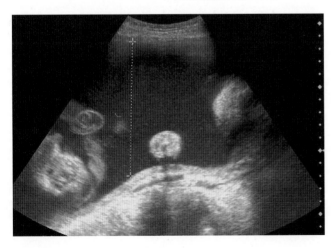

Reproduced with permission from Cunningham FG, Leveno KJ, Bloom SL, et al (eds): Fetal imaging. In Williams Obstetrics, 23rd ed. New York, McGraw-Hill, 2010, Figure 16-5.

    a. 6 cm

    b. 8 cm

    c. 10 cm

    d. 12 cm

10–12. Which of the following fetal anomalies has few sonographic findings and is typically not diagnosed antenatally?

    a. Anencephaly

    b. Hydrocephalus

    c. Gastroschisis

    d. Choanal atresia

10–13. Absence of the cavum septum pellucidum, as shown in this ultrasound image, may be associated with all **EXCEPT** which of the following conditions?

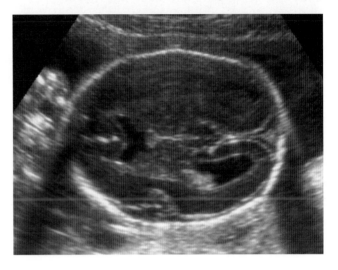

Reproduced with permission from Cunningham FG, Leveno KJ, Bloom SL, et al (eds): Fetal imaging. In Williams Obstetrics, 24th ed. New York, McGraw-Hill, 2014, eFigure 10-4.

    a. Porencephaly

    b. Septo-optic dysplasia

    c. Lobar holoprosencephaly

    d. Agenesis of the corpus callosum

10–14. What is the most common class of fetal malformations?

    a. Cardiac

    b. Oral cleft

    c. Neural tube

    d. Ventral wall

10–15. In fetuses with spina bifida defects, the associated cranial abnormalities include all **EXCEPT** which of the following?

    a. Ventriculomegaly

    b. Dandy-Walker malformation

    c. Scalloping of the frontal bones

    d. Effacement of the cisterna magna

10–16. A 19-year-old primigravida presents at 20 weeks' gestation for a dating sonographic examination. The following fetal head image is obtained in the transatrial view. Overt or severe ventriculomegaly is diagnosed when the lateral ventricular atrial width exceeds what measurement threshold?

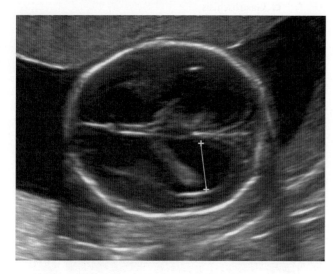

Reproduced with permission from Cunningham FG, Leveno KJ, Bloom SL, et al (eds): Fetal imaging. In Williams Obstetrics, 24th ed. New York, McGraw-Hill, 2014, Figure 10-8.

  a. 5 mm

  b. 10 mm

  c. 12 mm

  d. 15 mm

10–17. Again referring to the patient in Question 10-16, which of the following are appropriate as a part of the subsequent evaluation?

  a. Fetal karyotyping

  b. Tests for congenital infections

  c. Fetal magnetic resonance imaging

  d. All of the above

10–18. Shown in the image below are the intracranial findings of alobar holoprosencephaly. Fetal karyotyping is most likely to identify which aneuploidy? V= ventricle, Th = thalami.

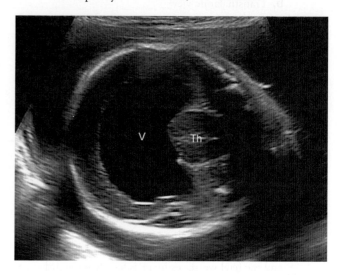

Reproduced with permission from Cunningham FG, Leveno KJ, Bloom SL, et al (eds): Fetal imaging. In Williams Obstetrics, 24th ed. New York, McGraw-Hill, 2014, Figure 10-10A.

  a. Trisomy 13

  b. Trisomy 18

  c. Trisomy 21

  d. Monosomy X

10–19. Caudal regression sequence, which is characterized by absence of the sacral spine, is associated with which of the following maternal conditions?

  a. Epilepsy

  b. Diabetes mellitus

  c. Sickle-cell anemia

  d. Systemic lupus erythematosus

10–20. Which of the following cleft abnormalities are most associated with aneuploidy?

  a. Unilateral cleft lip

  b. Bilateral cleft lip and palate

  c. Unilateral cleft lip and palate

  d. All are equally associated with aneuploidy

10–21. The following image depicts a 15-week fetus with massive cystic hygromas. When associated with aneuploidy, which of the following fetal karyotypes is most likely?

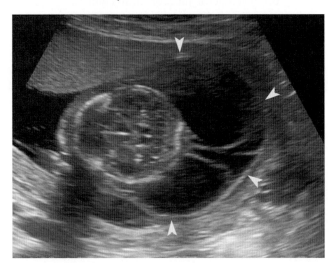

Reproduced with permission from Cunningham FG, Leveno KJ, Bloom SL, et al (eds): Fetal imaging. In Williams Obstetrics, 24th ed. New York, McGraw-Hill, 2014, Figure 10-16B.

    a. 45,X

    b. 47,XY,+21

    c. 47,XX,+18

    d. 47,XX,+16

10–22. Where do most congenital diaphragmatic hernia defects protrude into the fetal thorax?

    a. Midline

    b. Left side

    c. Bilateral

    d. Right side

10–23. The vascular supply to an extralobar pulmonary sequestration originates from which of the following blood vessels?

    a. Aorta

    b. Vena cava

    c. Pulmonary artery

    d. None of the above

10–24. The following ultrasound image demonstrates a normal four-chamber view of the fetal heart. Which of the following cardiac malformations may not be detected when only this view is obtained? LV = Left ventricle, RV = right ventricle, LA = left atrium, RA = right atrium, Ao = aorta.

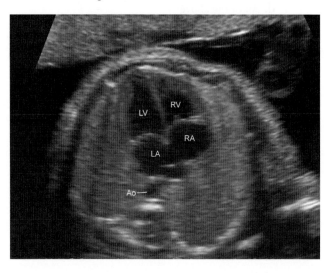

Reproduced with permission from Cunningham FG, Leveno KJ, Bloom SL, et al (eds): Fetal imaging. In Williams Obstetrics, 24th ed. New York, McGraw-Hill, 2014, Figure 10-20B.

    a. Ebstein anomaly

    b. Hypoplastic left heart

    c. Transposition of the great vessels

    d. Atrioventricular septal defect (endocardial cushion defect)

10–25. Endocardial cushion defects are associated with which of the following conditions?

    a. Trisomy 21

    b. Heterotaxy syndromes

    c. Third-degree atrioventricular block

    d. All of the above

10–26. Approximately 50 percent of cardiac rhabdomyomas are associated with which of the following genetic conditions?

    a. Tay-Sachs

    b. Cystic fibrosis

    c. Tuberous sclerosis

    d. Infantile polycystic kidney disease

10–27. Maternal risk factors for fetal gastroschisis defects include which of the following?

a. Young age

b. Pregestational diabetes

c. Phenytoin administration

d. All of the above

10–28. Gastrointestinal atresia in which of the following portions of the bowel is most likely to be associated with polyhydramnios?

a. Ileum

b. Jejunum

c. Sigmoid colon

d. Transverse colon

10–29. Amnionic fluid production is largely from the placenta and membranes until the fetal kidney assumes this role at what gestational age?

a. 12 weeks

b. 14 weeks

c. 18 weeks

d. 22 weeks

10–30. What is the most common abnormality associated with renal pelvis dilatation?

a. Bladder outlet obstruction

b. Ureteropelvic junction obstruction

c. Duplicated renal collecting system

d. Ureterovesical junction obstruction

10–31. Only which of the following types of polycystic kidney disease (PKD) may be reliably diagnosed prenatally?

a. X-linked PKD

b. Autosomal dominant PKD

c. Autosomal recessive PKD

d. None of the above

10–32. What is the most common nonlethal skeletal dysplasia?

a. Hypophosphatasia

b. Thanatophoric dysplasia

c. Heterozygous achondroplasia

d. Type IIa osteogenesis imperfecta

CHAPTER 10 ANSWER KEY

Question number	Letter answer	Page cited	Header cited
10–1	a	p. 194	Technology and Safety
10–2	b	p. 195	Fetal Safety
10–3	a	p. 195	Fetal Safety
10–4	a	p. 195	First Trimester Sonography
10–5	b	p. 195	First Trimester Sonography
10–6	d	p. 195	First Trimester Sonography
10–7	b	p. 196	Nuchal Translucency
10–8	b	p. 198	Fetal Biometry
10–9	d	p. 198	Fetal Biometry
10–10	c	p. 198	Fetal Biometry
10–11	b	p. 199	Amnionic Fluid
10–12	d	p. 199	Second-Trimester Fetal Anomaly Detection
10–13	a	p. 200	Brain and Spine
10–14	a	p. 201	Neural Tube Defects
10–15	b	p. 201	Neural Tube Defects
10–16	d	p. 202	Ventriculomegaly
10–17	d	p. 202	Ventriculomegaly
10–18	a	p. 203	Holoprosencephaly
10–19	b	p. 204	Caudal Regression Sequence—Sacral Agenesis
10–20	b	p. 205	Facial Clefts
10–21	a	p. 205	Cystic Hygromas
10–22	b	p. 206	Congenital Diaphragmatic Hernia
10–23	a	p. 208	Extralobar Pulmonary Sequestration
10–24	c	p. 208	Basic Cardiac Examination
10–25	d	p. 209	Endocardial Cushion Defects
10–26	c	p. 211	Cardiac Rhabdomyomas
10–27	a	p. 212	Gastroschisis
10–28	b	p. 213	Gastrointestinal Atresia
10–29	c	p. 214	Kidneys and Urinary Tract
10–30	b	p. 215	Ureteropelvic Junction Obstruction
10–31	c	p. 216	Polycystic Kidney Disease
10–32	c	p. 217	Skeletal Dysplasias

CHAPTER 11

Amnionic Fluid

11–1. Which of the following conditions is not related to an absence or diminution of amnionic fluid volume during fetal development?

    a. Contractures

    b. Pulmonary hypoplasia

    c. Abdominal wall defects

    d. Gastrointestinal tract development

11–2. What is the normal amnionic fluid volume at term?

    a. 300 mL

    b. 800 mL

    c. 1200 mL

    d. 1500 mL

11–3. Which of the following is **NOT** a significant source for fluid in the amnionic cavity in the first trimester?

    a. Fetal skin

    b. Fetal urine

    c. Flow across amnion

    d. Flow across fetal vessels

11–4. In a normal fetus at term, what is the daily volume of fetal urine that contributes to the amount of amnionic fluid present?

    a. 250 mL

    b. 500 mL

    c. 750 mL

    d. 1000 mL

11–5. A 28-year-old primigravida presents with a 3-day history of fever, vomiting, and diarrhea at 28 weeks' gestation. Several family members are also sick at home with similar complaints. During sonographic evaluation, her fetus is appropriately grown, but her amnionic fluid index is below the 10th percentile for the gestational age. What is the most likely explanation for this finding?

    a. Increased fetal swallowing

    b. Decreased fetal serum osmolality

    c. Increased maternal serum osmolality

    d. Probable premature rupture of membranes

11–6. Amnionic fluid volume is a balance between production and resorption. What is the primary mechanism of fluid resorption?

    a. Fetal breathing

    b. Fetal swallowing

    c. Absorption across fetal skin

    d. Absorption and filtration by fetal kidneys

11–7. All **EXCEPT** which of the following are acceptable methods of sonographic amnionic fluid volume evaluation?

    a. Subjective estimate

    b. Amnionic fluid index

    c. Dye-dilution measurement

    d. Two-dimension single-pocket measurement

11–8. Which of the following is associated with the single deepest pocket measurement seen below?

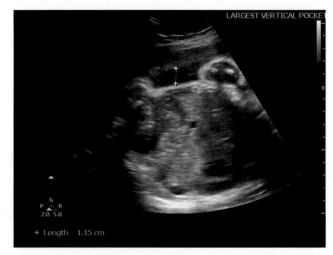

    a. Increased perinatal mortality rate

    b. Increased rate of bronchopulmonary dysplasia

    c. Increased rate of operative vaginal delivery

    d. Decreased rate of nonreassuring fetal heart rate tracings

11–9. Oligohydramnios is defined as which of the following?

  a. Amnionic fluid index < 5 cm

  b. Single deepest pocket < 2 cm

  c. Amnionic fluid index < 90th percentile

  d. All of the above

11–10. What technique for amnionic fluid evaluation in multifetal gestations is used in the image below?

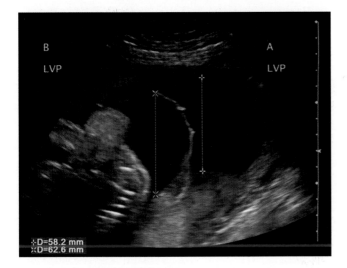

  a. Amnionic fluid index

  b. Single deepest pocket

  c. Subjective evaluation

  d. Two-dimension single pocket measurement

11–11. Concurrent use of this imaging technique with amnionic fluid index measurements leads to which of the following?

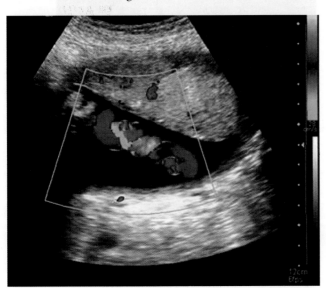

  a. Improved fetal outcomes

  b. Overdiagnosis of hydramnios

  c. Overdiagnosis of oligohydramnios

  d. More accurate estimation of amnionic fluid volume

11–12. Which of the following is a clinical sign of polyhydramnios?

  a. Tense uterus

  b. Increase in fundal height measurement

  c. Inability to palpate fetal small parts

  d. All of the above

11–13. Using the technique demonstrated in this figure, what is the lower threshold for diagnosing hydramnios?

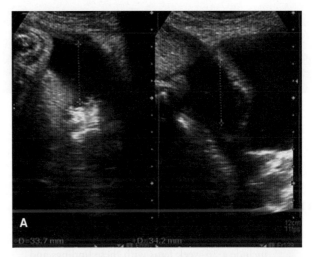

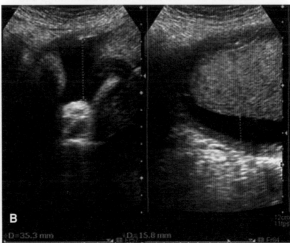

  a. 18 cm

  b. 20 cm

  c. 24 cm

  d. 28 cm

11–14. How would the amnionic fluid be categorized based on the following image of a single deepest pocket?

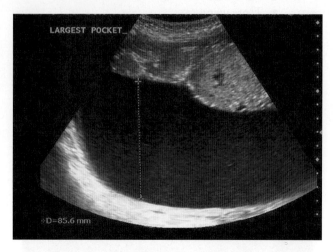

a. Normal

b. Mild polyhydramnios

c. Severe polyhydramnios

d. Moderate polyhydramnios

11–15. A new patient presents for her first prenatal visit at 26 weeks' gestation. She has no complaints other than rapid abdominal growth. Sonographic findings include a 26-week fetus with these findings and a pleural effusion. Potential associated maternal complications may include all **EXCEPT** which of the following?

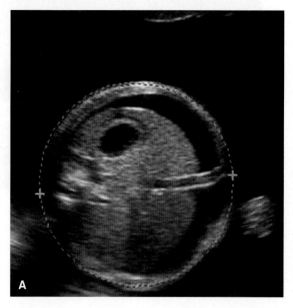
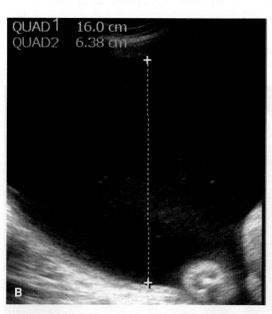

a. Dyspnea

b. Oliguria

c. Seizures

d. Vulvar edema

11–16. Which of the following laboratory studies is **NOT** currently indicated in evaluation of the patient in Question 11–15?

a. Creatinine

b. Indirect Coombs

c. Cytomegalovirus IgM and IgG titers

d. Venereal Disease Research Laboratory (VDRL)

11–17. What is the etiology of hydramnios in the condition depicted in the following image? Arrows point to the fetal eye and nose.

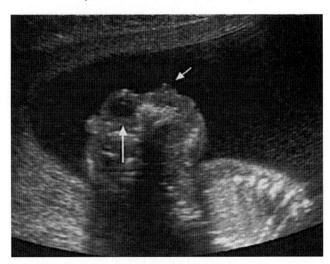

Reproduced with permission from Cunningham FG, Leveno KJ, Bloom SL, et al (eds): Fetal imaging. In Williams Obstetrics, 23rd ed. New York, McGraw-Hill, 2010, Figure 16-8.

a. Reduced fetal swallowing

b. Increased maternal glucose levels

c. Increased production of fetal urine

d. High frequency of associated tracheal-esophageal fistula

11–18. Which of the following congenital anomalies is **NOT** associated with polyhydramnios?

a. Pierre Robin sequence

b. Infantile polycystic kidney

c. Congenital diaphragmatic hernia

d. Ureteropelvic junction obstruction

11–19. What placental abnormality, seen in the following image, is associated with polyhydramnios?

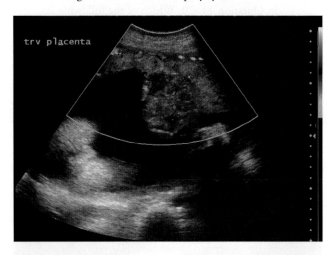

Reproduced with permission from Hoffman BL, Dashe JS: Placental chorioangioma (update) in Cunningham FG, Leveno KL, Bloom SL, et al (eds): Williams Obstetrics, 22nd ed. Online. New York, McGraw-Hill, 2009. http://www.accessmedicine.com. Figure 10.

a. Chorioangioma

b. Choriocarcinoma

c. Placenta previa

d. Placenta accreta

11–20. A 30-year-old patient had an sonographic evaluation for a uterine size-date discrepancy. The amnionic fluid index was 36 cm. Without any other information, what is the risk of congenital malformation in this patient's fetus?

a. 1%

b. 5%

c. 10%

d. 25%

11–21. The following image depicts the fetal abdomen seen during sonographic evaluation of the patient in Question 11–20. Which of the following is appropriate in the evaluation of this fetus?

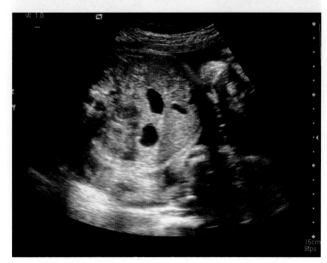

    a. Glucose tolerance test

    b. Fetal magnetic resonance imaging

    c. Amniocentesis with fetal karyotype

    d. None of the above

11–22. A patient with a known monozygotic twin gestation presents at 26 weeks' gestation for sonographic evaluation of fetal growth. Twin A has an estimated fetal weight of 804 g, whereas twin B's estimated fetal weight is 643 g. The largest pocket of amnionic fluid around twin A is 9.6 cm and 2.2 cm for twin B. Which of the following conditions most likely explains these findings?

    a. Gestational diabetes

    b. Congenital anomaly in twin A

    c. Twin-twin transfusion syndrome

    d. Twin B with premature membrane rupture

11–23. Idiopathic hydramnios is associated with which of the following conditions?

    a. Congenital infection

    b. Birthweight > 4000 g

    c. Neonatal diabetes mellitus

    d. Increased perinatal mortality rate

11–24. Which of the following is **NOT** a recognized maternal complication associated with hydramnios?

    a. Postpartum atony

    b. Placental abruption

    c. Ureteral obstruction

    d. Gestational hypertension

11–25. Fetal-growth restriction and polyhydramnios are associated with which of the following chromosomal abnormalities?

    a. Triploidy

    b. Trisomy 18

    c. Trisomy 21

    d. Turner syndrome (Monosomy X)

11–26. Use of the amnionic fluid index rather than single deepest pocket for defining oligohydramnios is associated with which of the following?

    a. Improved pregnancy outcomes

    b. Increased diagnosis of oligohydramnios

    c. Improved detection of congenital anomalies

    d. Increased detection of fetal-growth restriction

11–27. Second-trimester oligohydramnios may be attributed to which of the following conditions?

    a. Poor placental perfusion

    b. Rupture of fetal membranes

    c. Fetal bladder outlet obstruction

    d. All of the above

11–28. An obstetric patient presents at 35 weeks' gestation with a complaint of decreased fetal movement. Variable decelerations are present on a nonstress test, so an amnionic fluid index (AFI) is performed. The result is seen below. What subsequent evaluation is recommended?

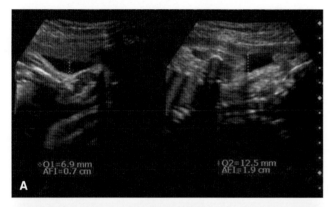

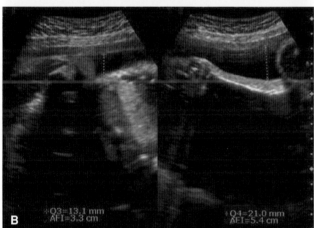

a. Sterile speculum examination

b. Umbilical artery Doppler studies

c. Sonographic measurement of fetal growth

d. All of the above

11–29. The evaluation of the patient in Question 11–28 is normal. What is the most appropriate step in the management of her pregnancy?

a. Immediate cesarean delivery

b. Induction of labor in 1 week

c. Administration of antenatal corticosteroids

d. Expectant management with fetal surveillance

11–30. Which of the following medications is associated with oligohydramnios when taken in the latter half of pregnancy?

a. Hydralazine

b. Beta blockers

c. Calcium-channel blockers

d. Angiotensin-receptor blockers

11–31. Oligohydramnios is **NOT** associated with which of the following pregnancy complications?

a. Stillbirth

b. Neonatal sepsis

c. Congenital malformations

d. Meconium aspiration syndrome

11–32. A borderline amnionic fluid index (AFI), defined as an AFI between 5 and 8 cm, is associated with increased rates of all **EXCEPT** which of the following?

a. Preterm birth

b. Neonatal mortality

c. Fetal-growth restriction

d. Cesarean delivery for nonreassuring fetal heart rate pattern

CHAPTER 11 ANSWER KEY

Question number	Letter answer	Page cited	Header cited
11–1	c	p. 231	Introduction
11–2	b	p. 231	Normal Amnionic Fluid Volume
11–3	b	p. 231	Physiology
11–4	d	p. 231	Physiology
11–5	c	p. 231	Physiology
11–6	b	p. 231	Physiology
11–7	c	p. 232	Sonographic Assessment
11–8	a	p. 232	Single Deepest Pocket
11–9	d	p. 231	Single Deepest Pocket
11–10	b	p. 232	Single Deepest Pocket
11–11	c	p. 233	Amnionic Fluid Index (AFI)
11–12	d	p. 233	Hydramnios
11–13	c	p. 233	Normal AFI
11–14	b	p. 233	Hydramnios
11–15	c	p. 235	Complications
11–16	a	p. 236	Etiology
11–17	a	p. 237	Congenital Anomalies
11–18	b	p. 237	Congenital Anomalies
11–19	a	p. 237	Congenital Anomalies
11–20	c	p. 237	Congenital Anomalies
11–21	c	p. 237	Congenital Anomalies
11–22	c	p. 235	Multifetal Gestation
11–23	b	p. 235	Idiopathic Hydramnios
11–24	d	p. 235	Complications
11–25	b	p. 235	Pregnancy Outcomes
11–26	b	p. 236	Oligohydramnios
11–27	d	p. 236	Etiology
11–28	d	p. 236	Oligohydramnios after Midpregnancy
11–29	d	p. 238	Management
11–30	d	p. 237	Medication
11–31	b	p. 238	Pregnancy Outcomes
11–32	b	p. 238	"Borderline" Oligohydramnios

CHAPTER 12

Teratology, Teratogens, and Fetotoxic Agents

12–1. What percentage of all birth defects is caused by exposure to medications during pregnancy?

 a. 1%

 b. 7%

 c. 11%

 d. 17%

12–2. What is the strict definition of a trophogen?

 a. An agent that alters growth

 b. An agent that interferes with normal function of an organ

 c. An agent that interferes with normal maturation of an organ

 d. All of the above

12–3. Which of the following drawbacks is typical of case-control studies when studying potential teratogens?

 a. Recall bias

 b. Lack of a control group

 c. Only causality can be established

 d. All of the above

12–4. What is the background rate of major congenital anomalies diagnosed at birth?

 a. 0.5%

 b. 3%

 c. 6%

 d. 9%

12–5. Which of the following criteria is not required to prove teratogenicity of a particular agent?

 a. The agent must cross the placenta.

 b. Exposure to the agent must occur during organogenesis.

 c. The association with the teratogen must be biologically plausible.

 d. Two or more high-quality epidemiological studies must report similar findings.

12–6. If discordant among fetuses, which of the following can render certain fetuses more susceptible to a teratogen?

 a. Fetal genome

 b. Folic acid pathway disturbances

 c. Paternal exposures to certain drugs

 d. All of the above

12–7. What is the leading cause of preventable birth defects in the United States?

 a. Maternal smoking

 b. Maternal alcohol consumption

 c. Maternal anticonvulsant treatment

 d. Continued inadvertent use of birth control pills during early pregnancy

12–8. In addition to having dysmorphic facial features and postnatal growth restriction, which of the following would have to be present for a diagnosis of fetal alcohol syndrome?

 a. Scoliosis

 b. Dysplastic kidney

 c. Ventricular septal defect

 d. Head size < 10th percentile

12–9. Increased rates of which complication have been linked to binge drinking during pregnancy?

 a. Stillbirth

 b. Preterm birth

 c. Postpartum depression

 d. Fetal-growth restriction

12–10. A 32-week fetus is growth restricted and has oligohydramnios and an abnormal calvarium. Which antihypertensive agent taken by the mother may have caused this problem?

 a. Verapamil

 b. Nifedipine

 c. Lisinopril

 d. Methyldopa

12–11. Which of the following associations regarding anticonvulsants and their risk of birth defects has not been reported?

   a. Hydantoin exposure can cause midfacial hypoplasia.

   b. Valproic acid exposure can cause neural-tube defects.

   c. Topiramate exposure increases the risk of orofacial clefts.

   d. Valproic acid exposure increases the risk of abdominal wall defects.

12–12. What fetal complication is associated with the nonsteroidal antiinflammatory agent indomethacin?

   a. Hydramnios

   b. Pulmonary valve atresia

   c. Bronchopulmonary dysplasia

   d. Premature closure of the ductus arteriosus

12–13. Considered Category X in pregnancy, which antiviral causes skull, palate, jaw, eye, limb, and gastrointestinal anomalies in rodent models?

   a. Ribavirin

   b. Efavirenz

   c. Zidovudine

   d. Nevirapine

12–14. Which of the following associations between first-trimester antibiotic exposure and the given birth defect is true?

   a. Aminoglycosides may cause ototoxicity.

   b. Chloramphenicol may cause ashen-gray skin coloration.

   c. Tetracyclines may cause deciduous teeth discoloration.

   d. Nitrofurantoin may cause hypoplastic left heart syndrome.

12–15. Prenatal exposure to which of the following agents is associated with the sonographic finding shown here?

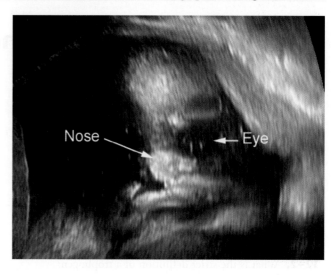

   a. Tamoxifen

   b. Topiramate

   c. Trastuzumab

   d. Methotrexate

12–16. Which of the following genitourinary anomalies is not typically associated with prenatal exposure to diethylstilbestrol?

   a. Microphallus

   b. Hooded cervix

   c. Bicornuate uterus

   d. Testicular hypoplasia

12–17. Which of the following statements is true regarding corticosteroids and the risk of birth defects?

   a. They may cause orofacial fetal clefts.

   b. They may cause clitoromegaly in the female fetus.

   c. They may cause phallic enlargement in the male fetus.

   d. They may cause labioscrotal fusion in the female fetus.

12–18. For fetuses exposed to mycophenolate mofetil during pregnancy, which of the following is the most likely outcome?

   a. Spontaneous abortion

   b. Born at term with ear abnormalities

   c. Born at term without evidence of abnormalities

   d. Born prematurely without evidence of abnormalities

12–19. Which prenatal exposure is associated with an increased risk of childhood thyroid cancer?

   a. Lead

   b. Lithium

   c. Mercury

   d. Radioiodine

12–20. Which drug is associated with the rare cardiac anomaly shown in this fetal sonogram?

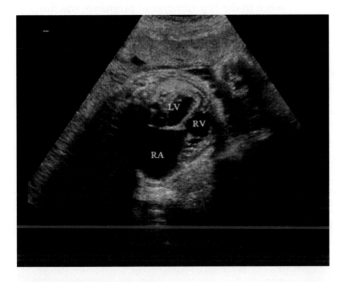

   a. Lithium

   b. Leflunomide

   c. Indomethacin

   d. Cyclophosphamide

12–21. Prenatal exposure near term to which of the following agents can lead to neonatal toxicity that manifests as hypothyroidism, diabetes insipidus, cardiomegaly, bradycardia, and hypotonia?

   a. Lithium

   b. Fluoxetine

   c. Paroxetine

   d. Escitalopram

12–22. Which of the following selective serotonin-reuptake inhibitors (SSRIs) is most strongly associated with the cardiac defect shown in this sonogram?

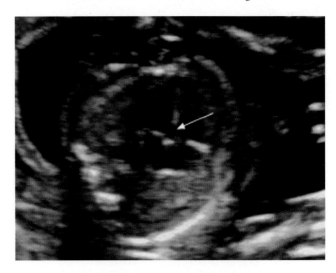

   a. Paroxetine

   b. Fluoxetine

   c. Sertraline

   d. Escitalopram

12–23. The *severe* form of the neonatal behavioral syndrome associated with prenatal exposure to serotonin-reuptake inhibitors includes all **EXCEPT** which of the following?

   a. Seizures

   b. Hyperpyrexia

   c. Respiratory failure

   d. Persistent pulmonary hypertension

12–24. Prenatal exposure to which of the following agents is most likely responsible for the congenital malformations seen in these photographs?

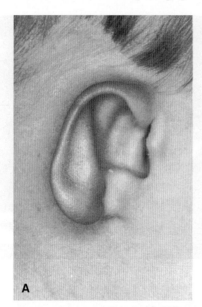

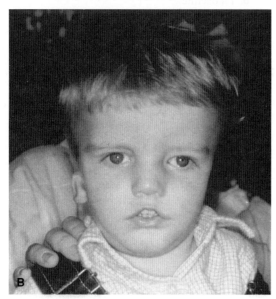

Reproduced with permission from Cunningham FG, Leveno KJ, Bloom SL, et al (eds): Teratology, teratogens, and fetotoxic agents. In Williams Obstetrics, 24th ed. New York, McGraw-Hill, 2014, Figure 12-4.

a. Alcohol

b. Warfarin

c. Isotretinoin

d. Valproic acid

12–25. Severe malformations may be seen with use of all **EXCEPT** which of the following vitamin A-derived compounds?

a. Acitretin

b. Bexarotene

c. Isotretinoin

d. Beta carotene

12–26. With the upper limb defect seen in this photograph, when in the first trimester of pregnancy was this infant most likely exposed to the causative drug?

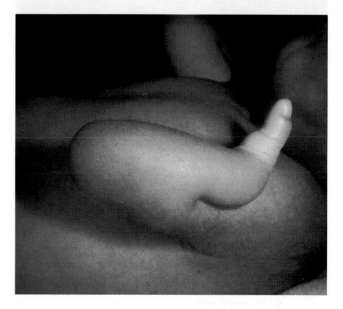

Reproduced with permission from Walsh Ra, O'Rourke RA, Shaver JA: The history, physical examination, and cardiac auscultation. In Fuster V, Walsh RA, Harrington RA, et al (eds): Hurst's The Heart, 13th ed. New York, McGraw-Hill, 2011, Figure 14-6.

a. Days 27–30

b. Days 30–33

c. Days 40–47

d. Days 42–43

12–27. The nasal hypoplasia seen in this prenatal sonogram is consistent with exposure to which of the following agents?

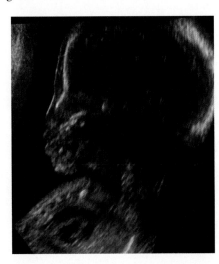

Reproduced with permission from Cunningham FG, Leveno KJ, Bloom SL, et al (eds): Teratology, teratogens, and fetotoxic agents. In Williams Obstetrics, 24th ed. New York, McGraw-Hill, 2014, Figure 12-5B.

a. Warfarin

b. Corticosteroids

c. Diethylstilbestrol

d. Mycophenolate mofetil

12–28. When used in the second and third trimesters, which drug may lead to central nervous system defects such as agenesis of the corpus callosum, Dandy-Walker malformation, and midline cerebellar malformations?

a. Heroin

b. Cocaine

c. Warfarin

d. Isotretinoin

12–29. Which of the following herbal remedies is associated with increased risk of bleeding by inhibiting cyclooxygenase?

a. Garlic

b. Ginger

c. Ginseng

d. Gingko biloba

12–30. Among recreational drugs, which one has been linked to cleft palate, cardiovascular abnormalities, and urinary tract abnormalities?

a. Heroin

b. Cocaine

c. Methadone

d. Methamphetamine

12–31. Cigarette smoking in pregnancy has been associated with an increased risk for all **EXCEPT** which of the following?

a. Microcephaly

b. Cleft lip and palate

c. Neonatal hypoglycemia

d. Congenital heart disease

12–32. Which of the following agents has not been shown to be a human teratogen?

a. Toluene

b. Marijuana

c. Methadone

d. Phencyclidine

CHAPTER 12 ANSWER KEY

Question number	Letter answer	Page cited	Header cited
12–1	a	p. 240	Introduction
12–2	a	p. 240	Teratology
12–3	a	p. 241	Case-Control Studies
12–4	b	p. 241	Criteria for Determining Teratogencity
12–5	b	p. 241	Criteria for Determining Teratogencity
12–6	d	p. 244	Genetic and Physiological Susceptibility to Teratogens
12–7	b	p. 245	Alcohol
12–8	d	p. 245	Alcohol; Table 12-4
12–9	a	p. 245	Alcohol
12–10	c	p. 247	Angiotensin-Converting Enzyme Inhibitors and Angiotensin-Receptor Blocking Drugs
12–11	d	p. 246	Anticonvulsant Medications
12–12	d	p. 247	Nonsteroidal Antiinflammatory Drugs
12–13	a	p. 249	Ribavirin
12–14	d	p. 248	Nitrofurantoin
12–15	b	p. 246	Anticonvulsant Medications
12–16	c	p. 249	Diethylstilbestrol
12–17	a	p. 250	Corticosteroids
12–18	a	p. 250	Mycophenolate Mofetil
12–19	d	p. 250	Radioiodine
12–20	a	p. 250	Lithium
12–21	a	p. 250	Lithium
12–22	a	p. 250	Selective Serotonin- and Norepinephrine- Reuptake Inhibitors
12–23	d	p. 250	Selective Serotonin- and Norepinephrine- Reuptake Inhibitors
12–24	c	p. 251	Isotretinoin; Figure 12-4
12–25	d	p. 251	Retinoids
12–26	a	p. 252	Thalidomide and Lenalidomide
12–27	a	p. 252	Warfarin
12–28	c	p. 252	Warfarin
12–29	b	p. 253	Herbal Remedies; Table 12-5
12–30	b	p. 253	Cocaine
12–31	c	p. 254	Miscellaneous Drugs
12–32	b	p. 255	Tobacco

CHAPTER 13

Genetics

13-1. What percentage of individuals will experience a disease with a genetic component during the course of their lifetime?

    a. 10%

    b. 33%

    c. 66%

    d. 85%

13-2. When correctly reporting a karyotype, where should the sex chromosomes be listed?

    a. First, before the total number of chromosomes

    b. Second, after the total number of chromosomes

    c. Last, after any description of structural abnormalities

    d. None of the above

13-3. Which of the following karyotypes accurately describes a female with a deletion on the long arm of chromosome 17 at band q3?

    a. 46,XY,del(17)(q3)

    b. 46,del(17)(q3)

    c. 46,XX,del(17)(q3)

    d. XX,46,del(17)(q3)

13-4. What is the most common cause of the abnormality depicted in the karyotype below?

    a. Dispermy

    b. Mitotic nondisjunction

    c. Meiotic nondisjunction

    d. Unbalanced translocation

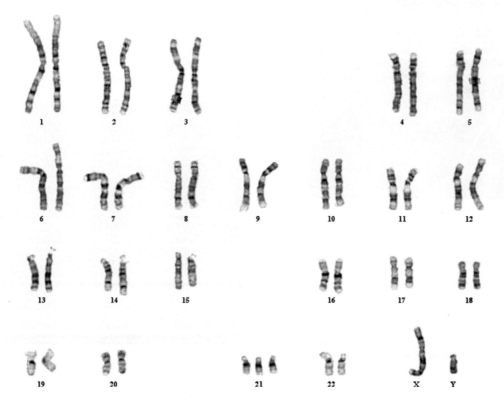

Reproduced with permission from Cunningham FG, Leveno KJ, Bloom SL, et al (eds): Genetics. In Williams Obstetrics, 24th ed. New York, McGraw-Hill, 2014, Figure 13-3.

13–5. Trisomy of which of the following autosomal chromosomes is **LEAST** likely to result in a term pregnancy?

    a. 8

    b. 13

    c. 18

    d. 21

13–6. Which of the following generalizations is true regarding the reproductive capacity of adults with Down syndrome?

    a. Both males and females are sterile.

    b. Both males and females are fertile.

    c. Males are fertile, and females are sterile.

    d. Males are sterile, and females are fertile.

13–7. Characteristic features of infants with Down syndrome, as depicted in this image, include all **EXCEPT** which of the following?

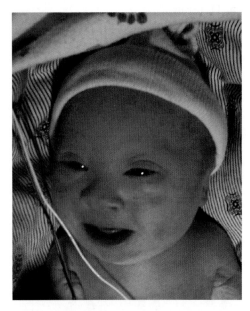

Reproduced with permission from Cunningham FG, Leveno KJ, Bloom SL, et al (eds): Genetics. In Williams Obstetrics, 24th ed. New York, McGraw-Hill, 2014, Figure 13-4A.

    a. Brachycephaly

    b. Epicanthal folds

    c. Flat nasal bridge

    d. Down-slanting palpebral fissures

13–8. Which of the following is not an acrocentric chromosome?

    a. 13

    b. 14

    c. 18

    d. 22

13–9. This sonographic image depicts a fetal head in the midtrimester of pregnancy. Cysts are noted within the choroid plexus. This finding, when associated with other fetal abnormalities, raises suspicion for which genetic condition?

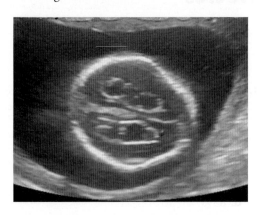

Reproduced with permission from Cunningham FG, Leveno KJ, Bloom SL, et al (eds): Genetics. In Williams Obstetrics, 24th ed. New York, McGraw-Hill, 2014, Figure 13-5A.

    a. Down syndrome

    b. Patau syndrome

    c. Edwards syndrome

    d. Turner syndrome

13–10. A 22-year-old G2P1 undergoes a routine sonographic evaluation of fetal anatomy at 18 weeks' gestation. Alobar holoprosencephaly is noted and shown in the image below. Which of the following genetic conditions is frequently associated with this finding?

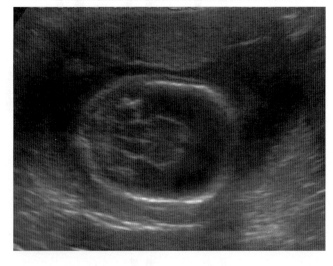

Used with permission from Dr. Jodi Dashe.

    a. Trisomy 13

    b. Trisomy 16

    c. Trisomy 21

    d. Monosomy X

13–11. Amniocentesis is elected by the patient described in Question 13-10 and confirms the suspected genetic abnormality. What is the likelihood of survival of her infant at 1 year of age?

a. 95%

b. 50%

c. 25%

d. Less than 5%

13–12. The patient described in Question 13-10 would be at an increased risk for which particular pregnancy-related complication?

a. Preeclampsia

b. Gestational diabetes

c. Postpartum hemorrhage

d. Acute fatty liver of pregnancy

13–13. The overwhelming majority of monosomy X conceptions result in what outcome?

a. Early first-trimester spontaneous abortion

b. Small cystic hygromas and live birth at term

c. Large cystic hygromas, hydrops fetalis, and second-trimester fetal death

d. None of the above

13–14. All **EXCEPT** which of the following are clinical features associated with Turner syndrome?

a. Hypothyroidism

b. Mental retardation

c. Renal abnormalities

d. Coarctation of the aorta

13–15. What is the most common sex chromosome abnormality?

a. 45,X

b. 47,XXX

c. 47,XYY

d. 47,XXY

13–16. Carriers of Robertsonian translocations involving which of the following chromosomes could produce only unbalanced gametes?

a. 13 and 14

b. 14 and 21

c. 21 and 22

d. 21 and 21

13–17. All **EXCEPT** which of the following statements regarding Robertsonian translocations are correct?

a. They are not a major cause of miscarriage.

b. The most common of them is between chromosomes 13 and 14.

c. Offspring are more likely to be abnormal if the father is the translocation carrier.

d. When a child is found to have one, both parents should be offered karyotype testing.

13–18. The most common isochromosome involves the long arm of what chromosome?

a. 6

b. X

c. Y

d. 21

13–19. What term is used to refer to two or more cytogenetically distinct cell lines that are derived from a single zygote?

a. Chimerism

b. Mosaicism

c. Polygenic

d. Genetic blending

13–20. Gonadal mosaicism may explain what type of de novo mutations in offspring of normal parents?

a. Mitochondrial

b. Autosomal recessive

c. Autosomal dominant

d. None of the above

13–21. What term is used to describe the degree to which an individual with an autosomal dominant condition demonstrates the phenotype?

a. Penetrance

b. Variability

c. Concordance

d. Expressivity

13–22. Which of the following genetic disorders would be expected to occur more frequently in the setting of advanced paternal age?

a. Turner syndrome

b. Cystic fibrosis

c. Sickle-cell anemia

d. Tuberous sclerosis

13–23. A 22-year-old G1P0 at 12 weeks' gestation who has sickle-cell anemia requests genetic counseling to learn about the risk of transmission to her fetus. If her partner is a heterozygous carrier for this condition, what is the risk that their offspring will be affected?

a. 25%

b. 50%

c. 75%

d. 100%

13–24. Consanguinity increases the risk for what types of genetic syndromes?

a. X-linked dominant

b. Autosomal dominant

c. X-linked recessive

d. Autosomal recessive

13–25. All **EXCEPT** which of the following statements regarding X-linked diseases are true?

a. Most are X-linked recessive.

b. X-linked dominant disorders mainly affect females.

c. Female carriers of X-linked recessive conditions may demonstrate some clinical features.

d. All statements are true.

13–26. A couple is referred for genetic counseling because the woman has several relatives with the same unusual genetic condition. A pedigree of her family reveals that both males and females are equally affected but transmission occurs only though females. Which pattern of inheritance is suggested?

a. Mitochondrial

b. Multifactorial

c. X-linked dominant

d. Autosomal dominant

13–27. According to the American College of Obstetricians and Gynecologists, how many CGG triplet repeats are required to have the *premutation* for fragile-X syndrome?

a. < 45

b. 45–54

c. 55–200

d. > 200

13–28. Females who are premutation carriers for fragile-X syndrome are at increased risk for which of the following conditions?

a. Breast cancer

b. Endometriosis

c. Hypothyroidism

d. Primary ovarian failure

13–29. All **EXCEPT** which of the following conditions are considered to have multifactorial inheritance?

a. Beta-thalassemia

b. Diabetes mellitus

c. Neural-tube defects

d. Coronary heart disease

13–30. Hyperthermia has been associated with what specific type of neural-tube defect?

a. Anencephaly

b. Lumbar defects

c. Sacral defects

d. Cervical defects

13–31. The image below represents amnionic fluid analyzed with fluorescence in situ hybridization (FISH). If the green probe is directed at the X chromosome and the red probe is directed at chromosome 21, which karyotype is correct?

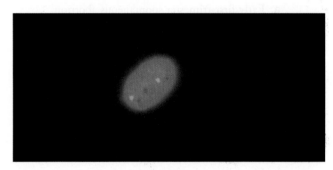

Reproduced with permission from Hassold TJ, Schwartz S: Chromosome disorders. In Fauci AS, Braunwald E, Kasper DL (eds): Harrison's Principles of Internal Medicine, 17th ed. New York, McGraw-Hill, 2008, Figure 63-2B.

a. 46,XX,+21

b. 47,XX,+21

c. 46,XY,+21

d. 47,XY,+21

13–32. Chromosomal microarray analysis can identify DNA deletions and duplications as small as how many kilobases?

a. 1

b. 3

c. 5

d. 10

CHAPTER 13 ANSWER KEY

Question number	Letter answer	Page cited	Header cited
13–1	**c**	p. 259	Introduction
13–2	**b**	p. 260	Standard Nomenclature
13–3	**c**	p. 260	Standard Nomenclature
13–4	**c**	p. 260	Autosomal Trisomies
13–5	**a**	p. 260	Autosomal Trisomies
13–6	**d**	p. 261	Trisomy 21—Down Syndrome
13–7	**d**	p. 261	Trisomy 21—Down Syndrome; Clinical Findings
13–8	**c**	p. 263	Trisomy 18—Edwards Syndrome
13–9	**c**	p. 263	Trisomy 18—Edwards Syndrome
13–10	**a**	p. 263	Trisomy 13—Patau Syndrome
13–11	**d**	p. 263	Trisomy 13—Patau Syndrome
13–12	**a**	p. 263	Trisomy 13—Patau Syndrome
13–13	**a**	p. 264	45,X—Turner Syndrome
13–14	**b**	p. 264	45,X—Turner Syndrome
13–15	**d**	p. 265	47,XXY—Klinefelter Syndrome
13–16	**d**	p. 267	Robertsonian Translocations
13–17	**c**	p. 267	Robertsonian Translocations
13–18	**b**	p. 268	Isochromosomes
13–19	**b**	p. 269	Chromosomal Mosaicism
13–20	**c**	p. 269	Gonadal Mosaicism
13–21	**d**	p. 270	Expressivity
13–22	**d**	p. 270	Advanced Paternal Age
13–23	**b**	p. 271	Autosomal Recessive Inheritance
13–24	**d**	p. 271	Consanguinity
13–25	**d**	p. 272	X-Linked and Y-Linked Inheritance
13–26	**a**	p. 272	Mitochondrial Inheritance
13–27	**c**	p. 272	Fragile X Syndrome
13–28	**d**	p. 272	Fragile X Syndrome
13–29	**a**	p. 274	Multifactorial Inheritance
13–30	**a**	p. 275	Neural-Tube Defects
13–31	**b**	p. 276	Fluorescence in-Situ Hybridization
13–32	**a**	p. 277	Chromosomal Microarray Analysis

CHAPTER 14

Prenatal Diagnosis

14–1. A 36-year-old primigravida at 20 weeks' gestation presents to her obstetrician's office with a complaint of leaking fluid. Sonographic examination performed confirms markedly decreased fluid, and midtrimester rupture of membranes is suspected. The patient elects to continue her pregnancy, and minimal amnionic fluid is present around the fetus. At term, her fetus is born with a right-sided clubbed foot. This is an example of which of the following?

a. Sequence

b. Disruption

c. Deformation

d. Malformation

14–2. The finding seen below was identified prenatally during sonographic examination and is an example of which of the following?

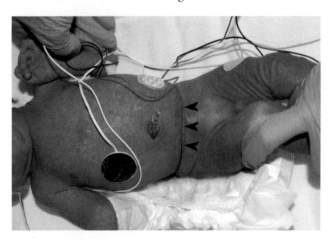

Used with permission from Dr. Dina Chamsy.

a. Syndrome

b. Disruption

c. Association

d. Malformation

14–3. The infant shown below was also born with a cleft palate. These findings are consistent with which of the following processes?

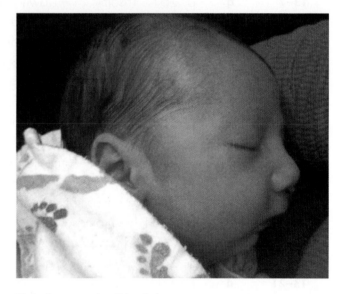

Used with permission from Valorie Butler.

a. Syndrome

b. Sequence

c. Association

d. Chromosome abnormality

14–4. A pregnant 25-year-old postdoctoral student presents for genetic counseling following a multiple marker screen that revealed an increased risk for an open neural-tube defect and trisomy 18. She is from France and her husband is from Great Britain. Her medical history is significant for a seizure disorder well controlled on phenytoin. Which of the following is **NOT** an expected possible contributing factor in her elevated risk for an open neural-tube defect?

a. Ethnicity

b. Medication exposure

c. Chromosome abnormality

d. None of the above

14–5. What is the recurrence risk for an open neural-tube defect after a couple has had one child born with anencephaly?

a. 3% to 5%

b. 10%

c. 25%

d. Unknown

14–6. Four-milligram folic acid supplementation before conception and in the first trimester of pregnancy would be most indicated in which of the following scenarios?

a. Maternal pregestational diabetes

b. A personal history of open neural-tube defect

c. Maternal valproic acid use for seizure disorder

d. Maternal paroxetine use for depression

14–7. Which of the following maternal factors does not affect the maternal serum alpha fetoprotein (AFP) multiples of the median calculation?

a. Race

b. Parity

c. Weight

d. Gestational age

14–8. Which of the following is **NOT** an indication for sonographic evaluation of an elevated maternal serum AFP level result?

a. Determination of fetal sex

b. Estimation of gestational age

c. Determination of fetal number

d. Documentation of fetal viability

14–9. During routine sonographic examination, the abnormality seen below was detected. This condition is associated with which of the following conditions?

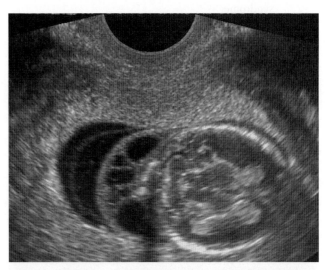

a. Twin gestation

b. Low maternal inhibin level

c. Maternal pregestational diabetes

d. Elevated maternal serum AFP level

14–10. Your patient has a 1:100 risk for a fetal open neural-tube defect based on serum screening at 18 weeks' gestation. She undergoes targeted sonographic examination, which documents a singleton fetus and a marginal placenta previa. No fetal abnormalities are detected. Following this examination, how should she be counseled regarding her fetus's risk for having an open neural-tube defect?

a. Reduced by 25%

b. Reduced by 50%

c. Reduced by 95%

d. Unchanged from the 1% risk

14–11. Which of the following obstetric complications is the patient in Question 14–10 **NOT** at increased risk for?

a. Fetal death

b. Fetal macrosomia

c. Placenta abruption

d. Preterm rupture of membranes

14–12. Multiple screening strategies exist to detect Down syndrome during pregnancy. Which of the following tests has the highest detection rate for Down syndrome?

   a. Maternal serum AFP

   b. Integrated screening

   c. Quadruple marker test

   d. Combined first-trimester screening

14–13. A 38-year-old woman presents for first-trimester screening for Down syndrome at a gestational age of 12 weeks and 1 day. The ultrasound image below was seen. What is the next step in evaluating this finding?

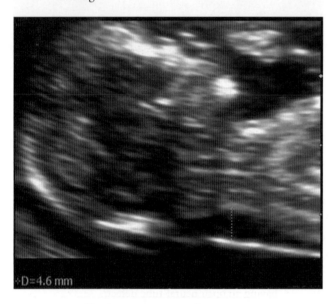

   a. Offer diagnostic prenatal testing

   b. Repeat the ultrasound measurement in 1 week

   c. Complete the first-trimester screen and wait for her numeric risk assessment

   d. Offer a sequential test as it has a high sensitivity for Down syndrome detection

14–14. Which of the following correctly identifies the second-trimester analyte level abnormalities in a pregnancy at increased risk for Down syndrome?

   a. Decreased MSAFP, increased unconjugated estriol, increased inhibin, increased beta hCG

   b. Decreased MSAFP, decreased unconjugated estriol, increased inhibin, increased beta hCG

   c. Increased MSAFP, increased unconjugated estriol, decreased inhibin, decreased beta hCG

   d. Decreased MSAFP, decreased unconjugated estriol, decreased inhibin, increased beta hCG

14–15. The American College of Obstetricians and Gynecologists recommends a strategy using first- and second-trimester screening for what reason?

   a. Earlier results

   b. Improved Down syndrome detection rates

   c. Reduced false-positive rate compared with second trimester screening

   d. None of the above

14–16. Testing for the most common trisomies that complicate pregnancies can be accomplished by isolating which of the following substances from maternal blood?

   a. Fetal RNA

   b. Free fetal cells

   c. Mitochondrial DNA

   d. Cell-free fetal DNA

14–17. The congenital anomaly seen in the ultrasound image below was discovered during routine evaluation at 20 weeks' gestation and was an isolated finding. What should your patient be told regarding the risk of a chromosome abnormality in her fetus?

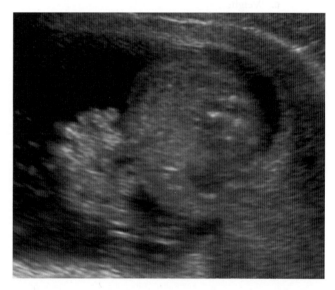

Reproduced with permission from Cunningham FG, Leveno KJ, Bloom SL, et al (eds): Fetal imaging. In Williams Obstetrics, 24th ed. New York, McGraw-Hill, 2014, eF10-22A.

   a. 10%

   b. 22%

   c. 30%

   d. No increase in risk

14–18. A 25-year-old primigravida from China has a Down syndrome risk of 1:5000 based on her first-trimester screening results. The finding shown is noted during a routine sonographic examination performed at 17 weeks' gestation. How should she be counseled regarding this finding?

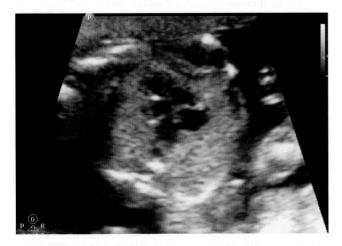

a. Schedule a fetal echocardiogram at 22 weeks' gestation

b. Offer an amniocentesis since she is now considered "high-risk"

c. Inform her that this finding is seen in up to 30% of fetuses of Asian descent

d. Inform her that her Down syndrome risk has now increased from 1 in 5000 to 1 in 500

14–19. Which of the following fetal conditions or events is **NOT** associated with the finding of echogenic bowel during a second-trimester sonographic examination?

a. Down syndrome

b. Cystic fibrosis

c. Toxoplasmosis infection

d. Intraamniotic hemorrhage

14–20. Which of the following skeletal findings during sonographic examination suggest an increased fetal risk for Down syndrome?

a. Observed:expected femur ratio ≤ .90

b. Observed:expected humerus ratio ≤ .90

c. Femur length:abdominal circumference ratio < .20

d. Observed:expected biparietal diameter ratio < .89

14–21. What chromosome is the cystic fibrosis conductance transmembrane regulator (CFTR) gene located on?

a. 7

b. 14

c. 17

d. None of the above

14–22. A white couple presents for preconceptional counseling regarding cystic fibrosis. She has a prior child affected with the disease; he has two unaffected children. What is their risk of having an affected fetus?

a. 1:50

b. 1:100

c. 1:200

d. 1:2500

14–23. What is the appropriate screening test for hemoglobinopathies in patients of African descent?

a. Complete blood count

b. Peripheral blood smear

c. Hemoglobin electrophoresis

d. Hemoglobin S mutation analysis

14–24. An Asian patient presents for prenatal care. Her complete blood count reveals a microcytic anemia. What is the most appropriate next step in the evaluation of her anemia?

a. Iron studies

b. Hemoglobin electrophoresis

c. Alpha thalassemia molecular genetic testing

d. None of the above

14–25. Hexosaminidase A activity levels should be used in testing for carrier status for Tay-Sachs disease in which of the following samples?

a. Blood from a pregnant woman

b. Blood from a male of Indian descent

c. Blood from a male of Ashkenazi Jewish descent

d. Amnionic fluid from a suspected affected fetus

14–26. Which of the following is **NOT** a reason for the decreased prevalence of fetal blood sampling in the last decade?

a. Increase in procedure-related loss rate with fetal blood sampling

b. Increased availability of DNA-based tests for amnionic fluid

c. Increased use of fluorescence in situ hybridization (FISH) on amnionic fluid samples

d. Increased use of middle cerebral artery Doppler studies in the evaluation of suspected fetal anemia

14–27. There is an increased pregnancy loss rate following amniocentesis in all **EXCEPT** which of the following conditions?

   a. Twin gestation

   b. Maternal BMI $\geq$ 40 kg/m^2

   c. Transplacental puncture with needle

   d. All of the above

14–28. A 40-year-old infertility patient underwent an amniocentesis at 17 weeks' gestation. She calls 1 day later and reports that she is leaking amnionic fluid. What should she be told about this postamniocentesis complication?

   a. Fetal survival is > 90%.

   b. The risk of fetal death is 25%.

   c. The risk for chorioamnionitis is 2%.

   d. Fluid leakage occurs in approximately 10% of patients.

14–29. Early amniocentesis is defined as amniocentesis that is performed during which of the following gestational age windows?

   a. 9–11 weeks

   b. 11–14 weeks

   c. 12–15 weeks

   d. 14–16 weeks

14–30. A woman undergoes a chorionic villus sampling (CVS) at 11 weeks' gestation. The result shows two cell lines—46,XY and 47,XY,+21. What is the appropriate next step?

   a. Repeat CVS at 13 weeks' gestation

   b. Plan no further evaluation or treatment

   c. Offer amniocentesis for clarification of results

   d. Provide the patient with appropriate information regarding Down syndrome

14–31. Chorionic villus sampling has been associated with limb reduction defects under what condition?

   a. Multiple needle passes are made.

   b. Performed at a gestational age < 10 weeks

   c. Performed using a transabdominal approach

   d. Larger volumes of chorionic villi are sampled.

14–32. Fetal blood sampling performed at the placental insertion site is associated with which of the following?

   a. Shorter procedure duration

   b. Increased pregnancy loss rate

   c. Increased procedure success rate

   d. Decreased maternal blood contamination

14–33. Which of the following statements correctly describes polar body analysis when used for preimplantation genetic testing?

   a. It involves sampling one cell of the embryo on day 3.

   b. It is associated with decreased pregnancy success rates.

   c. It can be used to determine paternally inherited genetic disorders.

   d. None of the above

14–34. Preimplantation genetic diagnosis may be used for which of the following scenarios?

   a. Determine fetal gender

   b. Diagnose single gene mutations

   c. Human leukocyte antigen (HLA) typing

   d. All of the above

14–35. Which of the following is **NOT** a limitation of preimplantation genetic screening using fluorescence in situ hybridization?

   a. The result may not reflect the embryonic karyotype.

   b. Genomic hybridization arrays have a high failure rate.

   c. Mosaicism is common in cleavage-stage embryo blastomeres.

   d. Pregnancy rates are lower following preimplantation genetic screening.

14–36. What is the most common cause of infant death in the United States?

   a. Preterm birth

   b. Motor vehicle accidents

   c. Major congenital anomalies

   d. Complications from maternal hypertension

CHAPTER 14 ANSWER KEY

Question number	Letter answer	Page cited	Header cited
14–1	c	p. 283	Introduction
14–2	b	p. 283	Introduction
14–3	b	p. 283	Introduction
14–4	b	p. 284	Table 14-1
14–5	a	p. 284	Risk Factors
14–6	b	p. 284	Prevention
14–7	b	p. 284	Maternal Serum Alpha-Fetoprotein Screening
14–8	a	p. 285	MSAFP Elevation
14–9	d	p. 287	Table 14-2
14–10	c	p. 285	Targeted Sonography
14–11	b	p. 287	Unexplained Maternal Serum AFP Level Evaluation
14–12	b	p. 291	Combined First- and Second-Trimester Screening
14–13	a	p. 289	Nuchal Translucency
14–14	b	p. 290	Second-Trimester Screening
14–15	b	p. 291	Combined First- and Second-Trimester Screening
14–16	d	p. 291	Cell-Free Fetal DNA Screening
14–17	d	p. 292	Table 14-6
14–18	c	p. 292	Second-Trimester Sonographic Markers—"Soft Signs"
14–19	c	p. 292	Second-Trimester Sonographic Markers—"Soft Signs"
14–20	a	p. 292	Second-Trimester Sonographic Markers—"Soft Signs"
14–21	a	p. 295	Cystic Fibrosis
14–22	c	p. 295	Cystic Fibrosis
14–23	c	p. 296	Sickle Hemoglobinopathies
14–24	a	p. 296	Alpha-Thalassemia
14–25	b	p. 296	Tay-Sachs Disease
14–26	a	p. 297	Prenatal and Preimplantation Diagnostic Testing
14–27	c	p. 299	Complications
14–28	a	p. 299	Complications
14–29	b	p. 299	Early Amniocentesis
14–30	c	p. 300	Complications
14–31	b	p. 300	Complications
14–32	a	p. 300	Complications
14–33	d	p. 301	Preimplantation Genetic Testing
14–34	d	p. 301	Preimplantation Genetic Diagnosis (PGD)
14–35	b	p. 302	Preimplantation Genetic Screening (PGS)
14–36	c	p. 283	Introduction

CHAPTER 15

Fetal Disorders

15–1. What is the most common cause of fetal anemia?

   a. Alpha thalassemia

   b. Fetomaternal hemorrhage

   c. Parvovirus B19 infection

   d. Red cell alloimmunization

15–2. What is the approximate prevalence of red cell alloimmunization in pregnancy?

   a. 0.1%

   b. 1%

   c. 5%

   d. 8%

15–3. Most cases of severe fetal anemia secondary to alloimmunization are due to all **EXCEPT** which of the following antibodies?

   a. Anti-c

   b. Anti-d

   c. Anti-D

   d. Anti-Kell

15–4. What is the critical titer for anti-D antibody alloimmunization?

   a. 1:4

   b. 1:8

   c. 1:16

   d. 1:32

15–5. What is the minimum amount of fetal erythrocytes needed in the maternal circulation to provoke sensitization to D antigen?

   a. 0.01 mL

   b. 0.1 mL

   c. 1 mL

   d. 5 mL

15–6. A mother whose blood type is A negative labors and delivers a B-positive child at term. She does not receive anti-D immune globulin postpartum. What are the chances that the patient will become alloimmunized?

   a. 2%

   b. 8%

   c. 20%

   d. 33%

15–7. All **EXCEPT** which of the following antibodies are harmless in pregnancy?

   a. Anti-I

   b. Anti-Lu^a

   c. Anti-Fy^b

   d. Anti-Lewis

15–8. What percentage of Kell-sensitized cases is due to prior transfusion?

   a. 60%

   b. 70%

   c. 80%

   d. 90%

15–9. What is the most common cause of hemolytic disease in newborns?

   a. Alpha-thalassemia

   b. ABO incompatibility

   c. Rh alloimmunization

   d. Glucose-6-phosphate dehydrogenase (G6PD) deficiency

15–10. Why can ABO incompatibility manifest in firstborn children, even though there has been no prior exposure to pregnancy?

    a. Fetal red cells have more antigenic sites than adult cells.

    b. Anti-A and anti-B antibodies can cross the placenta early in the first trimester.

    c. Most group O women have been previously exposed to bacteria possessing A- or B-like antigens.

    d. None of the above

15–11. What percentage of fetuses from Rh D alloimmunized pregnancies will develop mild to moderate anemia?

    a. 5%

    b. 15%

    c. 25%

    d. 50%

15–12. Of these, what percentage will progress to hydrops if left untreated?

    a. 0.1%

    b. 5%

    c. 15%

    d. 25%

15–13. A 42-year-old G3P2 presents for prenatal care at 12 weeks' gestation. She is Rh D-negative and has a positive antibody screen with anti-D antibodies. She has a firstborn child who needed a blood transfusion at birth for mild anemia. What management strategy would you implement next?

    a. Test the patient for titers of anti-D antibodies

    b. Test the father of the baby for red-cell antigens

    c. Perform amniocentesis to assess fetal antigen type

    d. Perform fetal blood sampling to assess fetal hematocrit

15–14. The patient from Question 15–13 confirms paternity, and the patient's husband is a heterozygote at the D locus. Which of the following is an appropriate next step?

    a. Expectant management

    b. Amniocentesis to assess fetal antigen type

    c. Serial measurement of maternal anti-D titers

    d. Fetal blood sampling to assess fetal hematocrit

15–15. The patient from Question 15–13 declines invasive testing. Which of the following can you offer to serially assess the fetus's risk for anemia?

    a. Maternal anti-D titers

    b. Peak systolic velocity of the umbilical artery

    c. Peak systolic velocity of the middle cerebral artery

    d. All of the above

15–16. The patient from Question 15–13 returns for sonographic surveillance. The peak systolic velocity of the middle cerebral artery is 52 cm/sec at 23 weeks. Based on this graph by Oepkes and colleagues (2006), what is your next management step?

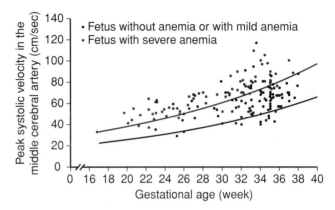

Reproduced with permission from Cunningham FG, Leveno KJ, Bloom SL, et al (eds): Fetal disorders. In Williams Obstetrics, 24th ed. New York, McGraw-Hill, 2014, Figure 15-1.

    a. Perform fetal blood transfusion

    b. Perform fetal blood sampling to assess fetal hematocrit

    c. Perform amniocentesis to measure amnionic fluid bilirubin concentration

    d. Continue serial measurement of the peak systolic velocity of the middle cerebral artery

15–17. What is the main reason that peak systolic velocity of the middle cerebral artery increases as fetal anemia worsens?

    a. Cardiac output increases.

    b. Blood viscosity decreases.

    c. Fetus shunts blood preferentially to the brain.

    d. All of the above

15–18. What should be the next management step if fetal anemia is suspected by noninvasive methods at 36 weeks' gestation?

    a. Proceed with delivery

    b. Perform fetal blood transfusion

    c. Administer corticosteroids for fetal lung maturation

    d. Continue serial measurement of the peak systolic velocity of the middle cerebral artery

15–19. Compared with Doppler measurement of the peak systolic velocity of the middle cerebral artery (MCA), which of the following is true regarding the Liley curve for evaluation of fetal anemia?

    a. It is a less invasive assessment tool.

    b. It leads to lower pregnancy loss rates.

    c. It is less sensitive to identify fetal anemia.

    d. It leads to lower rates of further alloimmunization.

15–20. Red cells used for fetal transfusion should have which of the following characteristics?

    a. Irradiated

    b. Leukocyte enriched

    c. Same ABO group as the mother

    d. An approximate hematocrit of 50%

15–21. What is the risk of death after fetal blood transfusion for the fetus of an alloimmunized pregnancy?

    a. 0.1%

    b. 3%

    c. 11%

    d. 22%

15–22. What is the overall survival rate after fetal blood transfusion for fetuses of alloimmunized pregnancies that are similar to the one seen in these sonograms?

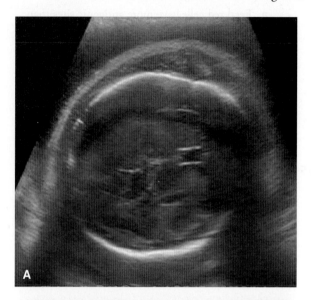

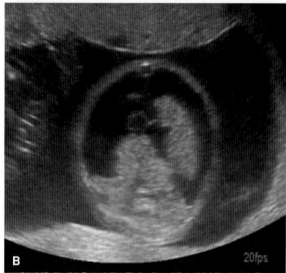

    a. 15%

    b. 40%

    c. 75%

    d. 90%

15–23. Which of the following statements is true regarding a 300-μg dose of anti-D immunoglobulin?

    a. It has a half-life of 6 weeks.

    b. It reduces the risk of alloimmunization to less than 2%.

    c. It will worsen alloimmunization if given to a previously D-sensitized patient.

    d. It will provide protection from a fetomaternal hemorrhage of approximately 30 mL of fetal red cells.

15–24. An Rh D-negative pregnant patient most likely may become alloimmunized after all **EXCEPT** which of the following situations?

   a. Amniocentesis

   b. Abdominal trauma

   c. Platelet transfusion

   d. Administration of anti-D immune globulin

15–25. Which test should be performed to quantify the appropriate dose of anti-D immune globulin needed to treat an at-risk patient?

   a. Rosette test

   b. Indirect coombs

   c. Kleihauer-Betke test

   d. All of the above

15–26. A patient at 29 weeks' gestation presents with heavy vaginal bleeding after a motor vehicle accident. The fetal heart rate tracing is shown here. Ultimately, what procedure could be helpful in the management of this patient?

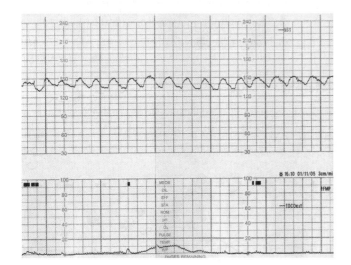

Reproduced with permission from Cunningham FG, Leveno KJ, Bloom SL, et al (eds): Fetal assessment. In Williams Obstetrics, 24th ed. New York, McGraw-Hill, 2014, Figure 24-10.

   a. Kleihauer-Betke test

   b. Fetal blood transfusion

   c. Sonographic measurement of the peak systolic velocity of the middle cerebral artery

   d. All of the above

15–27. The image here shows a test used to assess fetomaternal hemorrhage. Which of the following is **NOT** a limitation of this test?

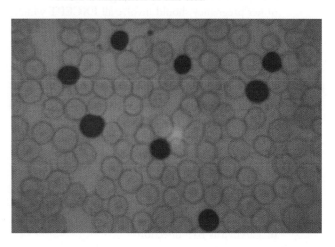

Reproduced with permission from Cunningham FG, Leveno KJ, Bloom SL, et al (eds): Fetal disorders. In Williams Obstetrics, 24th ed. New York, McGraw-Hill, 2014, Figure 15-4.

   a. It is labor intensive.

   b. It is only qualitative.

   c. It is less accurate at term.

   d. It is less accurate in the setting of maternal hemoglobinopathy.

15–28. What is the most common cause of severe neonatal thrombocytopenia?

   a. Neonatal viral infection

   b. Alloimmune thrombocytopenia

   c. Idiopathic thrombocytopenia

   d. Gestational thrombocytopenia

15–29. Which human platelet antigen (HPA) is the most common in cases of neonatal alloimmune thrombocytopenia?

   a. HPA-1a

   b. HPA-1b

   c. HPA-3a

   d. HPA-5b

15–30. What is the approximate risk of fetal or neonatal intracranial hemorrhage in the setting of alloimmune thrombocytopenia?

   a. 0.5%

   b. 7%

   c. 18%

   d. 33%

15–31. Your pregnant patient has a firstborn child affected by neonatal alloimmune thrombocytopenia and associated intracranial hemorrhage. The management of her pregnancy should involve all **EXCEPT** which of the following interventions?

    a. Prednisone

    b. Cesarean delivery

    c. Intravenous immunoglobulins

    d. Maternal platelet transfusion

15–32. All **EXCEPT** which of the following are treatable causes of nonimmune hydrops?

    a. Monosomy X

    b. Chylothorax

    c. Tachyarrhythmia

    d. Parvovirus B19 infection

15–33. What is the aneuploidy risk for a hydropic fetus detected in the first trimester?

    a. 25%

    b. 33%

    c. 50%

    d. 66%

15–34. An Rh D-positive patient is referred for evaluation because of the sonographic fetal finding shown here. If this finding is isolated, which of the following statements is true?

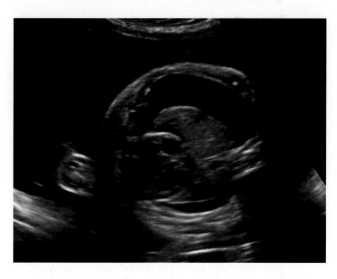

    a. The risk of aneuploidy is decreased.

    b. The fetus can be considered hydropic.

    c. The condition may resolve with treatment.

    d. None of the above

Reference

Oepkes D, Seaward PG, Vandenbussche FP, et al: Doppler ultrasonography versus amniocentesis to predict fetal anemia. N Engl J Med 355:156, 2006

CHAPTER 15 ANSWER KEY

Question number	Letter answer	Page cited	Header cited
15–1	d	p. 306	Fetal Anemia
15–2	b	p. 306	Red Cell Alloimmunization
15–3	b	p. 306	Red Cell Alloimmunization
15–4	c	p. 307	Alloimmunization Detection
15–5	b	p. 307	CDE (Rh) Blood Group Incompatibility
15–6	a	p. 307	CDE (Rh) Blood Group Incompatibility
15–7	b	p. 308	Table 15-1
15–8	d	p. 308	Kell Alloimmunization
15–9	b	p. 308	ABO Blood Group Incompatibility
15–10	c	p. 308	ABO Blood Group Incompatibility
15–11	c	p. 309	Management of the Alloimmunized Pregnancy
15–12	d	p. 309	Management of the Alloimmunized Pregnancy
15–13	b	p. 309	Determining Fetal Risk
15–14	b	p. 309	Determining Fetal Risk
15–15	c	p. 309	Determining Fetal Risk
15–16	b	p. 310	Middle Cerebral Artery Doppler Velocimetry; Figure 15-1
15–17	d	p. 310	Middle Cerebral Artery Doppler Velocimetry
15–18	a	p. 310	Fetal Blood Transfusion
15–19	c	p. 310	Amniotic Fluid Spectral Analysis
15–20	a	p. 310	Fetal Blood Transfusion
15–21	b	p. 311	Outcomes
15–22	c	p. 311	Outcomes
15–23	b	p. 311	Prevention of Rh D Alloimmunization
15–24	d	p. 311	Prevention of Rh D Alloimmunization; Table 15-2
15–25	c	p. 311	Prevention of Rh D Alloimmunization
15–26	d	p. 312	Fetomaternal Hemorrhage
15–27	b	p. 313	Tests for Fetomaternal Hemorrhage
15–28	b	p. 313	Alloimmune Thrombocytopenia
15–29	a	p. 313	Alloimmune Thrombocytopenia
15–30	b	p. 313	Alloimmune Thrombocytopenia
15–31	d	p. 313	Alloimmune Thrombocytopenia
15–32	a	p. 315	Nonimmune Hydrops
15–33	c	p. 315	Nonimmune Hydrops
15–34	c	p. 316	Isolated Effusion or Edema

CHAPTER 16

Fetal Therapy

16–1. All **EXCEPT** which of the following are examples of fetal conditions that may be amendable to medical therapy delivered transplacentally?

a. Dandy-Walker malformation

b. Supraventricular tachycardia

c. Congenital adrenal hyperplasia

d. Congenital cystic adenomatoid malformation

16–2. When a fetal rhythm disturbance is suspected, what type of sonography should be performed to determine the relationship between the atrial and ventricular rates?

a. M-mode

b. Power Doppler

c. 3-dimensional

d. Color Doppler

16–3. What is the most common fetal arrhythmia?

a. Atrial flutter

b. Congenital heart block

c. Supraventricular tachycardia

d. Premature atrial contraction

16–4. A 16-year-old primigravida is referred for sonographic examination because of a suspected fetal arrhythmia. The following image is obtained and demonstrates a premature atrial contraction (*blue arrow*). What is the most appropriate treatment for this condition?

a. Digoxin

b. Amiodarone

c. Corticosteroids

d. None of the above

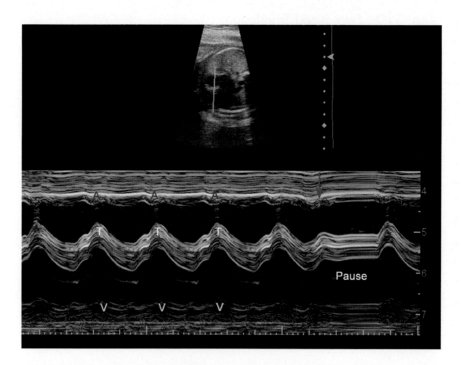

Reproduced with permission from Cunningham FG, Leveno KJ, Bloom SL, et al (eds): Fetal imaging. In Williams Obstetrics, 24th ed. New York, McGraw-Hill, 2014, Figure 10-24.

16–5. For the patient in Question 16-4, you counsel her that this condition can progress to supraventricular tachycardia in approximately what percentage of fetuses?

    a. 2%

    b. 5%

    c. 15%

    d. 35%

16–6. All **EXCEPT** which of the following are characteristic of fetal supraventricular tachycardia?

    a. Can be caused by an ectopic focus

    b. Displays a varying degree of atrioventricular block

    c. Has a ventricular rate of 180 to 300 beats per minute

    d. All are characteristic

16–7. All **EXCEPT** which of the following conditions can cause fetal sinus tachycardia?

    a. Fetal anemia

    b. Maternal fever

    c. Fetal accessory pathway

    d. Maternal thyrotoxicosis

16–8. A fetal tachyarrhythmia is defined as *sustained* if it is present for what percentage of the time?

    a. 10%

    b. 25%

    c. 50%

    d. 75%

16–9. A 28-year-old G2P1 at 25 weeks' gestation is referred for fetal echocardiography for a suspected tachyarrhythmia. The image below is obtained confirming atrial flutter with a 2:1 atrioventricular block. What is typically used as first-line treatment in this situation? A = atrial contractions, V = ventricular contractions.

    a. Digoxin

    b. Flecainide

    c. Amiodarone

    d. Procainamide

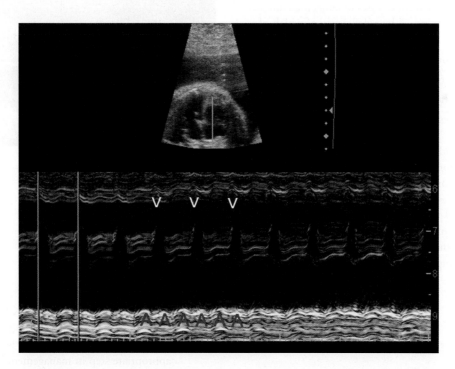

Reproduced with permission from Cunningham FG, Leveno KJ, Bloom SL, et al (eds): Fetal therapy. In Williams Obstetrics, 24th ed. New York, McGraw-Hill, 2014, Figure 16-1.

16–10. For the patient in Question 16-9, what additional sonographic finding in the fetus would make the treatment of this condition less effective?

a. Hydramnios

b. Hydrops fetalis

c. An associated atrial-septal defect

d. A ventricular rate of 220 beats per minute

16–11. What is the most common cause of congenital heart block in a structurally normal fetal heart?

a. Congenital syphilis

b. Maternal diabetes mellitus

c. Maternal anti-SSA or anti-SSB antibodies

d. Maternal administration of beta-blocking medications

16–12. Third-degree heart block in a fetus can be successfully reversed with maternal administration of which of the following medications?

a. Sotalol

b. Dexamethasone

c. Betamethasone

d. None of the above

16–13. More than 90 percent of cases of congenital adrenal hyperplasia are caused by a deficiency of which of the following enzymes?

a. 21-Hydroxylase

b. 11β-Hydroxylase

c. 17α-Hydroxylase

d. 3β-Hydroxysteroid dehydrogenase

16–14. A 28-year-old G1P1 presents with her husband for preconceptional counseling since her daughter was born with nonclassic congenital adrenal hyperplasia (CAH) and evidence of genital virilization. Her husband was the father of that child also. You discuss the inheritance pattern of this condition and inform her that approximately what proportion of their offspring would be at risk for CAH?

a. ½

b. ¼

c. ⅛

d. ¹⁄₁₆

16–15. The couple in Question 16-14 plan to conceive soon and understand that dexamethasone has been used in pregnant women to prevent virilization of a female fetus. You inform them that treatment, if elected, needs to be initiated by what gestational age?

a. 6 weeks

b. 9 weeks

c. 12 weeks

d. 15 weeks

16–16. A 22-year-old primigravida presents at 29 weeks' gestation for prenatal care enrollment. During routine sonographic examination, the following fetal chest mass (*C*) is identified. You suspect a congenital cystic adenomatoid malformation. You counsel her that if these masses become large enough, the fetus is at risk for which of the following?

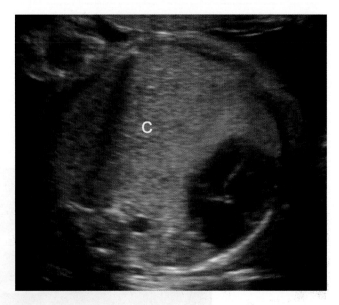

Reproduced with permission from Cunningham FG, Leveno KJ, Bloom SL, et al (eds): Fetal imaging. In Williams Obstetrics, 24th ed. New York, McGraw-Hill, 2014, Figure 10-18A.

a. Hydrops fetalis

b. Mediastinal shift

c. Depressed cardiac output

d. All of the above

16–17. For the patient in Question 16-16, you calculate a congenital cystic adenomatoid malformation-volume-ratio (CVR) of 1.9. What is the next most appropriate step in management based on this calculation?

a. Observation

b. Open fetal surgery

c. Medical therapy in pregnancy

d. Percutaneous thoraco-amnionic shunt placement

16–18. Once a fetal goiter is identified, it is important to guide therapy to determine whether this finding is associated with hyper- or hypothyroidism. Sampling which of the following is the preferred method to make this determination?

   a. Placenta

   b. Fetal blood

   c. Maternal blood

   d. Amnionic fluid

16–19. What is the clinical goal of treating fetal thyroid disorders associated with a goiter?

   a. Prevent hydramnios

   b. Decrease the risk of labor dystocia

   c. Correct the underlying physiological abnormality

   d. All of the above

16–20. Which of the following conditions has been successfully treated with fetal stem-cell transplantation?

   a. Beta thalassemia

   b. Sickle-cell anemia

   c. Maple-syrup urine disease

   d. Severe combined immunodeficiency syndrome

16–21. Consideration for fetal surgery should be limited to those situations in which all **EXCEPT** which of the following criteria are met?

   a. The defect is isolated.

   b. The defect results in a high likelihood of death.

   c. The safety and efficacy of the procedure is proven.

   d. There is an animal model for the defect and procedure.

16–22. What is the first nonlethal birth defect for which fetal surgery has been offered?

   a. Spina bifida

   b. Sacrococcygeal teratoma

   c. Extralobar pulmonary sequestration

   d. Congenital cystic adenomatoid malformation

16–23. A 28-year-old G2P1 at 19 weeks' gestation is referred for a targeted sonographic evaluation because of an elevated maternal serum alpha-fetoprotein level. The following spinal defect is appreciated and is consistent with a myelomeningocele (*arrowheads indicate nerve roots; arrow marks the cephalad junction of skin and bulging meningeal sac*). She inquires about possible fetal surgery. You counsel her that infants who underwent prenatal surgery in the Management of Myelomeningocele Study (MOMS) had which of the following outcomes compared with those that had postnatal surgery?

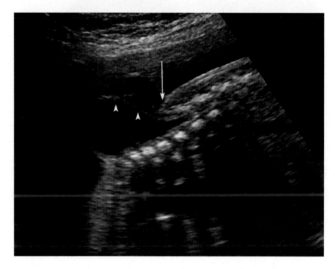

Reproduced with permission from Cunningham FG, Leveno KJ, Bloom SL, et al (eds): Fetal imaging. In Williams Obstetrics, 24th ed. New York, McGraw-Hill, 2014, Figure 10-7.

   a. They experienced lower hindbrain herniation rates.

   b. They were more likely to walk independently at 30 months.

   c. They were less likely to require ventriculoperitoneal shunting by 1 year of age.

   d. All of the above

16–24. The patient in Question 16–23 asks about the risks of fetal surgery. You counsel her that in the MOMS trial, all **EXCEPT** which of the following morbidities occurred more frequently in the prenatal surgery group compared with the postnatal surgery group?

   a. Preterm delivery

   b. Placental abruption

   c. Maternal hypertension

   d. Maternal pulmonary edema

16–25. Shown in the figure is a large sacrococcygeal teratoma. Hydrops fetalis can occur in these situations as a result of which of the following?

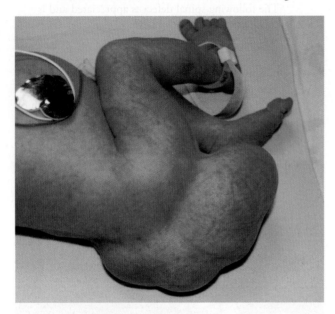

Used with permission from Dr. Michael Zaretsky.

a. Lymphatic obstruction

b. Congestive heart failure

c. High-output heart failure

d. None of the above

16–26. In the United States, which of the following twin pregnancies would be candidates for fetoscopic laser ablation therapy for twin-twin transfusion syndrome (TTTS)?

a. Monochorionic diamnionic twins at 23 weeks' gestation with stage I TTTS

b. Dichorionic diamnionic twins at 19 weeks' gestation with stage II TTTS

c. Monochorionic diamnionic twins at 15 weeks' gestation with stage IV TTTS

d. Monochorionic diamnionic twins at 21 weeks' gestation with stage III TTTS

16–27. Reasonable expectations of laser ablation for severe twin-twin transfusion syndrome include what anticipated fetal mortality rate following therapy?

a. 5–10%

b. 10–25%

c. 30–50%

d. 60–80%

16–28. What is the most significant risk factor for mortality in fetuses with isolated congenital diaphragmatic hernia?

a. Bowel herniation

b. Liver herniation

c. Mediastinal shift

d. Low residual lung volumes

16–29. The lung-to-head ratio is a measurement used to predict survival in fetuses with isolated left-sided congenital diaphragmatic hernia. This ratio is calculated by dividing the right lung area by which of the following?

a. Brain volume

b. Head circumference

c. Biparietal diameter

d. Occipitofrontal diameter

16–30. What is the most common etiology of a primary pulmonary effusion in the fetus?

a. Aneuploidy

b. Chylothorax

c. Viral infection

d. Extralobar pulmonary sequestration

16–31. What is the most common cause of bladder outlet obstruction?

a. Urethral cysts

b. Urethral atresia

c. Prune-belly syndrome

d. Posterior urethral valves

16–32. All **EXCEPT** which of the following would generally be considered contraindications to vesicoamnionic shunt placement in fetuses with bladder outlet obstruction?

a. Female sex

b. Aneuploidy

c. Presence of renal cysts

d. Urinary sodium of 80 mmol/L

CHAPTER 16 ANSWER KEY

Question number	Letter answer	Page cited	Header cited
16–1	a	p. 321	Medical Therapy
16–2	a	p. 321	Arrhythmias
16–3	d	p. 321	Premature Atrial Contractions
16–4	d	p. 321	Premature Atrial Contractions
16–5	a	p. 321	Premature Atrial Contractions
16–6	b	p. 321	Tachyarrhythmias
16–7	c	p. 321	Tachyarrhythmias
16–8	c	p. 321	Tachyarrhythmias
16–9	a	p. 321	Tachyarrhythmias
16–10	b	p. 321	Tachyarrhythmias
16–11	c	p. 322	Bradyarrhythmia
16–12	d	p. 322	Bradyarrhythmia
16–13	a	p. 323	Congenital Adrenal Hyperplasia
16–14	c	p. 323	Congenital Adrenal Hyperplasia
16–15	b	p. 323	Congenital Adrenal Hyperplasia
16–16	d	p. 323	Congenital Cystic Adenomatoid Malformation
16–17	c	p. 323	Congenital Cystic Adenomatoid Malformation
16–18	b	p. 324	Thyroid Disease
16–19	d	p. 324	Thyroid Disease
16–20	d	p. 324	Fetal Stem Cell Transplantation
16–21	c	p. 324	Surgical Therapy; Table 16-1
16–22	a	p. 325	Myelomeningocele Surgery
16–23	d	p. 325	Myelomeningocele Surgery
16–24	c	p. 325	Myelomeningocele Surgery; Table 16-3
16–25	c	p. 327	Sacrococcygeal Teratoma
16–26	d	p. 327	Twin-Twin Transfusion Syndrome
16–27	c	p. 327	Twin-Twin Transfusion Syndrome; Complications
16–28	b	p. 328	Congenital Diaphragmatic Hernia
16–29	b	p. 328	Lung-Head Ratio
16–30	b	p. 329	Thoracic Shunts
16–31	d	p. 330	Urinary Shunts
16–32	d	p. 330	Urinary Shunts; Table 16-4

CHAPTER 17

Fetal Assessment

17–1. What are the goals of antepartum fetal surveillance?
  a. Prevent fetal death
  b. Indicate timing of intervention
  c. Improve negative predictive values for antepartum testing
  d. All of the above

17–2. Concerning antepartum testing, positive predictive values for true-positive abnormal test results approximate which of the following?
  a. 5–10%
  b. 10–40%
  c. 40–60%
  d. 60–80%

17–3. Regarding sleep cyclicity (sleep-wake cycles), which of the following is true?
  a. It varies from 5 to 120 minutes.
  b. Mean length of inactive state for term fetuses is 23 minutes.
  c. In normal term pregnancies, the longest period of inactivity is 68 minutes.
  d. None of the above

17–4. Common fetal movement counting protocols include which of the following?
  a. 10 movements in 1 hour
  b. 10 movements in 2 hours
  c. Informal maternal perceptions of fetal activity are clinically meaningless.
  d. Monitor 2 hours daily; an accepted count equals or exceeds a previously established baseline count.

17–5. The figure below illustrates which of the following?
  a. Minimal counts of fetal movement occur at term.
  b. Maximal counts of fetal movement occur at 32 weeks.
  c. Daily movement counts reach approximately 16 at 29 weeks.
  d. Declining amnionic fluid volume and space account for decreased fetal movements at 32 weeks.

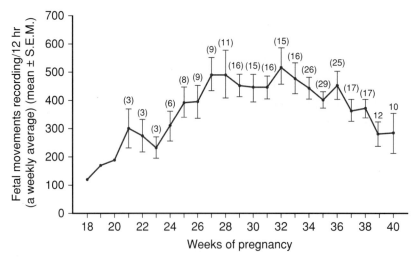

Reproduced with permission from Cunningham FG, Leveno KJ, Bloom SL, et al (eds): Antepartum assessment. In Williams Obstetrics, 23rd ed. New York, McGraw-Hill, 2010, Figure 15-2.

17–6. Which of the following is true regarding fetal breathing motions measured in this figure?

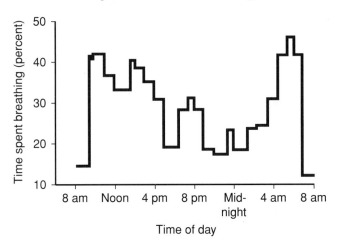

Reproduced with permission from Cunningham FG, Leveno KJ, Bloom SL, et al (eds): Antepartum assessment. In Williams Obstetrics, 24th ed. New York, McGraw-Hill, 2014, Figure 17-4.

   a. There is clear diurnal variation.

   b. They occur randomly during 24 hours.

   c. There is a sharp increase in the early morning hours while the mother sleeps.

   d. B and C

17–7. Concerning contraction stress testing, which of the following is true?

   a. Is positive if late decelerations follow at least 40% of contractions.

   b. Is unsatisfactory if there are fewer than three contractions in 10 minutes.

   c. If done with oxytocin, uses a dilute intravenous infusion initiated at 1 mU/min.

   d. Is reactive if two fetal heart rate accelerations are noted in 10 minutes.

17–8. Using nipple stimulation for contraction stress testing has which of the following advantages?

   a. No side effects

   b. Shorter duration of testing time

   c. Cheaper than oxytocin contraction stress testing

   d. B and C

17–9. The type of breathing displayed below has been called which of the following?

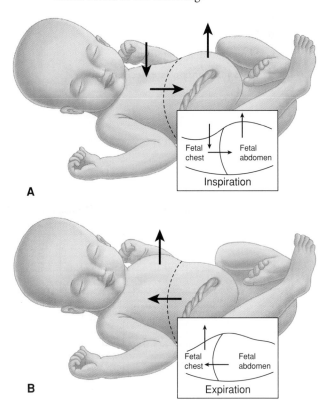

Reproduced with permission from Cunningham FG, Leveno KJ, Bloom SL, et al (eds): Antepartum assessment. In Williams Obstetrics, 24th ed. New York, McGraw-Hill, 2014, Figure 17-3.

   a. Anatomical

   b. Paradoxical

   c. Diaphragmatic

   d. Late term fetal breathing

17–10. Which of the following describes the fetal heart rate tracing in panel A?

    a. Has good variability

    b. Has a baseline of 150

    c. Shows good accelerations

    d. Does not contain late decelerations

17–12. In one study at Parkland Hospital, when accelerations were absent for 80 minutes on a continuous fetal heart rate tracing, which finding(s) had a > 50 percent prevalence?

    a. Fetal acidemia

    b. Oligohydramnios

    c. Fetal-growth restriction

    d. B and C

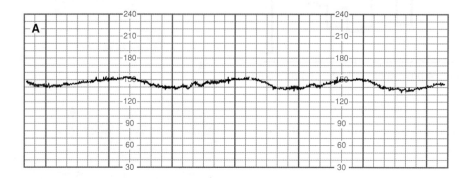

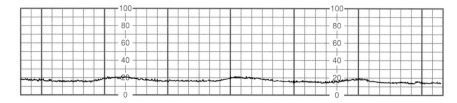

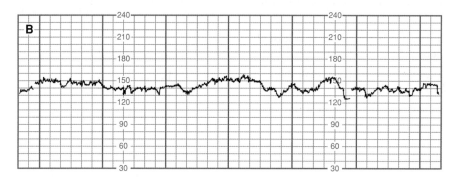

Reproduced with permission from Cunningham FG, Leveno KJ, Bloom SL, et al (eds): Antepartum assessment. In Williams Obstetrics, 24th ed. New York, McGraw-Hill, 2014, Figure 17-8.

17–11. A "terminal cardiotocogram" includes which of the following?

    a. Occasional accelerations

    b. Spontaneous decelerations

    c. Late decelerations with spontaneous contractions

    d. Baseline oscillation greater than 5 beats per minute

17–13. Biophysical profiles are composed of all **EXCEPT** which of the following?

    a. Fetal tone

    b. Fetal breathing

    c. Contraction stress test

    d. Amnionic fluid volume measurement

17–14. This graphic illustrates which of the following concepts regarding the biophysical profile?

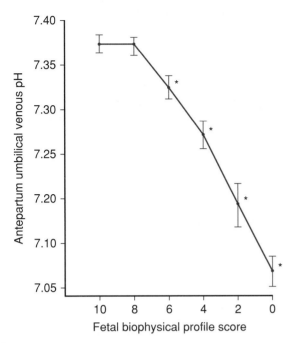

Reproduced with permission from Cunningham FG, Leveno KJ, Bloom SL, et al (eds): Antepartum assessment. In Williams Obstetrics, 24th ed. New York, McGraw-Hill, 2014, Figure 17-9.

a. Score of 2/10 is associated with acidemia.

b. Score of 6/10 is indication to proceed with delivery.

c. Score of 4/10 is similar to 6/10 in regard to umbilical venous pH.

d. Score of 8/10 is associated with an umbilical venous pH ≤ 7.30.

17–15. Which of the following is true of a modified biophysical profile?

a. Is superior to other forms of fetal surveillance

b. Combines nonstress testing (NST) with fetal breathing assessment

c. Is normal if the amnionic fluid index (AFI) = 5.1 cm and NST is reactive

d. Has a false-negative rate of 4.8 per 1000 and a false-positive rate of 1.5%

17–16. Which of the following statements is true regarding the modified biophysical profile?

a. It is associated with a false-negative rate of 4.8 per 1000.

b. It is associated with a false-positive rate of 1.5 per 1000.

c. The American College of Obstetricians and Gynecologists agrees that it is as good as any other fetal test of well-being.

d. None of the above

17–17. Which of the following is true of Doppler velocimetry, as applied to fetal surveillance?

a. Characterizes downstream impedance

b. Is superior to other modes of fetal surveillance

c. Focuses primarily on the systolic waveform of blood flow

d. Is recommended by the American College of Obstetricians and Gynecologists in the presence of other abnormal fetal tests

17–18. Of these three umbilical artery velocimetry waveforms, which is normal?

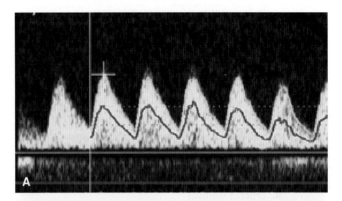

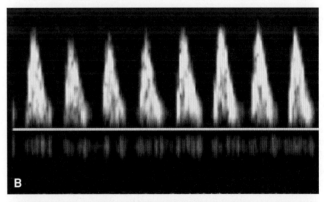

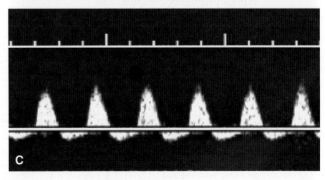

Reproduced with permission from Cunningham FG, Leveno KJ, Bloom SL, et al (eds): Fetal imaging. In Williams Obstetrics, 24th ed. New York, McGraw-Hill, 2014, Figure 10-39.

a. A

b. B

c. C

d. None of the above

17–19. In the image in Question 17-18, which waveform demonstrates reversed end-diastolic flow?

   a. A

   b. B

   c. C

   d. None of the above

17–20. Concerning middle cerebral artery Doppler velocimetry, which of the following is true?

   a. It is useful for detection and management of fetal anemia of any cause.

   b. It is superior to the modified biophysical profile in forecasting pregnancy outcomes.

   c. In those with brain sparing, decreased blood flow from reduced cerebrovascular impedance is detected.

   d. It was found to be inferior to amniocentesis and amnionic fluid spectral analysis for predicting fetal anemia.

17–21. Doppler interrogation of which of the following is the best predictor of perinatal outcome at 26 to 33 weeks' gestation in growth-restricted fetuses?

   a. Ductus venosus

   b. Uterine artery

   c. Umbilical artery

   d. Middle cerebral artery

17–22. Concerning uterine artery Doppler velocimetry, which of the following is true?

   a. Vascular resistance decreases in the first half of pregnancy.

   b. Low-resistance patterns are associated with preeclampsia.

   c. Low-resistance patterns have been linked to various pregnancy complications.

   d. It is not helpful in assessing pregnancies at high risk due to uteroplacental insufficiency.

17–23. Concerning antenatal fetal testing, which of the following is true?

   a. It is clearly beneficial.

   b. It should be considered experimental.

   c. The American College of Obstetricians and Gynecologists recommends contraction stress testing as the best test to evaluate fetal well-being.

   d. Despite its widespread use, the nonstress test is inferior to uterine artery Doppler velocimetry at predicting marginally poor cognitive outcomes.

17–24. During acoustic stimulation testing, which fetal response is measured?

   a. Breathing

   b. Heart rate

   c. Eye movement

   d. Body movement

17–25. What controls fetal heart rate accelerations?

   a. Aortic baroreceptor reflexes

   b. Carotid baroreceptor reflexes

   c. Autonomic function at the brainstem level

   d. Humoral factors such as atrial natriuretic peptide

17–26. Your patient is a 24-year-old G1P0 at 33 weeks' gestation who comes to Labor and Delivery obtunded with the following fetal hear rate tracing. After obtaining intravenous access and ordering laboratory tests, you obtain the following initial results: glucose 400 mg/dL, hematocrit 28 volume percent. Which of the following best explains this tracing?

   a. Abruption

   b. Fetal immaturity

   c. Maternal acidosis

   d. Sinusoidal pattern from fetal anemia

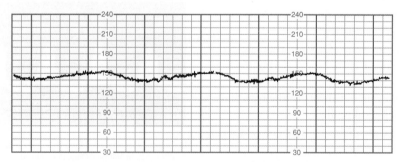
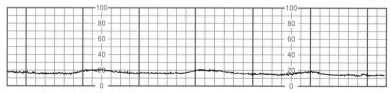

Reproduced with permission from Cunningham FG, Leveno KJ, Bloom SL, et al (eds): Antepartum assessment. In Williams Obstetrics, 24th ed. New York, McGraw-Hill, 2014, Figure 17-8A.

17–27. What should your clinical response be to these findings?

   a. Initiate management of diabetic ketoacidosis

   b. Transfuse packed red blood cells for maternal anemia

   c. Induce labor for nonreassuring fetal heart rate tracing

   d. Perform cesarean delivery for nonreassuring fetal heart rate tracing

17–28. Your patient is a 23-year-old African American woman at 27 weeks' gestation. Sonographic evaluation reveals no structural abnormalities, normal amnionic fluid index, and an estimated fetal weight measuring below the 3rd centile. During umbilical artery Doppler interrogation, the following waveform is obtained. What pattern is displayed here?

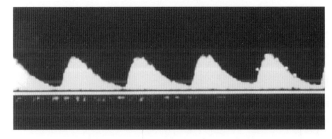

Reproduced with permission from Cunningham FG, Leveno KJ, Bloom SL, et al (eds): Antepartum assessment. In Williams Obstetrics, 23rd ed. New York, McGraw-Hill, 2010, Figure 15-11B.

   a. Absent end-diastolic flow

   b. Reversed end-diastolic flow

   c. Elevated systolic/diastolic (S/D) ratio

   d. None of the above

17–29. For the patient in Question 17-28, a nonstress test is obtained. It demonstrates 10 × 10 beat-per-minute accelerations and minimal variability. Your next best step is which of the following?

   a. Emergency cesarean delivery

   b. Neuroprophylaxis with magnesium sulfate

   c. Ward rest with fetal surveillance that includes at least weekly umbilical artery Doppler evaluations

   d. None of the above

17–30. The following week, umbilical artery Doppler studies appear as shown here for the patient in Question 17-28. The nonstress test now has no variability and no accelerations. The best course of action is which of the following?

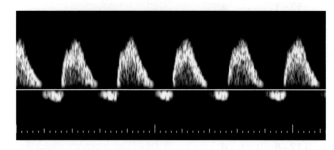

Reproduced with permission from Cunningham FG, Leveno KJ, Bloom SL, et al (eds): Antepartum assessment. In Williams Obstetrics, 23rd ed. New York, McGraw-Hill, 2010, Figure 15-11C.

   a. Move toward delivery

   b. Continue ward rest with intensified surveillance

   c. Neuroprophylaxis with magnesium sulfate and corticosteroids for fetal maturity if not previously given

   d. B and C

17–31. The risk of fetal death with elevated resistance in uterine artery Doppler studies is increased when associated with all **EXCEPT** which of the following?

   a. Preeclampsia

   b. Placental abruption

   c. Chronic hypertension

   d. Fetal-growth restriction

17–32. The most important consideration when deciding to begin antepartum fetal testing is which of the following?

   a. Age of fetus

   b. Severity of maternal condition

   c. Prognosis for neonatal survival

   d. Associated complication, such preeclampsia or fetal-growth restriction

17–33. Which of the following statements is true regarding antepartum fetal testing?

   a. Has evolved continually, exposing an inability to find a "best" test

   b. Definitely associated with decreased incidence of cerebral palsy

   c. Has been used to forecast fetal "wellness" rather than fetal "illness"

   d. A and C

CHAPTER 17 ANSWER KEY

Question number	Letter answer	Page cited	Header cited
17–1	a	p. 335	Introduction
17–2	b	p. 335	Introduction
17–3	b	p. 335	Fetal Movements
17–4	b	p. 336	Clinical Application
17–5	c	p. 335	Fetal Movements
17–6	d	p. 337	Fetal Breathing
17–7	b	p. 338	Contraction Stress Testing
17–8	d	p. 338	Contraction Stress Testing
17–9	b	p. 337	Fetal Breathing
17–10	b	p. 340	Abnormal Nonstress Tests
17–11	c	p. 340	Abnormal Nonstress Tests
17–12	d	p. 340	Abnormal Nonstress Tests
17–13	c	p. 341	Biophysical Profile
17–14	a	p. 341	Biophysical Profile
17–15	c	p. 341	Biophysical Profile
17–16	c	p. 343	Modified Biophysical Profile
17–17	a	p. 344	Umbilical Artery Velocimetry
17–18	a	p. 344	Umbilical Artery Velocimetry
17–19	c	p. 344	Umbilical Artery Velocimetry
17–20	a	p. 344	Middle Cerebral Artery
17–21	a	p. 345	Ductus Venosus
17–22	a	p. 345	Uterine Artery
17–23	b	p. 345	Significance of Fetal Testing
17–24	b	p. 341	Acoustic Stimulation Tests
17–25	c	p. 339	Fetal Heart Rate Acceleration
17–26	c	p. 340	Abnormal Nonstress Tests
17–27	a	p. 340	Abnormal Nonstress Tests
17–28	a	p. 344	Umbilical Artery Velocimetry
17–29	c	p. 339	Fetal Heart Rate Acceleration
17–30	d	p. 344	Umbilical Artery Velocimetry
17–31	c	p. 345	Uterine Artery
17–32	c	p. 345	Current Antenatal Testing Recommendations
17–33	d	p. 345	Significance of Fetal Testing

EARLY PREGNANCY COMPLICATIONS

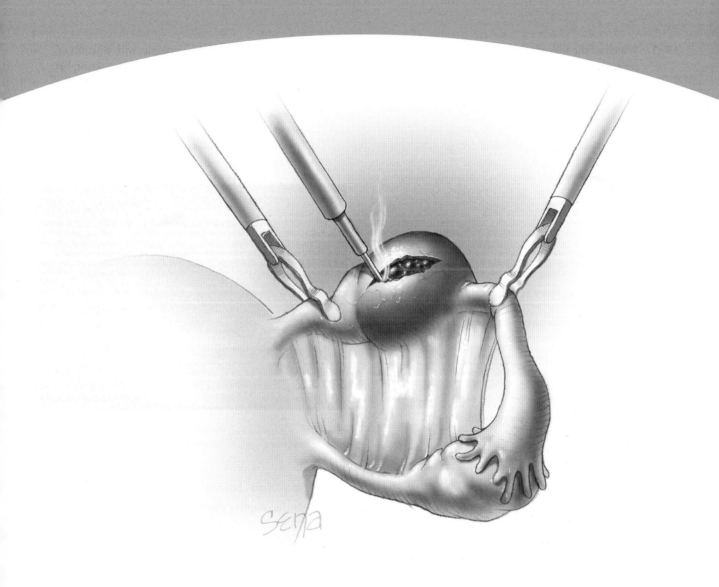

CHAPTER 18

Abortion

18–1. Which of the following gestational ages and weights are typically used to define abortion?

    a. Less than 12 weeks, less than 100 g

    b. Less than 12 weeks, less than 250 g

    c. Less than 16 weeks, less than 500 g

    d. Less than 20 weeks, less than 500 g

18–2. Approximately what percentage of spontaneous miscarriages occur in the first 12 weeks of pregnancy?

    a. 20%

    b. 40%

    c. 60%

    d. 80%

18–3. Which of the following is the most common cause of first-trimester pregnancy loss?

    a. Uterine anomalies

    b. Incompetent cervix

    c. Intrauterine infection

    d. Fetal chromosomal abnormalities

18–4. Which of the following factors is least likely to be linked with higher first-trimester miscarriage rates?

    a. Obesity

    b. Diabetes mellitus

    c. Parvovirus infection

    d. Maternal age older than 40 years

18–5. A 24-year-old G3P0A2 presents with 8 weeks of amenorrhea and vaginal bleeding. Her serum beta human chorionic gonadotropin (β-hCG) level is 68,000 mIU/mL, and her internal cervical os is closed. The sonographic uterine findings are shown below, and fetal heart motion is noted. Normal adnexal anatomy is seen. Your diagnosis is which of the following?

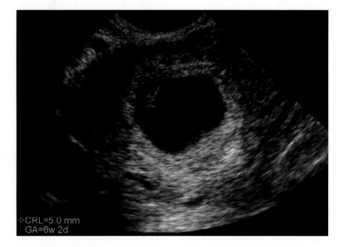

Reproduced with permission from Werner CL, Moschos E, Griffith WF, et al (eds): Abortion. In Williams Gynecology, 2nd Edition Study Guide. New York, McGraw-Hill, 2012, Q6–10.

    a. Missed abortion

    b. Incomplete abortion

    c. Threatened abortion

    d. Inevitable abortion

18–6. Effective prevention of miscarriage in women with threatened abortion includes which of the following?

    a. Bed rest

    b. McDonald cerclage

    c. Human chorionic gonadotropin injection

    d. None of the above

18–7. Anti-D immunoglobulin should be considered for Rh-negative women in which of the following settings?

    a. Threatened abortion

    b. Following complete hydatidiform mole evacuation

    c. After first-trimester elective pregnancy termination

    d. All of the above

18–8. The same patient in Question 18–5 represents 2 weeks later with light bleeding and strong, painful cramps. Her blood pressure is 132/78, pulse is 72, and she is afebrile. Her cervical os is closed, and hematocrit is 40 volume percent. Transvaginal sonography reveals the sagittal uterine image below. Appropriate management includes which of the following?

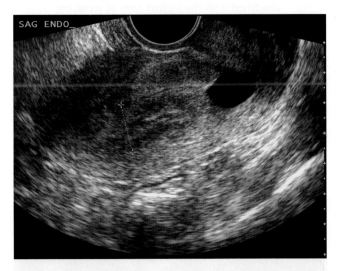

SAG ENDO_

Reproduced with permission from Werner CL, Moschos E, Griffith WF, et al (eds): Abortion. In Williams Gynecology, 2nd Edition Study Guide. New York, McGraw-Hill, 2012, Q6–11.

    a. Perform rescue cerclage

    b. Await spontaneous miscarriage

    c. Excision of cesarean scar pregnancy

    d. Administer intramuscular injection of methotrexate

18–9. While in your emergency department, the patient in Question 18–8 passes tissue, shown here in a cup filled with formalin. Her bleeding and pain have now subsided significantly. Her cervical os is closed. Your diagnosis is which of the following?

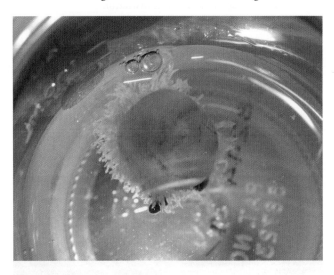

Used with permission from Dr. Heather Lytle.

    a. Missed abortion

    b. Complete abortion

    c. Threatened abortion

    d. None of the above

18–10. Appropriate management of the patient from Question 18–9 now includes which of the following?

    a. Diagnostic laparoscopy

    b. Transvaginal sonography

    c. Dilatation and curettage

    d. Administration of Rho [D] immunoglobulin, if the patient is Rh negative

18–11. An 18-year-old G1P0 presents with 12 weeks of amenorrhea and heavy vaginal bleeding. Her urine pregnancy test is positive. Tissue with the appearance of placenta is seen through an open cervical os. Your diagnosis and management plan include which of the following?

    a. Threatened abortion, plan bed rest

    b. Incomplete abortion, plan dilatation and curettage

    c. Ectopic tubal pregnancy, plan laparoscopic resection

    d. Complete abortion, plan subsequent β-hCG testing in 48 hours

18–12. Incomplete abortion may be treated successfully with which of the following?

　　a. Observation

　　b. Dilatation and curettage

　　c. Prostaglandin E_1 administration

　　d. All of the above

18–13. A 40-year-old G3P2 presents with 10 weeks of amenorrhea. Her serum β-hCG level is 25,000 mIU/mL, and her internal cervical os is closed. The following uterine sonographic findings are noted, and the anechoic intrauterine area measures 40 mm. Normal adnexal anatomy is seen. Your diagnosis is which of the following?

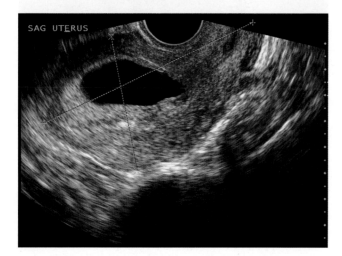

　　a. Missed abortion

　　b. Complete abortion

　　c. Threatened abortion

　　d. Complete hydatidiform mole

18–14. Missed abortion may be treated successfully with which of the following?

　　a. Observation

　　b. Dilatation and curettage

　　c. Prostaglandin E_1 administration

　　d. All of the above

18–15. Your patient with a pregnancy at 16 weeks' gestation presents with fever (38.5°C) and lower abdominal pain, but without bleeding. She describes a small leakage of vaginal fluid yesterday. Appropriate primary management includes intravenous antibiotics and which of the following?

　　a. Labor induction

　　b. Bed rest and observation

　　c. Tocolytic administration

　　d. Hysterotomy and evacuation

18–16. For the treatment of septic abortion, which of the following antibiotic coverages is most suitable?

　　a. Gram-positive

　　b. Gram-negative

　　c. Broad-spectrum

　　d. Anaerobic, gram-positive

18–17. With recurrent abortion, which of the following is a commonly found parental chromosomal abnormality?

　　a. X chromosome mosaicism

　　b. Robertsonian translocations

　　c. Balanced reciprocal translocations

　　d. All of the above

18–18. As shown in this 3-dimensional sonogram, which of the following müllerian anomalies has been associated with the highest rates of recurrent miscarriage?

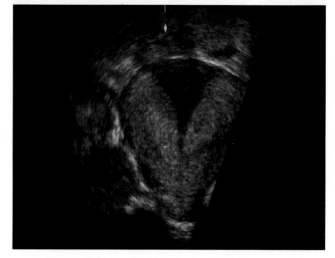

　　a. Septate uterus

　　b. Arcuate uterus

　　c. Uterine didelphys

　　d. Longitudinal vaginal septum

18–19. Which of the following tests would be the most effective in identifying an underlying cause of recurrent miscarriage?

　　a. Antithrombin III assay

　　b. Serum progesterone level

　　c. Lupus anticoagulant assay

　　d. Luteinizing hormone assay

18–20. All **EXCEPT** which of the following statements is true regarding cervical incompetence?

  a. Prior cervical conization is a risk factor.

  b. It is characterized by painless, second-trimester cervical dilatation.

  c. Rupture of membranes is not a contraindication to rescue cerclage placement.

  d. It may be suspected sonographically by membranes funneling past the internal os and shortening of the cervix to <25 mm.

18–21. Which of the following statements is true regarding cerclage?

  a. The Shirodkar procedure is most often selected.

  b. Broad-spectrum antibiotic prophylaxis is required.

  c. It is ideally performed at 10 to 12 weeks' gestation.

  d. Prolapsing membranes may be reduced with Trendelenburg positioning and bladder filling prior to cerclage placement.

18–22. Your patient underwent McDonald cerclage placement 3 days ago at 13 weeks' gestation and presents with complaints of strong cramps. Her temperature is 38.6°C, pulse 118, and blood pressure 98/66. Speculum examination reveals no pooling fluid, and her cerclage is in place. Her uterus is tender, and fetal heart rate is 160 beats per minute. Laboratory and physical examination exclude urinary, respiratory, or gastrointestinal sources of fever. In addition to broad-spectrum antibiotics, antipyretics, and intravenous fluids, how is this patient best managed?

  a. Bed rest

  b. Tocolysis

  c. Hysterotomy for uterine evacuation

  d. Cerclage removal and uterine evacuation

18–23. Which of the following may lower complications associated with dilatation and curettage?

  a. Perioperative oral antibiotics

  b. Preoperative cervical laminaria

  c. Preoperative bimanual examination

  d. All of the above

18–24. You place several laminaria in preparation for pregnancy termination at 16 week' gestation. An example is seen on the left, below. The next day your patient chooses NOT to proceed with the abortion. You remove the swollen laminaria (one example is on the right, below) and counsel her which of the following?

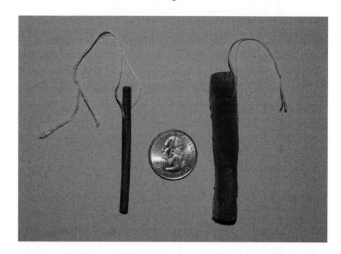

Reproduced with permission from Word L, Hoffman BL. Surgeries for benign gynecologic disorders. In Hoffman BL, Schorge JO, Schaffer JI, et al (eds): Williams Gynecology, 2nd ed. New York, McGraw-Hill, 2012, Figure 41-16.1.

  a. Observation is recommended.

  b. Abortion will spontaneously occur in most cases.

  c. Oral antimicrobials are required to prevent infection.

  d. Cerclage placement is required to sustain the pregnancy.

18–25. During D&C, if the uterine fundus is perforated with one of the instruments shown here, which of the following is the most appropriate primary management?

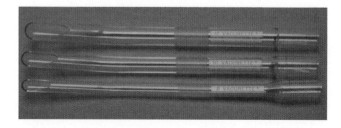

Reproduced with permission from Hoffman BL: Surgeries for benign gynecologic conditions. In Schorge JO, Schaffer JI, Halvorson LM, et al (eds): Williams Gynecology. New York, McGraw-Hill, 2008, Figure 41-17.3.

  a. Observation

  b. Hysterectomy

  c. Abdominal exploration

  d. Uterine artery embolization

18–26. Effective and safe combinations used for pregnancy termination include all **EXCEPT** which of the following?

    a. Misoprostol alone

    b. Mifepristone and misoprostol

    c. Methotrexate and misoprostol

    d. Mifepristone and methotrexate

18–27. The American College of Obstetricians and Gynecologists supports outpatient medical abortion as an acceptable alternative to surgical abortion for pregnancies below what menstrual age threshold?

    a. 5 weeks

    b. 7 weeks

    c. 9 weeks

    d. 11 weeks

18–28. In most cases of elective pregnancy termination, all **EXCEPT** which of the following is true regarding medical regimens compared with surgical techniques?

    a. Avoids anesthesia

    b. Requires one visit

    c. Comparable success rate

    d. Avoids invasive procedure

18–29. All **EXCEPT** which of the following are contraindications to medical abortion?

    a. Anticoagulant use

    b. Type 2 diabetes mellitus

    c. In situ intrauterine device

    d. Concurrent glucocorticoid use

18–30. Accepted options for second-trimester abortion include which of the following?

    a. Intravenous oxytocin

    b. Dilatation and evacuation

    c. Intravaginal prostaglandin E_2

    d. All of the above

18–31. A common side effect of prostaglandin E_2 includes which of the following?

    a. Fever

    b. Dysuria

    c. Arthralgias

    d. Somnolence

18–32. Postoperatively, elective abortion is associated with subsequent increased rates of which of the following?

    a. Infertility

    b. Mental illness

    c. Ectopic pregnancy

    d. None of the above

CHAPTER 18 ANSWER KEY

Question number	Letter answer	Page cited	Header cited
18–1	d	p. 350	Nomenclature
18–2	d	p. 351	Pathogenesis
18–3	d	p. 351	Figure 18-1
18–4	c	p. 352	Maternal Factors
18–5	c	p. 354	Threatened Abortion
18–6	d	p. 355	Management
18–7	d	p. 355	Anti-D Immunoglobulin
18–8	b	p. 356	Complete Abortion
18–9	b	p. 356	Complete Abortion
18–10	d	p. 356	Complete Abortion
18–11	b	p. 356	Incomplete Abortion
18–12	d	p. 356	Incomplete Abortion
18–13	a	p. 356	Missed Abortion
18–14	d	p. 357	Table 18-3
18–15	a	p. 356	Septic Abortion
18–16	c	p. 356	Septic Abortion
18–17	d	p. 358	Parental Chromosomal Abnormalities
18–18	a	p. 359	Table 18-5
18–19	c	p. 359	Immunological Factors
18–20	c	p. 360	Cervical Insufficiency
18–21	d	p. 361	Evaluation and Treatment; Cerclage Procedures
18–22	d	p. 363	Complications
18–23	d	p. 364	Techniques for Abortion
18–24	a	p. 365	Cervical Preparation
18–25	c	p. 367	Complications
18–26	d	p. 369	Table 18-9
18–27	b	p. 368	Medical Abortion
18–28	b	p. 368	Medical Abortion
18–29	b	p. 368	Contraindications
18–30	d	p. 369	Table 18-10
18–31	a	p. 370	Prostaglandins E_2 (PGE$_2$) and E_1 (PGE$_1$)
18–32	d	p. 370	Health and Future Pregnancies

CHAPTER 19

Ectopic Pregnancy

19–1. Which of the following most accurately defines ectopic pregnancy?

    a. Composed solely of cytotrophoblast

    b. Implantation within the fallopian tube

    c. Implantation outside the uterine cavity

    d. Abnormally rising maternal serum β-human chorionic gonadotropin (β-hCG) level

19–2. As shown here, what is the most common site of tubal pregnancy implantation?

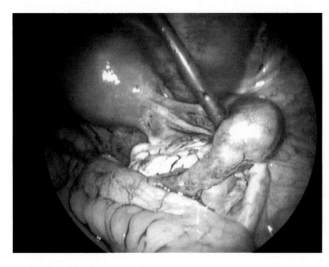

Used with permission from Dr. Kevin Doody. Reproduced with permission from Werner CL, Moschos E, Griffith WF (eds): Williams Gynecology, 2nd ed. Study Guide. New York, McGraw-Hill, 2012, p 39.

    a. Cornua

    b. Fimbria

    c. Isthmus

    d. Ampulla

19–3. Which of the following defines heterotopic pregnancy?

    a. One tubal and one abdominal pregnancy

    b. One ectopic and one intrauterine pregnancy

    c. Two pregnancies, one in each fallopian tube

    d. Two ectopic pregnancies in one fallopian tube

19–4. Which of the following is least likely to increase the risk for ectopic pregnancy?

    a. Prior pelvic infection

    b. Prior hydatidiform mole

    c. Prior ectopic pregnancy

    d. Salpingitis isthmica nodosum

19–5. With contraceptive failure, which method has a relative increased risk of ectopic pregnancy?

    a. Condoms

    b. Vasectomy

    c. Tubal sterilization

    d. All of the above

19–6. Which of the following clinical outcomes of tubal pregnancy is has the lowest potential for maternal morbidity?

    a. Tubal rupture

    b. Tubal abortion

    c. Chronic persistence

    d. Pregnancy resorption

19–7. Your patient is a 21-year-old nulligravida currently desiring pregnancy and attempting conception. Her last menstrual period was 6 weeks ago. She presents with complaints of vaginal spotting and right lower quadrant pain. She also provides you with tissue she passed just prior to coming to the emergency department. Without histological evaluation, what clinical term best describes this tissue that is shown in photograph A and opened in B?

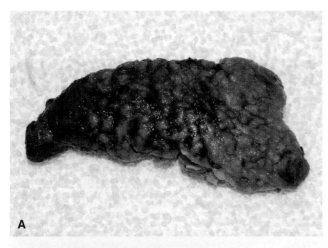

A

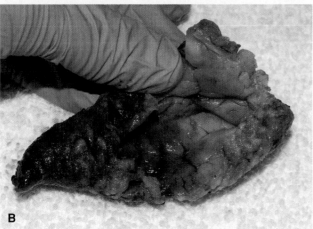

B

a. Decidual cast

b. Blighted ovum

c. Molar pregnancy

d. Products of conception

19–8. Regarding the patient in Question 19-7, her abdomen is soft and nontender. The cervical os is closed, scant blood is seen in the vagina, and uterine size approximates that of a lemon. What is the next best clinical step?

a. Obtain urine β-hCG assay

b. Perform transvaginal sonography

c. Perform dilatation and curettage

d. Discharge her home after assessing hematocrit and Rh status

19–9. For the patient from Question 19-7, her urine β-hCG assay is positive, vital signs are normal, hematocrit is 36 volume percent, and blood type is O negative. What is the next best clinical step?

a. Perform transvaginal sonography

b. Administer Rho(D) immunoglobulin

c. Perform dilatation and curettage

d. Discharge home with plans to reevaluate in 48 hours

19–10. For the patient from Question 19-7, during transvaginal sonographic examination, uterine images are obtained. In general, which of the following sagittal uterine images is most suggestive of an intrauterine pregnancy?

   a. A

   b. B

   c. C

   d. Both A and B

19–12. For the patient from Question 19-7, during her sonographic examination, in addition to the trilaminar endometrial lining seen in Figure 19-10C, other findings include normal myometrium, a cul-de-sac without free fluid, and normal adnexa. Her serum β-hCG level is 1400 mIU/mL. What is her diagnosis?

   a. Ectopic pregnancy

   b. Completed abortion

   c. Intrauterine pregnancy

   d. Pregnancy of unknown location

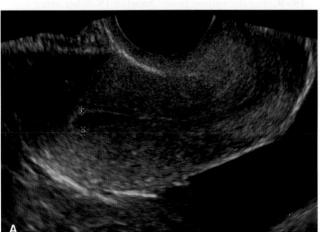

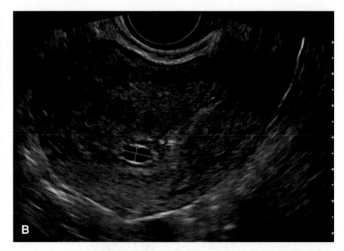

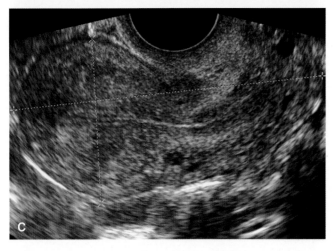

19–11. In Figure 19-10A, the hypoechoic, tear-shaped structure measured by calipers most likely represents which of the following?

   a. Gestational sac

   b. Intradecidual sign

   c. Double decidual sign

   d. Pseudogestational sac

19–13. For the patient from Question 19-7, with this diagnosis, which of the following is an appropriate next clinical step?

   a. Administer methotrexate

   b. Perform diagnostic laparoscopy

   c. Obtain second serum β-hCG level in 48 hours

   d. Discharge her home with follow-up appointment in 2 weeks

19–14. The patient from Question 19-7 returns in 48 hours with minimal right lower quadrant pain. Her vital signs are normal, and spotting has abated. Her clinical and laboratory findings are unchanged except for a serum β-hCG level now measuring 2100 mIU/mL and a progesterone level of 15 ng/mL. What is the next best clinical step for this patient?

   a. Administer methotrexate

   b. Repeat transvaginal sonography

   c. Perform dilatation and curettage

   d. Schedule repeat serum β-hCG level in 48 hours

19–15. For the patient from Question 19-7, her second transvaginal sonographic evaluation reveals a trilaminar endometrial stripe, no cul-de-sac fluid, and normal left adnexa. However, a paraovarian mass is seen on the right. Which of the following sonographic adnexal images would be most diagnostic of ectopic pregnancy?

   a. A

   b. B

   c. C

   d. D

19–16. Of the four images above, which is most commonly seen sonographically at the time ectopic pregnancy is diagnosed?

   a. A

   b. B

   c. C

   d. D

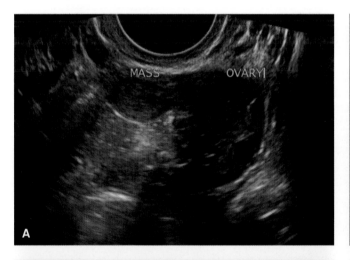

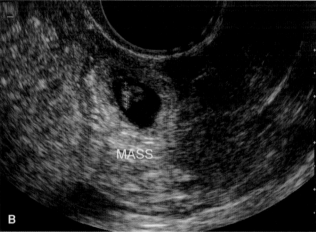

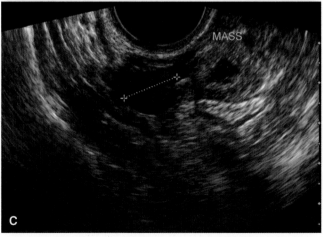

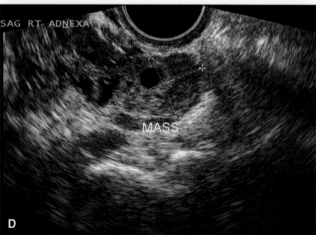

19–17. For the patient from Question 19-7, color Doppler is applied, and the following image is seen. This "ring of fire" may indicate ectopic pregnancy but may also be seen with which of the following?

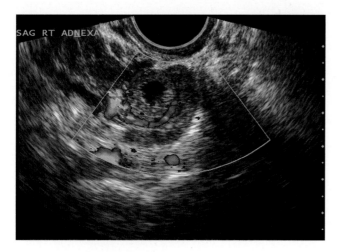

a. Corpus luteum

b. Ovarian endometrioma

c. Ovarian serous cystadenoma

d. Prior Filshie clip application

19–18. For the patient from Question 19-7, her sonographic images are seen below. Which of the following is the next best clinical step?

a. Perform dilatation and curettage

b. Obtain second serum β-hCG level in 48 hours

c. Discuss management of ectopic pregnancy with her

d. Discuss management of completed abortion with her

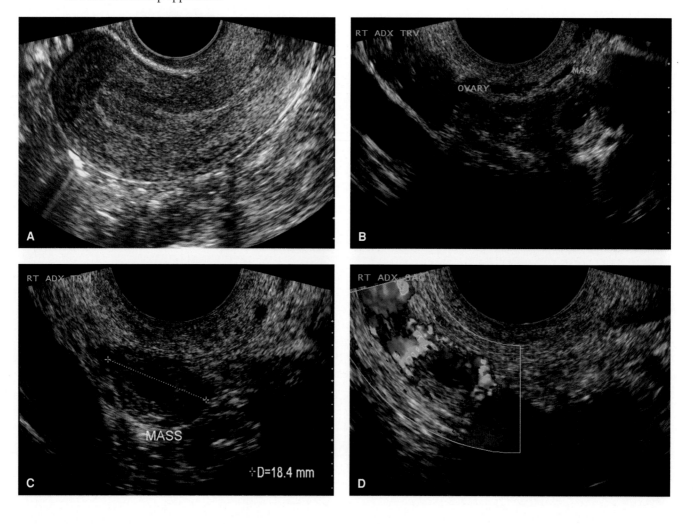

19–19. Which of the following would now be reasonable to offer the patient from Question 19-7.

    a. Salpingectomy

    b. Salpingostomy

    c. Methotrexate administration

    d. All the above

19–20. Contraindications for methotrexate therapy include all **EXCEPT** which of the following?

    a. Breast feeding

    b. Thrombocytopenia

    c. Migraine headache

    d. Intraabdominal hemorrhage

19–21. Which of the following would be most closely associated with methotrexate therapy failure during ectopic pregnancy treatment?

    a. Increased parity

    b. Ectopic size of 2.5 cm

    c. Prior ectopic pregnancy

    d. Serum β-hCG level of 9000 mIU/mL

19–22. Which of the following is **NOT** typically seen as a component of methotrexate embryopathy?

    a. Omphalocele

    b. Skeletal abnormalities

    c. Fetal-growth restriction

    d. Craniofacial abnormalities

19–23. Which of the following should be avoided during methotrexate therapy for ectopic pregnancy treatment?

    a. Folic acid

    b. Vaginal intercourse

    c. Nonsteroidal antiinflammatory drugs

    d. All of the above

19–24. Your patient from Question 19-7 elects to use methotrexate. Which of the following is **NOT** an expected possible complication of methotrexate therapy for ectopic pregnancy?

    a. Stomatitis

    b. Endocarditis

    c. Liver toxicity

    d. Gastroenteritis

19–25. Your patient from Question 19-7 returns on day 4 of methotrexate therapy for β-hCG level surveillance. Her serum β-hCG level is 2300 mIU/mL, and Hct is 35 volume percent. She notes aching right lower quadrant pain without vaginal bleeding. During abdominal and gentle bimanual examination, you note no peritoneal signs and minimal tenderness. Her vital signs are normal. What is the next clinical step for this rising serum β-hCG level?

    a. Plan laparoscopic salpingectomy

    b. Perform dilatation and curettage

    c. Administer second methotrexate dose

    d. Schedule her day 7 serum β-hCG level blood draw

19–26. The patient from Question 19-7 returns on day 7 and her serum β-hCG level is 2500 mIU/mL. Although you counsel her that a second methotrexate dose is an option, she now prefers definitive surgical intervention. In counseling, which of the following is true regarding salpingostomy?

    a. It poses a higher risk of persistent trophoblastic tissue compared with salpingectomy.

    b. Laparotomy is the preferred route due to higher associated subsequent pregnancy rates.

    c. Procedurally, it requires suture closure of the tubal incision with delayed-absorbable suture.

    d. It leads to lower future fertility rates in subsequent pregnancies compared with salpingectomy.

19–27. Persistent trophoblast following surgical treatment of ectopic pregnancy is unlikely if the serum β-hCG level falls by what minimum percentage on postoperative day 1?

    a. 10

    b. 25

    c. 50

    d. 75

SECTION 6

19–28. Criteria that may aid the sonographic diagnosis of interstitial ectopic pregnancy include which of the following?

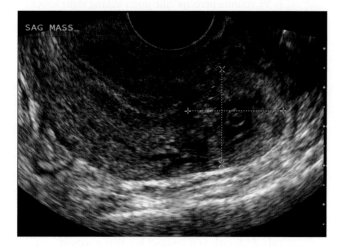

  a. Empty endometrial cavity
  b. Gestational sac separate from the endometrium
  c. Thin myometrial mantle surrounding the gestational sac
  d. All of the above

19–29. As shown in Figure 19-29B, during cornuectomy for interstitial ectopic pregnancy, what is the most compelling reason to resect the ipsilateral fallopian tube?

  a. Lower her ovarian cancer risk
  b. Avoid hydrosalpinx formation in the retained ipsilateral fallopian tube
  c. Avoid ectopic pregnancy in the retained ipsilateral fallopian tube
  d. None of the above

19–30. Sonographic findings that may suggest abdominal pregnancy include which of the following?

  a. Oligohydramnios
  b. Fetus outside and separate from the uterus
  c. Absent myometrium between the fetus and maternal anterior abdominal wall
  d. All of the above

19–31. As shown here, what adjunctive imaging modality may aid the diagnosis of abdominal pregnancy?

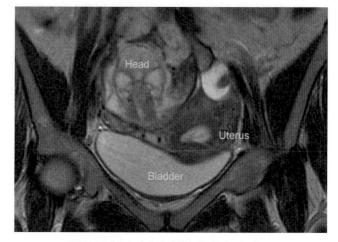

  a. Computed tomography
  b. Magnetic resonance imaging
  c. Saline infusion sonography
  d. 3-dimensional sonography

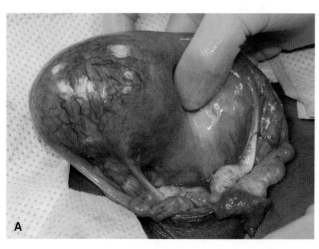

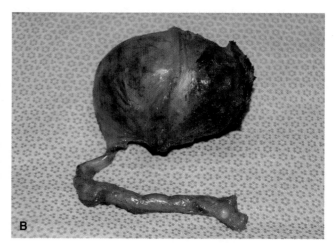

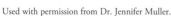
Used with permission from Dr. Jennifer Muller.

19–32. What is the most commonly used approach to treat an abdominal pregnancy at 16 weeks' gestation?

a. Intragestational sac methotrexate

b. Laparotomy with delivery of the fetus

c. Expectant management until fetal viability

d. Uterine artery embolization, then await fetal and placental resorption

19–33. Criteria proposed by Spiegelberg for the diagnosis of ovarian pregnancy include all **EXCEPT** which of the following?

a. The ectopic pregnancy occupies the affected ovary.

b. Trophoblast are seen histologically amid ovarian stroma.

c. The pregnancy is attached to the uterus via the round ligament.

d. An intact ipsilateral fallopian tube is seen distinct from the ovary.

19–34. Which of the following is an appropriate treatment of ovarian ectopic pregnancy?

a. Cystectomy

b. Oophorectomy

c. Ovarian wedge resection

d. All of the above

19–35. As shown by this sonogram image, which of the following is **NOT** a sonographic criterion for cervical pregnancy?

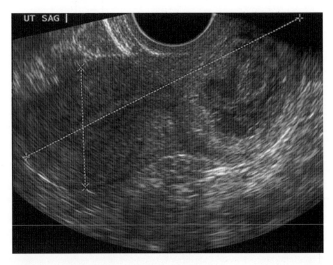

Reproduced with permission from Moschos E, Hoffman BL: Cervical ectopic pregnancy (update). In Cunningham FG, Leveno KL, Bloom SL, et al (eds): Williams Obstetrics, 22nd ed. Online. Accessmedicine.com. New York, McGraw-Hill, 2007, Figure 1.

a. Hourglass uterine shape

b. Ballooned cervical canal

c. Anterior uterine isthmic mass

d. Hyperechoic thin endometrial stripe

19–36. Which of the following most significantly increases the risk of cervical pregnancy?

a. Advanced maternal age

b. In vitro fertilization

c. Increased cesarean delivery rate

d. Increased incidence of cervical neoplasia

19–37. What is the preferred treatment for cervical pregnancy in a hemodynamically stable patient?

a. Methotrexate

b. Hysterectomy

c. Trachelectomy

d. Cerclage followed by dilatation and curettage

19–38. This represents which of the following ectopic pregnancy types?

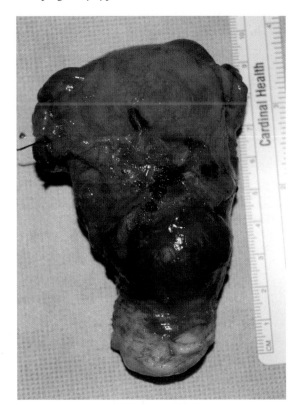

a. Isthmic

b. Cervical

c. Interstitial

d. Cesarean scar

19–39. As shown, which of the following is **NOT** a sonographic criterion for cesarean scar pregnancy?

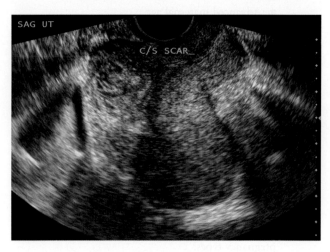

a. Empty cervical canal

b. Hourglass uterine shape

c. Anterior uterine isthmic mass

d. Hyperechoic thin endometrial stripe

19–40. Which of the following may be appropriate treatment of cesarean scar pregnancy in a hemodynamically stable patient?

a. Methotrexate

b. Hysterectomy

c. Anterior uterine isthmus resection

d. All of the above

CHAPTER 19 ANSWER KEY

Question number	Letter answer	Page cited	Header cited
19–1	c	p. 377	Introduction
19–2	d	p. 377	Classification
19–3	b	p. 377	Classification
19–4	b	p. 377	Risks
19–5	c	p. 377	Risks
19–6	d	p. 378	Evolution and Potential Outcomes
19–7	a	p. 379	Clinical Manifestations
19–8	a	p. 381	Beta Human Chorionic Gonadotropin
19–9	a	p. 380	Figure 19-4
19–10	b	p. 382	Endometrial Findings
19–11	d	p. 382	Endometrial Findings
19–12	d	p. 381	Beta Human Chorionic Gonadotropin
19–13	c	p. 381	Levels below the Discriminatory Zone
19–14	b	p. 381	Levels below the Discriminatory Zone
19–15	b	p. 383	Adnexal Findings
19–16	a	p. 383	Adnexal Findings
19–17	a	p. 383	Adnexal Findings
19–18	c	p. 383	Adnexal Findings
19–19	d	p. 384	Treatment Options
19–20	c	p. 384	Table 19-2
19–21	d	p. 385	Patient Selection
19–22	a	p. 384	Regimen Options
19–23	d	p. 384	Regimen Options
19–24	b	p. 385	Treatment Side Effects
19–25	d	p. 385	Monitoring Therapy Efficacy
19–26	a	p. 385	Surgical Management
19–27	c	p. 386	Persistent Trophoblast
19–28	d	p. 387	Interstitial Pregnancy
19–29	c	p. 387	Interstitial Pregnancy
19–30	d	p. 388	Abdominal Pregnancy
19–31	b	p. 388	Abdominal Pregnancy
19–32	b	p. 389	Management
19–33	c	p. 390	Ovarian Pregnancy
19–34	d	p. 390	Ovarian Pregnancy
19–35	c	p. 391	Figure 19-13
19–36	b	p. 390	Cervical Pregnancy
19–37	a	p. 390	Management
19–38	d	p. 391	Cesarean Scar Pregnancy
19–39	b	p. 391	Cesarean Scar Pregnancy
19–40	d	p. 391	Cesarean Scar Pregnancy

CHAPTER 20

Gestational Trophoblastic Disease

20–1. As a group, gestational trophoblastic disease is typified by which of the following?

    a. Scant cytotrophoblast

    b. Perivillous fibrin deposition

    c. Villous mesenchymal hyperplasia

    d. Abnormal trophoblast proliferation

20–2. As illustrated by differences seen here between invasive mole **(A)** and choriocarcinoma **(B)**, hydatidiform moles as a group are differentiated histologically from other nonmolar neoplasms by the presence of which of the following?

    a. Villi

    b. Cytotrophoblast

    c. Syncytiotrophoblast

    d. Marked angiogenesis

20–3. Gestational trophoblastic neoplasia includes all **EXCEPT** which of the following?

    a. Invasive mole

    b. Choriocarcinoma

    c. Partial hydatidiform mole

    d. Placental site trophoblastic tumor

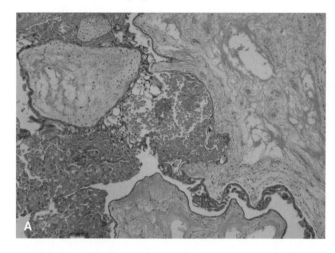
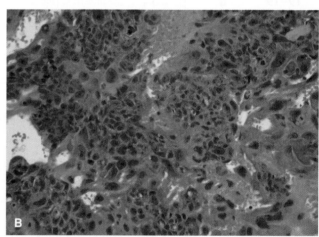

A. Used with permission from Dr. Ona Faye-Peterson. B. Reproduced with permission from Schorge JO: Gestational trophoblastic disease. In Hoffman BL, Schorge JO, Schaffer JI, et al (eds): Williams Gynecology, 2nd ed. New York, McGraw-Hill, 2012, Figure 37-8.

20–4. Which of the following histological changes, as shown here, are characteristic of hydatidiform moles?

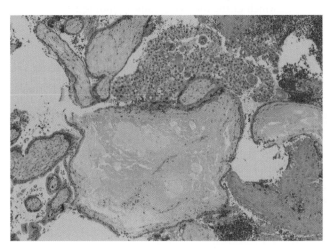

Used with permission from Dr. Y. Erika Fong. Reproduced with permission from Schorge JO: Gestational trophoblastic disease. In Hoffman BL, Schorge JO, Schaffer JI, et al (eds): Williams Gynecology, 2nd ed. New York, McGraw-Hill, 2012, Figure 37-1B.

   a. Chronic villitis and villous inclusion bodies

   b. Villous mesenchymal hyperplasia and acute villitis

   c. Villous lymphocytic infiltrates and syncytial knots

   d. Trophoblast proliferation and villous stromal edema

20–5. A predominant maternal risk factor for molar pregnancy includes which of the following?

   a. Advanced maternal age

   b. Prior cesarean delivery

   c. Type 2 diabetes mellitus

   d. African American ethnicity

20–6. Your patient has completed treatment for a complete hydatidiform mole. Compared with women without a prior molar pregnancy, those with one prior mole have which of the following risks of developing this condition again in a subsequent pregnancy?

   a. 2%

   b. 13%

   c. 26%

   d. 42%

20–7. This molar pregnancy lacked a fetal component. All **EXCEPT** which of the following features are also characteristic of this type of hydatidiform mole?

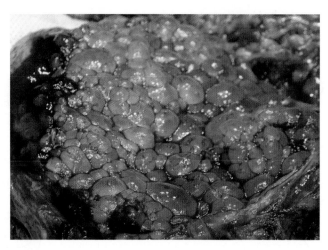

Used with permission from Dr. Sasha Andrews. Reproduced with permission from Schorge JO: Gestational trophoblastic disease. In Hoffman BL, Schorge JO, Schaffer JI, et al (eds): Williams Gynecology, 2nd ed. New York, McGraw-Hill, 2012, Figure 37-3.

   a. Diploid karyotype

   b. Focal villous edema

   c. Theca-lutein ovarian cysts are frequently associated

   d. Approximate 15% risk of subsequent gestational trophoblastic neoplasia

20–8. All **EXCEPT** which of the following features are characteristic of partial hydatidiform mole?

   a. Triploid karyotype

   b. Focal villous edema

   c. Fetal tissue present

   d. Approximate 15% risk of subsequent gestational trophoblastic neoplasia

20–9. With regard to molar pregnancies, what does the term "androgenesis" refer to?

   a. Increased placental androgen production that promotes villous edema

   b. Development of a zygote that contains only maternal chromosomes

   c. Increased placental androgen production that leads to maternal virilization

   d. None of the above

20–10. The pathogenesis of which of the following is shown in this diagram?

   a. Partial mole

   b. Complete mole

   c. Mature cystic teratoma

   d. Complete mole with coexistent twin

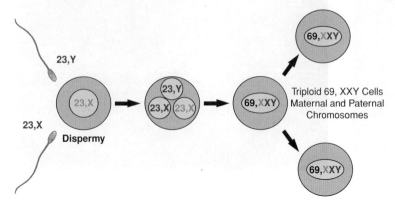

Reproduced with permission from Schorge JO: Gestational trophoblastic disease. In Schorge JO, Schaffer JI, Halvorson LM, et al (eds): Williams Gynecology. New York, McGraw-Hill, 2008, Figure 37-1B.

20–11. Your patient is a 39-year-old G2P1 with one prior uncomplicated pregnancy and vaginal delivery. Her current twin pregnancy is made up of a complete mole and a coexistent karyotypically normal fetus. Magnetic resonance imaging was completed, and one view is presented below. This cross-sectional image shows the complete mole (*asterisk*), a normal placenta above the mole, and a cross section of the normal fetus's abdomen on the left. Complications that may be reasonably anticipated during this pregnancy include all **EXCEPT** which of the following?

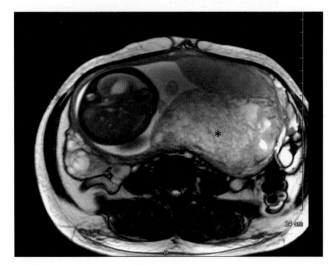

Used with permission from Dr. April Bleich.

   a. Preeclampsia

   b. Fetal demise

   c. Preterm delivery

   d. Placenta accreta

20–12. Patients with complete hydatidiform molar pregnancy frequently present with all **EXCEPT** which of the following clinical findings?

   a. Vaginal bleeding

   b. Multiple simple ovarian cysts

   c. Increased thyroid-stimulating hormone levels

   d. Greater than expected serum β-human chorionic gonadotropin (hCG) levels

20–13. Your patient is diagnosed with a complete hydatidiform mole. Sonographic examination of the adnexa reveals the findings below. The underlying etiology stems from increased placental production of which of the following?

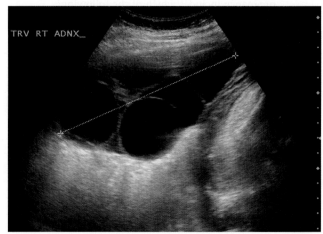

   a. Estrogen

   b. Thyroxine

   c. Progesterone

   d. β-Human chorionic gonadotropin

20–14. The condition shown in Question 20–13 is best managed by which of the following?

   a. Oophoropexy

   b. Oophorectomy

   c. Ovarian cystectomy

   d. Molar pregnancy uterine evacuation

20–15. Increased serum free thyroxine levels in women with hydatidiform moles stem from increases in which of the following?

   a. Maternal estrogen levels

   b. Fetal thyroxine production

   c. Maternal progesterone levels

   d. Maternal β-human chorionic gonadotropin levels

20–16. A 24-year-old G3P2 presents with vaginal bleeding, a β-human chorionic gonadotropin (β-hCG) level of 300,000 mIU/mL, uterine size consistent with a 12-week gestation, B negative blood type, and the sonographic findings below. What is the most appropriate management?

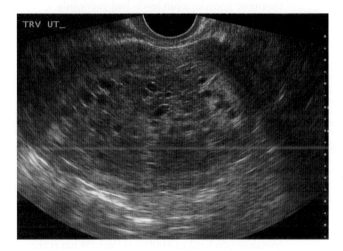

   a. Plan for hysterectomy

   b. Rhogam administration and bed rest

   c. Plan for dilatation and curettage

   d. Repeat a serum β-hCG level in 48 hours

20–17. Prior to surgical intervention for a hydatidiform mole, all **EXCEPT** which of the following are typically completed?

   a. Type and screen

   b. Complete blood count

   c. Chest computed tomography

   d. Serum testing of liver, renal, and thyroid function

20–18. Prior to molar pregnancy evacuation, a preoperative chest radiograph is typically obtained to exclude which of the following associated conditions?

   a. Cardiomegaly

   b. Pleural effusion

   c. Hilar lymphadenopathy

   d. Trophoblastic deportation

20–19. What is the treatment of choice for a 20-week size complete mole in a 28-year-old G2P1?

   a. Hysterectomy

   b. Hysterotomy and evacuation

   c. Dilatation and suction curettage

   d. Intramuscular systemic methotrexate

20–20. Steps during dilatation and curettage that may hasten evacuation and lessen intraoperative blood loss include which of the following?

   a. Preoperative laminaria

   b. Large-bore suction cannula

   c. Uterotonic administration during curettage

   d. All of the above

20–21. Which of the following uterotonics are contraindicated in the setting of molar pregnancy evacuation?

   a. Misoprostol

   b. Synthetic oxytocin

   c. Carboprost tromethamine

   d. None of the above

20–22. In the United States, routine postevacuation treatment of molar pregnancy typically includes which of the following?

   a. Methotrexate chemotherapy

   b. Intrauterine device insertion

   c. Rhogam administration to Rh-negative women

   d. All of the above

20–23. In the United States, a reasonable alternative to dilatation and curettage for the management of complete hydatidiform mole includes which of the following?

   a. Hysterectomy

   b. Hysterotomy and uterine evacuation

   c. Misoprostol labor induction following laminaria placement

   d. All of the above

20–24. Your patient, who is pregnant with an estimated gestational age of 8 weeks by last menstrual period, presents to the emergency department with heavy vaginal bleeding and passage of tissue. Sonographic examination reveals an endometrial cavity filled with blood and tissue exhibiting inhomogeneous echoes. You perform a dilatation and curettage with no complications. A week later, you receive the pathology report for the evacuated products of conception:

> Specimen: uterine contents
> DNA interpretation by image cytometry: diploid
> Immunostaining: p57KIP2 positive

These histological findings are consistent with which of the following diagnoses?

  a. Partial mole
  b. Complete mole
  c. Spontaneous abortion
  d. None of the above

20–25. Which of the statements below are true regarding surveillance practices following evacuation of a molar pregnancy?

  a. Endometrial biopsy and chest radiograph should be performed every 3 months for 1 year.
  b. Endometrial biopsy, chest radiographs, and β-human chorionic gonadotropin levels are obtained serially, but each at different intervals.
  c. Serum β-human chorionic gonadotropin levels should be monitored every 1 to 2 weeks until undetectable, after which monthly levels are drawn for the next 6 months.
  d. None of the above

20–26. Which of the following statements is true regarding contraceptive practices after evacuation of a molar pregnancy?

  a. Intrauterine devices should not be inserted until the β-human chorionic gonadotropin (β-hCG) level is undetectable.
  b. Pregnancies that occur during the monitoring period increase the risk of progression to gestational trophoblastic neoplasia.
  c. Hormonal contraception, such as oral contraceptive pills and injectable medroxyprogesterone acetate, should not be initiated until the β-hCG level is undetectable.
  d. All of the above

20–27. During surveillance, all **EXCEPT** which of the following portend a greater risk for development of gestational trophoblastic neoplasia?

  a. Maternal age > 40 years
  b. 8-cm theca lutein cysts
  c. Rapidly declining β-human chorionic gonadotropin level
  d. β-Human chorionic gonadotropin level > 100,000 mIU/mL prior to uterine evacuation

20–28. Your patient is a 32-year-old G1P0A1 who has undergone molar pregnancy evacuation and is using combination oral contraceptive pills. During postevacuation surveillance, her serum β-human chorionic gonadotropin levels had previously dropped to an undetectable level. Today, as part of her monthly surveillance, her value is 900 mIU/mL. Appropriate initial management includes which of the following?

  a. Preparation for dilatation and curettage
  b. Initiation of intramuscular methotrexate therapy
  c. Repeat β-human chorionic gonadotropin level in 48 hours
  d. International Federation of Gynecology and Obstetrics (FIGO) staging

20–29. The patient from Question 20–28 presents again in 48 hours and has a β-human chorionic gonadotropin level of 6000 mIU/mL. What is the next most appropriate step in her care?

  a. Transvaginal sonography
  b. Preparation for dilatation and curettage
  c. Initiation of intramuscular methotrexate therapy
  d. Chest and abdominopelvic computed tomography (CT) imaging and brain magnetic resonance imaging

20–30. The patient from Question 20–28 undergoes transvaginal sonography, which reveals no intrauterine or adnexal gestation. Appropriate management includes which of the following?

  a. Hysterectomy
  b. Initiation of intravenous dactinomycin therapy
  c. Initiation of intramuscular methotrexate therapy
  d. International Federation of Gynecology and Obstetrics (FIGO) staging

20–31. In practice, the diagnosis of gestational trophoblastic neoplasia typically is determined by which of the following?

  a. Histologic tissue evaluation

  b. Physical examination findings

  c. Computed tomography (CT) imaging

  d. Serum β-human chorionic gonadotropin levels

20–32. Criteria for the diagnosis of gestational trophoblastic neoplasia includes which of the following?

  a. Rising β-human chorionic gonadotropin levels

  b. Plateaued β-human chorionic gonadotropin levels

  c. Persistent β-human chorionic gonadotropin levels

  d. All of the above

20–33. Gestational trophoblastic neoplasia may develop after which of the following?

  a. Evacuation of a partial mole

  b. Delivery of a normal term pregnancy

  c. Miscarriage of a genetically normal abortus

  d. All of the above

20–34. The hallmark sign of gestational trophoblastic neoplasia is which of the following?

  a. Seizures

  b. Hemoptysis

  c. Uterine bleeding

  d. Pelvic vein thrombosis

20–35. Evaluation of abnormal bleeding for more than 6 weeks following any pregnancy may include which of the following?

  a. Transvaginal sonography

  b. Serum β-human chorionic gonadotropin level

  c. Endometrial sampling to exclude placental site trophoblastic tumor or epithelioid trophoblastic tumor

  d. All of the above

20–36. According to the World Health Organization (WHO) modified prognostic scoring system that was adapted by the International Federation of Gynecology and Obstetrics (FIGO), which of the following is assessed and assigned a rating score during staging of gestational trophoblastic neoplasia?

  a. Parity

  b. Severity of thyrotoxicosis

  c. Number of months from the antecedent pregnancy

  d. Presence and diameter of largest theca-lutein cyst

20–37. Following dilatation and curettage for a complete mole, your patient is surveilled with serial β-human chorionic gonadotropin (β-hCG) levels. For the past 3 weeks, the β-hCG values have plateaued. Diagnostic evaluation reveals a metastatic lesion in the liver (shown here). Given this extent of disease, what is the International Federation of Gynecology and Obstetrics (FIGO) stage?

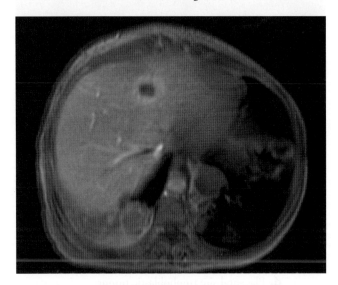

Used with permission from Dr. John Schorge.

  a. Stage I

  b. Stage II

  c. Stage III

  d. Stage IV

20–38. According to the World Health Organization (WHO) modified prognostic scoring system that was adapted by the International Federation of Gynecology and Obstetrics (FIGO), patients with scores below which of the following thresholds are assigned to the low-risk gestational trophoblastic neoplasia group?

  a. ≤ 4

  b. ≤ 6

  c. ≤ 8

  d. ≤ 10

20–39. Which of the following characteristics are most typical of invasive moles?

  a. Follows a term pregnancy

  b. Penetrates deeply into the myometrium

  c. Displays minimal trophoblastic growth

  d. Is almost invariably associated with widespread pulmonary metastasis

20–40. Metastatic disease, such as that shown here, is most commonly due to which of the following?

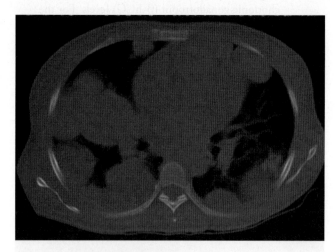

Reproduced with permission from Schorge JO: Gestational trophoblastic disease. In Schorge JO, Schaffer JI, Halvorson LM, et al (eds): Williams Gynecology. New York, McGraw-Hill, 2008, Figure 37-8.

a. Invasive mole

b. Choriocarcinoma

c. Epithelioid trophoblastic tumor

d. Placental site trophoblastic tumor

20–41. Metastatic spread of choriocarcinoma is most commonly by which of the following routes?

a. Lymphatic

b. Hematogenous

c. Peritoneal fluid

d. Cerebrospinal fluid

20–42. What is the most common site of metastatic spread of choriocarcinoma?

a. Brain

b. Liver

c. Lungs

d. Spleen

20–43. Your patient has International Federation of Gynecology and Obstetrics (FIGO) stage I gestational trophoblastic neoplasia. Preferred and effective treatment includes methotrexate or which of the following?

a. Radical hysterectomy

b. Combination chemotherapy

c. External beam pelvic radiation

d. Actinomycin-D single-agent chemotherapy

20–44. Your patient has International Federation of Gynecology and Obstetrics (FIGO) stage III gestational trophoblastic neoplasia. Which of the following is considered typical treatment?

a. Radical hysterectomy

b. Combination chemotherapy

c. Radical hysterectomy plus adjuvant methotrexate

d. External beam pelvic radiation plus adjuvant methotrexate

20–45. Chemotherapeutic agents in the EMA-CO regimen include all **EXCEPT** which of the following?

a. Cisplatin

b. Etoposide

c. Methotrexate

d. Actinomycin-D

20–46. True evidenced-based risks for future pregnancy following treatment of gestational trophoblastic disease include which of the following?

a. Decreased fertility

b. Increased risk of preterm labor

c. Increased risk of placenta accreta

d. Increased risk of a second molar pregnancy

CHAPTER 20 ANSWER KEY

Question number	Letter answer	Page cited	Header cited
20–1	**d**	p. 396	Introduction
20–2	**a**	p. 396	Introduction
20–3	**c**	p. 396	Introduction
20–4	**d**	p. 396	Hydatidiform Mole—Molar Pregnancy
20–5	**a**	p. 396	Epidemiology and Risk Factors
20–6	**a**	p. 397	Epidemiology and Risk Factors
20–7	**b**	p. 397	Table 20-1
20–8	**d**	p. 397	Table 20-1
20–9	**d**	p. 397	Pathogenesis
20–10	**a**	p. 398	Figure 20-2B
20–11	**d**	p. 398	Twin Pregnancy Comprising a Normal Fetus and Coexistent Complete Mole
20–12	**c**	p. 398	Clinical Findings
20–13	**d**	p. 398	Clinical Findings
20–14	**d**	p. 398	Clinical Findings
20–15	**d**	p. 398	Clinical Findings
20–16	**c**	p. 399	Sonography
20–17	**c**	p. 400	Table 20-2
20–18	**d**	p. 400	Termination of Molar Pregnancy
20–19	**c**	p. 400	Termination of Molar Pregnancy
20–20	**d**	p. 400	Termination of Molar Pregnancy
20–21	**d**	p. 400	Table 20-2
20–22	**c**	p. 400	Termination of Molar Pregnancy
20–23	**a**	p. 400	Termination of Molar Pregnancy
20–24	**c**	p. 400	Pathological Diagnosis
20–25	**c**	p. 401	Postevacuation Surveillance
20–26	**a**	p. 401	Postevacuation Surveillance
20–27	**c**	p. 401	Postevacuation Surveillance
20–28	**c**	p. 401	Postevacuation Surveillance
20–29	**a**	p. 401	Postevacuation Surveillance
20–30	**d**	p. 401	Postevacuation Surveillance
20–31	**d**	p. 401	Gestational trophoblastic Neoplasia
20–32	**d**	p. 402	Table 20-3
20–33	**d**	p. 401	Gestational Trophoblastic Neoplasia
20–34	**c**	p. 401	Clinical Findings
20–35	**d**	p. 402	Diagnosis, Staging, and Prognostic Scoring
20–36	**c**	p. 402	Table 20-4
20–37	**d**	p. 402	Table 20-4
20–38	**b**	p. 402	Diagnosis, Staging, and Prognostic Scoring
20–39	**b**	p. 402	Invasive Mole
20–40	**b**	p. 403	Gestational Choriocarcinoma
20–41	**b**	p. 403	Gestational Choriocarcinoma
20–42	**c**	p. 403	Gestational Choriocarcinoma
20–43	**d**	p. 403	Treatment
20–44	**b**	p. 403	Treatment
20–45	**a**	p. 403	Treatment
20–46	**d**	p. 404	Subsequent Pregnancy

LABOR

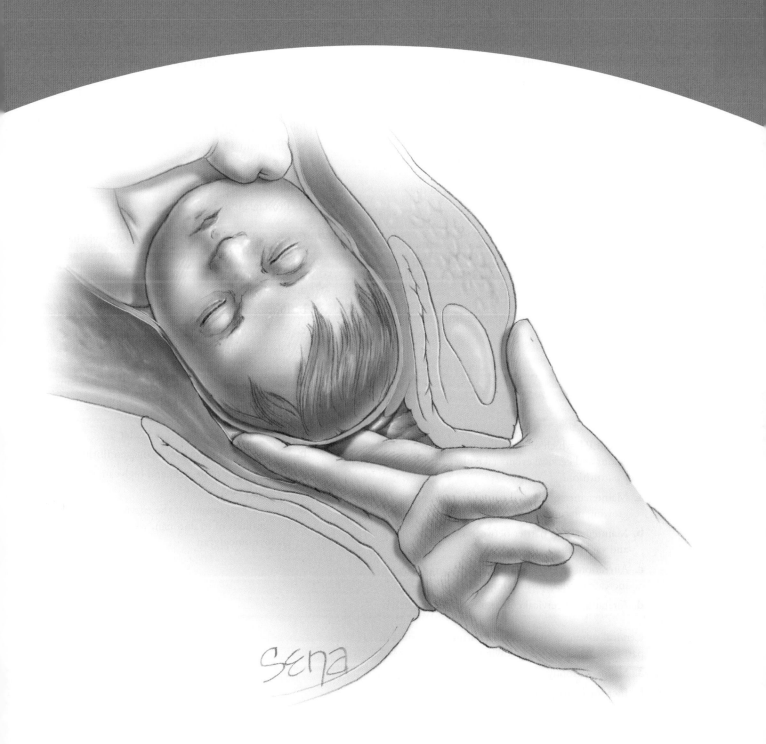

Physiology of Labor

21–1. Of the four phases of parturition, phase 2 is characterized by which of the following?

   a. Uterine activation, cervical ripening

   b. Uterine quiescence, cervical softening

   c. Uterine involution, cervical remodeling

   d. Uterine contraction, cervical dilatation

21–2. Which phase of parturition corresponds to the clinical stages of labor?

   a. Phase 1

   b. Phase 2

   c. Phase 3

   d. Phase 4

21–3. During which of the stages of labor is the fetus delivered?

   a. Stage 1

   b. Stage 2

   c. Stage 3

   d. Stage 4

21–4. All **EXCEPT** which of the following cervical functions and cervical events take place during phase 1 of parturition?

   a. Maintenance of cervical competence despite growing uterine weight

   b. Maintenance of barrier between uterine contents and vaginal bacteria

   c. Alterations in extracellular matrix to gradually increase cervical tissue compliance

   d. Alteration of cervical collagen to stiffen the cervix

21–5. Cervical softening in phase 1 of parturition results in part from which of the following?

   a. Stromal atrophy

   b. Increased stromal vascularity

   c. Increased collagen monomer cross-linking

   d. All of the above

21–6. Contraction-associated proteins (CAPs) within uterine smooth muscle prepare it to contract during labor. CAP concentrations increase during phase 2 of parturition and include all **EXCEPT** which of the following proteins?

   a. Connexin 43

   b. Oxytocin receptor

   c. Progesterone receptor A

   d. Prostaglandin F receptor

21–7. Compared with the uterine body, the cervix has a significantly lower percentage of which of the following?

   a. Collagen

   b. Proteoglycans

   c. Smooth muscle

   d. Glycosaminoglycans

21–8. All **EXCEPT** which of the following mechanisms lead in part to the cervical ripening that is characteristic of phase 2 of parturition?

   a. Decreased collagen fibril diameter

   b. Increased spacing between collagen fibrils

   c. Altered levels of decorin and biglycan, which are proteoglycans

   d. Increased expression of the enzymes responsible for synthesis of hyaluronan, which is a glycosaminoglycan

21–9. Your primigravid patient at 41 weeks' gestation presents for her weekly prenatal care visit with complaints of decreased fetal movement. Clinically, you are unable to ballot the fetal head, and the amnionic fluid index reflects oligohydramnios. Her Bishop score is only 4. The vaginal insert shown here is one of which class of agents used clinically to effect cervical ripening?

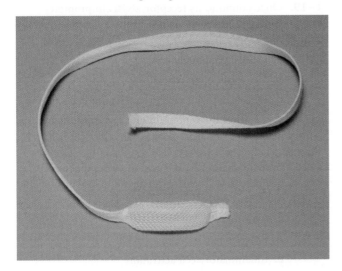

a. Oxytocin

b. Beta mimetics

c. Prostaglandins

d. Nonsteroidal antiinflammatory drugs

21–10. Which of the following are considered plausible causes of uterine contraction pain?

a. Myometrial hypoxia

b. Uterine peritoneum stretching

c. Compression of nerve ganglia in the cervix

d. All of the above

21–11. Which of the following best defines the Ferguson reflex?

a. Mechanical stretch of the cervix enhances uterine activity

b. Maternal ambulation augments contraction intensity and frequency

c. Fetal scalp stimulation leads to fetal heart rate acceleration

d. Maternal shifting to the left lateral recumbent position increases venous return

21–12. During cesarean delivery, the hysterotomy incision is ideally made in the lower uterine segment, shown here prior to bladder flap creation. Which of the following aids development of this uterine segment during phase 3 of parturition?

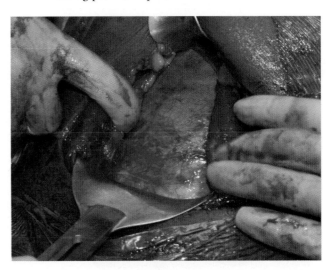

a. Progressive thickening of the upper uterine segment with labor progression

b. Smooth muscle fibers of the fundus relax to their original length after each contraction

c. Smooth muscle cell fibers of the lower uterine segment relax to their original length after each contraction

d. All of the above

21–13. Extreme development of both upper and lower uterine segments may be seen with obstructed labor and clinically may be reflected by which of the following?

a. Hegar sign

b. Bandl ring

c. Bloody show

d. Chadwick sign

21–14. As a result of contraction forces, the cervix effaces and dilates by mechanisms that include all **EXCEPT** which of the following?

a. Contraction forces create lateral pull against the cervix to open its canal.

b. Contraction forces are transferred directly through the presenting part to the cervix to dilate its canal.

c. Contraction forces pull smooth muscle fibers at the internal os up into the adjacent upper uterine segment to efface the cervix.

d. Contraction forces are translated into hydrostatic pressure within the amnionic sac, which presses against the cervix to dilate the cervical canal.

21–15. This image depicts stresses on the pelvic floor caused by fetal head delivery during phase 3 of parturition. All **EXCEPT** which of the following is true at this point in delivery?

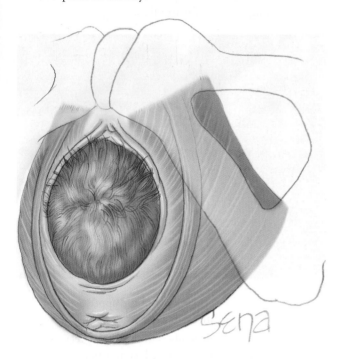

Reproduced with permission from Cunningham FG, Leveno KJ, Bloom SL, et al (eds): Maternal anatomy. In Williams Obstetrics, 23rd ed. New York, McGraw-Hill, 2010, Figure 2-26.

    a. The anus may dilate up to 3 cm.

    b. The perineal body becomes attenuated.

    c. The puborectalis muscle is markedly stretched.

    d. The coccygeus muscles receive the bulk of expulsive forces.

21–16. Which of the following is most important for initial placental separation from its uterine implantation site?

    a. Maternal pushing

    b. Gentle cord traction

    c. Uterine smooth muscle contraction

    d. Hematoma formation between the uterine wall and placenta

21–17. Compared with skeletal muscle, uterine smooth muscle offers which of the following advantages?

    a. Generates forces along one axis

    b. Has greater muscle fiber shortening

    c. Displays more structured alignment of muscle fibers

    d. All of the above

21–18. Which of the following can bring about myometrial contractions?

    a. Extracellular magnesium

    b. Actin-tubulin protein pairs

    c. G-protein-coupled receptors

    d. Gap junctions composed of decorin subunits

21–19. Once bound to its receptor, oxytocin promotes contraction through which of the following mechanisms?

    a. Opens calcium channels

    b. Generates nitric oxide

    c. Degrades 15-hydroxyprostaglandin dehydrogenase

    d. Activates the gene promoter region of the myosin light-chain kinase gene

21–20. In many mammals, suspension of the quiescence seen in phase 2 of parturition is due to which of the following?

    a. Cortisol withdrawal

    b. Progesterone withdrawal

    c. Inflammatory cell activation

    d. Increased oxytocin receptor concentration

21–21. Your patient presents with 6 weeks of amenorrhea. Transvaginal sonography reveals an intrauterine pregnancy. She elects to proceed with a medically induced abortion. For this, regimens of mifepristone and misoprostol are suitable. Mifepristone promotes cervical ripening and increased uterotonin sensitivity through which of the following mechanisms?

    a. Progesterone antagonism

    b. Calcium-channel blockade

    c. Adenyl cyclase activation

    d. Opening of maxi-K channels

21–22. For women with a prior preterm birth delivered at < 37 weeks' gestation, 17α-hydroxyprogesterone caproate may be used to prevent recurrent preterm birth. One mechanism by which progesterone maintains uterine quiescence is its ability to decrease expression of which of the following?

    a. Adenyl cyclase

    b. Progesterone receptor A

    c. Progesterone receptor B

    d. Contraction-associated proteins

21–23. A decline in progesterone's relative activity may be important for initiation of phase 2 of parturition in humans. This decline may be achieved through which of the following mechanisms?

a. Increased expression of progesterone receptor corepressors

b. Posttranslational modifications of the progesterone receptor

c. Changes in the expression of different progesterone isoforms

d. All of the above

21–24. Your patient presents at 39 weeks' gestation with a breech-presenting fetus. After a discussion of the risks and benefits, she agrees to an external cephalic version attempt. Prior to initiation, you administer 0.25 mg of terbutaline subcutaneously. This drug binds to beta-adrenergic receptors to create which of the following cellular responses to cause uterine relaxation?

a. Increased extracellular Mg^{2+} levels

b. Increased intracellular Ca^{2+} levels

c. Increased cyclic adenosine monophosphate (cAMP) levels

d. Decreased cyclic guanosine monophosphate (cGMP) levels

21–25. Human chorionic gonadotropin (hCG) shares the exact same receptor with which of the following hormones? Because of this, the high hCG levels seen with complete hydatidiform moles may lead to ovarian stimulation and formation of the theca-lutein cysts seen here.

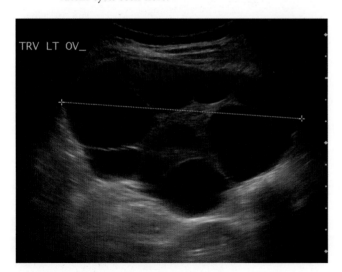

Used with permission from Dr. Sarah White.

a. Luteinizing hormone (LH)

b. Thyroid-stimulating hormone (TSH)

c. Follicle-stimulating hormone (FSH)

d. None of the above

21–26. Indomethacin, a nonsteroidal antiinflammatory drug (NSAID), has some tocolytic actions. As a group, NSAIDs target which enzyme in prostaglandin production?

a. Cyclooxygenase-1

b. Phospholipase A_2

c. Prostaglandin isomerase

d. Prostaglandin dehydrogenase

21–27. During phases 1 and 2 of parturition, uterine quiescence is maintained in part through inhibition of smooth muscle's response to oxytocin. Which of the following is a primary regulator of oxytocin receptor expression?

a. Calcium

b. Progesterone

c. Prostaglandin dehydrogenase

d. Corticotropin-releasing hormone

21–28. Stretch is believed important for uterine activation in phase 1 of parturition. One result of myometrial stretch includes increased expression of which of the following?

a. Actin and myosin

b. Contraction-associate proteins

c. Corticotropin-releasing hormone

d. None of the above

21–29. Corticotropin-releasing hormone (CRH) is suggested to promote parturition progression. Which of the following is the main contributor to CRH levels in pregnancy?

a. Placenta

b. Fetal adrenal

c. Fetal hypothalamus

d. Maternal hypothalamus

21–30. Which of the following abnormalities of normal parturition has been associated with this neural-tube defect?

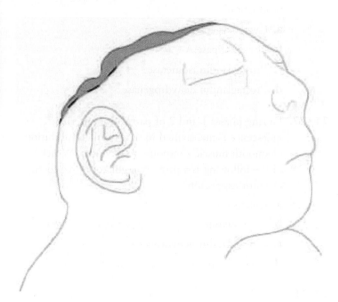

Reproduced with permission from Hoffman BL, Dashe JS, Snell K: Update in Cunningham FG, Leveno KL, Bloom SL, et al (eds): Williams Obstetrics, 23rd ed. Online. New York, McGraw-Hill, 2013. http://www.accessmedicine.com.

　　a. Preterm labor

　　b. Prolonged gestation

　　c. Uterine tachysystole

　　d. None of the above

21–31. Which group of agents is theorized to initiate phase 3 of parturition?

　　a. Uterotonins

　　b. Sex steroids

　　c. Beta mimetics

　　d. Calcium-channel blockers

21–32. Prostaglandins play a critical role in phase 3 of parturition. Levels of these are altered by which of the following?

　　a. Amnion

　　b. Decidua

　　c. Chorion

　　d. All of the above

CHAPTER 21 ANSWER KEY

Question number	Letter answer	Page cited	Header cited
21–1	a	p. 410	Phase 2 of Parturition: Preparation for Labor
21–2	c	p. 408	Phases of Parturition
21–3	b	p. 409	Figure 21-2
21–4	d	p. 409	Cervical Softening
21–5	b	p. 409	Structural Changes with Softening
21–6	c	p. 410	Myometrial Changes
21–7	c	p. 410	Cervical Ripening During Phase 2
21–8	a	p. 410	Cervical Connective Tissue
21–9	c	p. 412	Induction and Prevention of Cervical Ripening
21–10	d	p. 412	Uterine Labor Contractions
21–11	a	p. 412	Uterine Labor Contractions
21–12	a	p. 412	Distinct Lower and Upper Uterine Segments
21–13	b	p. 412	Distinct Lower and Upper Uterine Segments
21–14	c	p. 414	Cervical Changes
21–15	d	p. 415	Pelvic Floor Changes During Labor
21–16	c	p. 416	Third Stage of Labor: Delivery of Placenta and Membranes
21–17	b	p. 417	Anatomical and Physiological Considerations
21–18	c	p. 417	Regulation of Myometrial Contraction and Relaxation
21–19	a	p. 417	Intracellular Calcium
21–20	b	p. 419	Progesterone and Estrogen Contributions
21–21	a	p. 419	Progesterone and Estrogen Contributions
21–22	d	p. 421	Myometrial Cell-to-Cell Communication
21–23	d	p. 423	Functional Progesterone Withdrawal in Human Parturition
21–24	c	p. 421	Beta-adrenoreceptors
21–25	a	p. 421	Luteinizing Hormone (LH) and Human Chorionic Gonadotropin (hCG) Receptors
21–26	a	p. 422	Prostaglandins
21–27	b	p. 423	Oxytocin Receptor
21–28	b	p. 424	Uterine Stretch and Parturition
21–29	a	p. 424	Fetal Endocrine Cascades Leading to Parturition
21–30	b	p. 426	Fetal Anomalies and Delayed Parturition
21–31	a	p. 426	Phase 3: Uterine Stimulation
21–32	d	p. 428	Contributions of Intrauterine Tissues to Parturition

CHAPTER 22

Normal Labor

22–1. The relation of the fetal long axis to that of the mother is termed which of the following?

  a. Fetal lie

  b. Fetal angle

  c. Fetal position

  d. Fetal polarity

22–2. Which of the following is not a predisposing factor for transverse fetal lie?

  a. Multiparity

  b. Oligohydramnios

  c. Placenta previa

  d. Uterine anomalies

22–3. Which of the following fetal presentations is the least common?

  a. Breech

  b. Cephalic

  c. Compound

  d. Transverse lie

22–4. What percentage of fetuses are breech at 28 weeks' gestation?

  a. 1%

  b. 10%

  c. 25%

  d. 50%

22–5. When the anterior fontanel is the presenting part, which term is used?

  a. Brow

  b. Face

  c. Vertex

  d. Sinciput

22–6. This drawing shows a fetal head in which position?

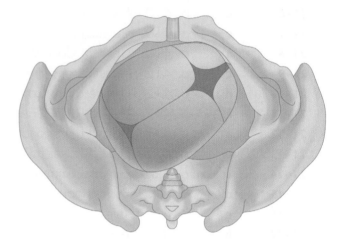

Reproduced with permission from Cunningham FG, Leveno KJ, Bloom SL, et al (eds): Normal labor. In Williams Obstetrics, 24th ed. New York, McGraw-Hill, 2014, Figure 22-3A.

  a. Left occiput anterior (LOA)

  b. Left occiput posterior (LOP)

  c. Right occiput anterior (ROA)

  d. Right occiput posterior (ROP)

22–7. The face presentation in this drawing is described as which of the following?

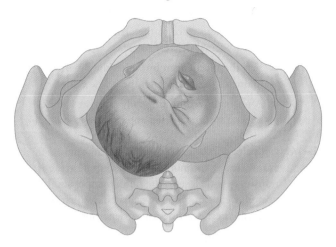

Reproduced with permission from Cunningham FG, Leveno KJ, Bloom SL, et al (eds): Normal labor. In Williams Obstetrics, 24th ed. New York, McGraw-Hill, 2014, Figure 22-5A.

a. Left mento-anterior

b. Left mento-posterior

c. Right mento-anterior

d. Right mento-posterior

22–8. The fetus in this drawing is breech. His position is best described as which of the following?

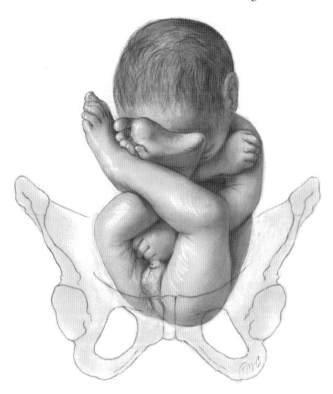

Reproduced with permission from Cunningham FG, Leveno KJ, Bloom SL, et al (eds): Breech delivery. In Williams Obstetrics, 24th ed. New York, McGraw-Hill, 2014, Figure 28-2.

a. Left sacrum anterior

b. Left sacrum posterior

c. Right sacrum anterior

d. Right sacrum posterior

22–9. The fetus in this drawing has a transverse lie. The position is best described as which of the following?

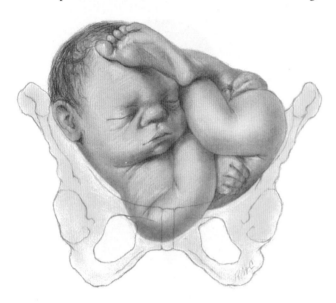

Reproduced with permission from Cunningham FG, Leveno KJ, Bloom SL, et al (eds): Normal labor. In Williams Obstetrics, 24th ed. New York, McGraw-Hill, 2014, Figure 22-7.

    a. Left acromidorsoanterior (LADA)

    b. Left acromidorsoposterior (LADP)

    c. Right acromidorsoanterior (RADA)

    d. Right acromidorsoposterior (RADP)

22–10. In shoulder presentations, the portion of the fetus chosen for orientation with the maternal pelvis is which of the following?

    a. Head

    b. Breech

    c. Scapula

    d. Umbilicus

22–11. Which of the following could inhibit performance of Leopold maneuvers?

    a. Oligohydramnios

    b. Maternal obesity

    c. Posterior placenta

    d. Supine maternal positioning

22–12. Which of the following is the correct order for the cardinal movements of labor?

    a. Descent, engagement, internal fixation, flexion, extension, external rotation, expulsion

    b. Descent, flexion, engagement, external fixation, extension, internal rotation, expulsion

    c. Engagement, descent, flexion, internal rotation, extension, external rotation, and expulsion

    d. Engagement, flexion, descent, internal rotation, straightening, extension, and expulsion

22–13. Regarding engagement of the fetal head, which of the following statements is true?

    a. It does not occur until labor commences.

    b. Engagement prior to the onset of labor does not affect vaginal delivery rates.

    c. It is the mechanism by which the biparietal diameter passes through the pelvic outlet.

    d. A normal-sized head usually engages with its sagittal suture directed anteroposteriorly.

22–14. On palpation of the fetal head during vaginal examination, you note that the sagittal suture is transverse and close to the pubic symphysis. The posterior ear can be easily palpated. Which of the following best describes this orientation?

    a. Anterior asynclitism

    b. Posterior asynclitism

    c. Mento-anterior position

    d. Mento-posterior position

22–15. Of the cardinal movements of labor, internal rotation achieves what goal?

    a. Flexes the fetal neck

    b. Brings the occiput to an anterior position

    c. Brings the anterior fontanel through the pelvic inlet

    d. None of the above

22–16. In what percentage of labors does the fetus enter the pelvis in an occiput posterior position?

    a. 0.5%

    b. 5%

    c. 20%

    d. 33%

22–17. Which of the following is not a risk factor for incomplete rotation of the posterior occiput?

    a. Macrosomia

    b. Poor contractions

    c. Lack of analgesia

    d. Inadequate head flexion

22–18. This photograph demonstrates which of the following?

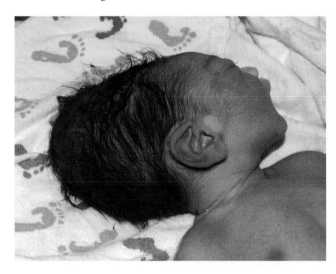

    a. Hydrocephalus

    b. Plagiocephaly

    c. Craniosynostosis

    d. Caput and molding

22–19. Which of the following statements regarding the preparatory division of labor is true?

    a. The cervix dilates very little.

    b. Connective tissue components of the cervix change considerably.

    c. Sedation and conduction analgesia are capable of arresting this labor division.

    d. All of the above

22–20. When does the latent phase of labor end for most women?

    a. 1–2 cm

    b. 2–3 cm

    c. 3–5 cm

    d. 7–8 cm

22–21. A 20-year-old G1P0 at 39 weeks' gestation presents complaining of strong contractions. Her cervix is dilated 1 cm. She is given sedation, and 4 hours later, her contractions have stopped. Her cervix is still 1 cm dilated. Which of the following is the most likely diagnosis?

    a. False labor

    b. Prolonged latent phase of labor

    c. Arrest of the latent phase of labor

    d. Arrest of the active phase of labor

22–22. According to Friedman, the minimum normal rate of active-phase labor in a multipara is which of the following?

    a. 1 cm/hr

    b. 1.2 cm/hr

    c. 1.5 cm/hr

    d. 3.4 cm/hr

22–23. Which stage of labor begins with complete cervical dilatation and ends with delivery of the fetus?

    a. First stage

    b. Second stage

    c. Third stage

    d. Fourth stage

22–24. A 24-year-old G1P0 at 27 weeks' gestation presents in active preterm labor to a hospital without delivery services or a neonatal intensive care unit. The physician in the emergency department evaluates the patient. He determines that her cervix is approximately 4 cm dilated and membranes are intact. He would like to transfer her to you because you are at the nearest hospital with obstetric and neonatal services qualified to handle this patient's complications. According to the Emergency Medical Treatment and Labor Act (EMTALA), which of the following is true?

    a. A woman complaining of contractions is not considered an emergency.

    b. A screening examination is not required because it will unreasonably slow the transfer of the patient.

    c. The patient cannot be transferred because a woman in true labor is considered "unstable" for interhospital transfer.

    d. This patient can be transferred if the physician certifies that the benefits of treatment at your facility outweigh the transfer risks.

22–25. When evaluating a pregnant woman for rupture of membranes, which of the following has been associated with a false-positive nitrazine test result?

    a. Blood

    b. Semen

    c. Bacterial vaginosis

    d. All of the above

22–26. When performing a bimanual examination on a pregnant woman, the position of the cervix is determined by the relationship of the cervical os to which of the following?

   a. Rectum

   b. Uterus

   c. Fetal head

   d. Pubic symphysis

22–27. Station describes the relationship between which of the following?

   a. The biparietal diameter and the pelvic outlet

   b. The biparietal diameter and the ischial spines

   c. The lowermost portion of the presenting fetal part and the pelvic inlet

   d. The lowermost portion of the presenting fetal part and the ischial spines

22–28. A 20-year-old G2P1 presents in active labor at term. The patient requires augmentation with oxytocin during her labor course. She has a forceps-assisted vaginal delivery and sustains a second-degree laceration. Which of the following is not a risk factor for urinary retention in this patient?

   a. Multiparity

   b. Perineal laceration

   c. Oxytocin-augmented labor

   d. Operative vaginal delivery

22–29. What is the median duration of second-stage labor in nulliparas without conduction analgesia?

   a. 20 minutes

   b. 40 minutes

   c. 50 minutes

   d. 90 minutes

22–30. What is the median duration of the second-stage labor in multiparas without conduction analgesia?

   a. 20 minutes

   b. 40 minutes

   c. 50 minutes

   d. 90 minutes

22–31. A 25-year-old G1P0 at 39 weeks' gestation presents in active labor. Her cervix is dilated 4 cm and is completely effaced, and the presenting fetal part has reached 0 station. Membranes are intact. With examination 2 hours later, you note that the cervix is still 4 cm dilated. At this point, which of the following is the best management?

   a. Cesarean delivery

   b. Rupture of membranes

   c. Insertion of a bladder catheter to assist fetal head descent

   d. Rupture of membranes, placement of internal monitors, and oxytocin augmentation

22–32. A 19-year-old G1P0 at term presents in active labor. Her cervix is 5 cm dilated, and fluid is leaking from spontaneously ruptured membranes. You examine her 2 hours later, and the cervix is still 5 cm dilated. At this point, which of the following is the best management?

   a. Cesarean delivery

   b. Placement of internal monitors and reassessment in 2 hours

   c. Placement of internal monitors, oxytocin augmentation, and reassessment in 2 hours

   d. Placement of internal monitors, oxytocin augmentation, antibiotics for prolonged rupture of membranes, and reassessment in 2 hours

CHAPTER 22 ANSWER KEY

Question number	Letter answer	Page cited	Header cited
22–1	a	p. 433	Fetal Lie
22–2	b	p. 433	Fetal Lie
22–3	c	p. 434	Table 22-1
22–4	c	p. 433	Cephalic Presentation
22–5	d	p. 434	Figure 22-1
22–6	d	p. 435	Figure 22-3
22–7	a	p. 436	Figure 22-5
22–8	b	p. 436	Figure 22-6
22–9	d	p. 437	Figure 22-7
22–10	c	p. 437	Varieties of Presentations and Positions
22–11	b	p. 437	Abdominal Palpation—Leopold Maneuvers
22–12	c	p. 438	Occiput Anterior Presentation
22–13	b	p. 439	Engagement
22–14	b	p. 439	Asynclitism
22–15	b	p. 442	Internal Rotation
22–16	c	p. 443	Occiput Posterior Presentation
22–17	c	p. 443	Occiput Posterior Presentation
22–18	d	p. 444	Figure 22-18
22–19	d	p. 445	First Stage of Labor
22–20	c	p. 445	Latent Phase
22–21	a	p. 446	Prolonged Latent Phase
22–22	c	p. 446	Active Labor
22–23	b	p. 447	Second Stage of Labor
22–24	d	p. 448	Emergency Medical Treatment and Labor Act—EMTALA
22–25	d	p. 448	Ruptured Membranes
22–26	c	p. 449	Cervical Assessment
22–27	d	p. 449	Cervical Assessment
22–28	a	p. 451	Urinary Bladder Function
22–29	c	p. 451	Management of the Second Stage of Labor
22–30	a	p. 451	Management of the Second Stage of Labor
22–31	b	p. 452	Figure 22-25
22–32	b	p. 452	Figure 22-25

CHAPTER 23

Abnormal Labor

23–1. Which of the following may be responsible for dystocia in labor?

    a. Bony-pelvis abnormalities

    b. Inadequate expulsive forces

    c. Soft-tissue abnormalities of the reproductive tract

    d. All of the above

23–2. Which of the following is true regarding cephalopelvic disproportion?

    a. It currently is responsible for 34% of dystocia cases.

    b. It is a term that originated in the 1960s to describe abnormal bony pelves.

    c. It was defined during a time when dystocia developed secondary to vitamin D deficiency or rickets, which is now rare in developed countries.

    d. B and C

23–3. In this diagram below, what represents the biggest obstacle to labor and delivery?

    a. Prominent coccyx

    b. Contraction band in the lower uterine segment

    c. Decreased anteroposterior diameter of the pelvic inlet

    d. A and C

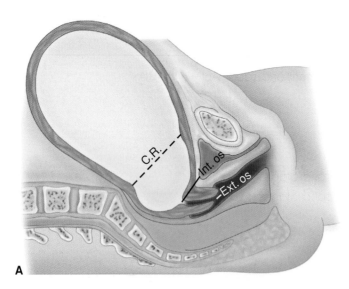

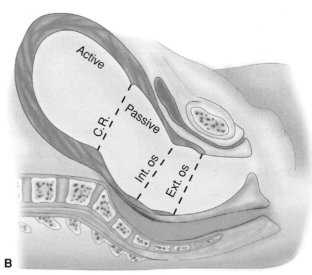

Reproduced with permission from Cunningham FG, Leveno KJ, Bloom SL, et al (eds): Abnormal labor. In Williams Obstetrics, 24th ed. New York, McGraw-Hill, 2014, Figure 23-1. C. R. = contraction ring, Ext. = external, Int. = internal.

23–4. The National Institute of Child Health and Human Development (NICHD) and American College of Obstetricians and Gynecologists (ACOG) have made recommendations concerning the diagnosis of arrested second-stage labor. Which of the following statements are consistent with their recommendations?

a. Arrested labor in the second stage should not be diagnosed until adequate time has elapsed.

b. Before this diagnosis is given, nulliparas without epidural anesthesia should be allowed 2 hours without progress.

c. Before this diagnosis is given, nulliparas without epidural anesthesia should be allowed 3 hours without progress.

d. A and C

23–5. At Parkland Hospital, neonates delivered from parturients whose second-stage labor lasted > 3 hours had which of the following adverse outcomes compared with neonates of mothers with shorter second-stage labor?

a. Neonates from each group of parturients had equivalent rates of perinatal morbidity.

b. The lowest prevalence of 5-minute Apgar scores ≤ 3 was noted in the group of parturients with longer second-stage labor.

c. The percentage of neonates requiring resuscitative efforts was higher in the group of parturients with longer second-stage labor.

d. B and C

23–6. Which of the following is among the advances in labor dysfunction management?

a. Use of oxytocin

b. Reliance on midforceps deliveries for transverse arrest

c. Realization that undue prolongation of labor leads to increased perinatal morbidity

d. A and C

23–7. Where are contraction forces the greatest during normal labor?

a. Fundus

b. Lower uterine segment

c. Midzone of the posterior uterine wall

d. Forces are equal throughout the uterus

23–8. The Montevideo group concluded that which of the following was the lowest contraction pressure necessary to cause cervical dilation?

a. 15 mm Hg

b. 25 mm Hg

c. 35 mm Hg

d. 45 mm Hg

23–9. Terms to describe specific active-phase abnormalities include which of the following?

a. Arrest disorders

b. Saltatory disorders

c. Protraction disorders

d. A and C

23–10. What is the total number of Montevideo units shown in this monitor strip?

    a. 235

    b. 242

    c. 196

    d. None of the above

23–14. Which of the following is true regarding epidural anesthesia during labor?

    a. It slows the first stage of labor.

    b. It slows the second stage of labor.

    c. It has no effect on the length of labor.

    d. A and B

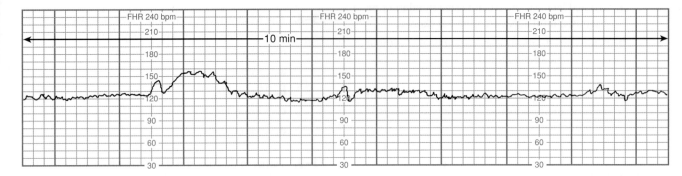

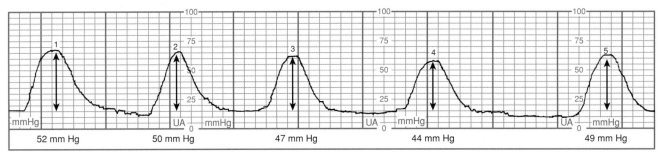

Reproduced with permission from Cunningham FG, Leveno KJ, Bloom SL, et al (eds): Abnormal labor. In Williams Obstetrics, 24th ed. New York, McGraw-Hill, 2014, Figure 23-3.

23–11. According to data from Menticoglou (1995a,b), approximately what percentage of parturients achieved spontaneous vaginal delivery in the subsequent hour once second-stage labor reached 5 hours?

    a. 0.5%

    b. 5%

    c. 15%

    d. 20%

23–12. Which of the following is true regarding coached maternal pushing efforts during second-stage labor?

    a. It has no effect on second-stage length.

    b. It significantly shortens the second stage.

    c. It shortens the second stage but has no effect on maternal or neonatal morbidity rates.

    d. B and C

23–13. In laboring nulliparas, fetal station above 0 is associated with which of the following?

    a. A 25% cesarean rate

    b. A 50% cesarean rate

    c. A higher cesarean rate than if the head is engaged

    d. A and C

23–15. Which of the following is true regarding chorioamnionitis and its effects on labor?

    a. Infection in early labor is a cause of labor dysfunction.

    b. Infection in late second-stage labor is a by-product of dysfunctional labor.

    c. Chorioamnionitis is most often associated with precipitous labor.

    d. A and C

23–16. For low-risk parturients, walking in the first stage of labor has which of the following effects?

    a. Has no effect on labor length

    b. Decreases second-stage labor length

    c. Decreases the neonatal 5-minute Apgar score

    d. Increases the length of the latent phase of labor

23–17. Compared with recumbent positioning, upright positions during second-stage labor are associated with which of the following?

    a. Less pain

    b. Slightly shorter labor duration

    c. Higher rates of blood loss exceeding 500 mL

    d. All of the above

23–18. Laboring in a birthing tub is associated with higher rates of which adverse neonatal outcome?

a. Waterborne infection

b. Neonatal hypocalcemia

c. Neonatal intensive care admission

d. A and C

23–19. According to research by Hannah (1996) and Peleg (1999), which of the following is true regarding premature rupture of membranes at term?

a. Cesarean delivery rates were lowest in those managed expectantly.

b. Oxytocin induction led to the lowest rates of chorioamnionitis.

c. Prophylactic antibiotics significantly lowered rates of chorioamnionitis.

d. A and C

23–20. Which of the following is true regarding precipitous labor?

a. Defined as delivery within 3 hours of labor onset

b. May result from diminished pelvic soft-tissue resistance

c. May result from a decreased sensation and awareness of active labor

d. All of the above

23–21. Which of the following is an associated complication of precipitous labor and delivery?

a. Uterine atony

b. Chorioamnionitis

c. Shoulder dystocia

d. A and B

23–22. In obstetrics, which of the following defines a contracted pelvic inlet?

a. A transverse diameter < 12 cm

b. A diagonal conjugate < 11.5 cm

c. An anteroposterior diameter < 10 cm

d. All of the above

23–23. The computed tomographic image shown here demonstrates which of the following?

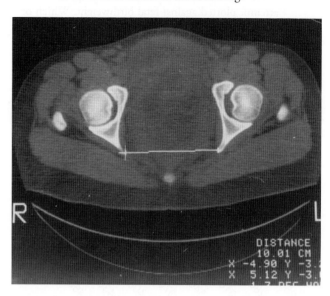

Reproduced with permission from Cunningham FG, Leveno KJ, Bloom SL, et al (eds): Abnormal labor. In Williams Obstetrics, 24th ed. New York, McGraw-Hill, 2014, Figure 23-4C.

a. Obstetrical conjugate

b. Intertuberous diameter

c. Transverse diameter of the midpelvis

d. Transverse diameter of the pelvic inlet

23–24. Which interischial tuberous diameter measurement serves as the threshold to define pelvic outlet contraction?

a. 7 cm

b. 8 cm

c. 9 cm

d. 10 cm

23–25. Your patient has a history of a prior pelvic fracture. Which of the following is true regarding this condition?

a. Most cases are caused by a fall.

b. It is a contraindication to vaginal delivery.

c. Bony anatomy must be reviewed with pelvimetry prior to allowing vaginal delivery.

d. A and C

23–26. The graphic below demonstrates the prevalence of cesarean deliveries after a failed forceps delivery attempt plotted against fetal birthweight. Which of the following is true regarding these data?

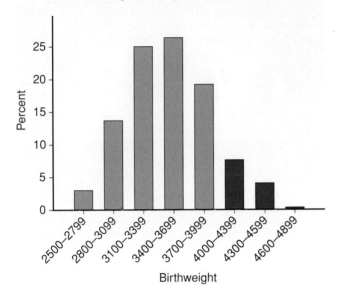

Reproduced with permission from Cunningham FG, Leveno KJ, Bloom SL, et al (eds): Abnormal labor. In Williams Obstetrics, 24th ed. New York, McGraw-Hill, 2014, Figure 23-5.

a. Most cesarean deliveries occurred in women with macrosomic babies.

b. Fetal size appears to be the significant contributor to failed forceps deliveries.

c. Nearly 20% of cesarean deliveries occurred in women whose newborns weighed < 3100 g.

d. None of the above

23–27. This image illustrates which fetal presentation?

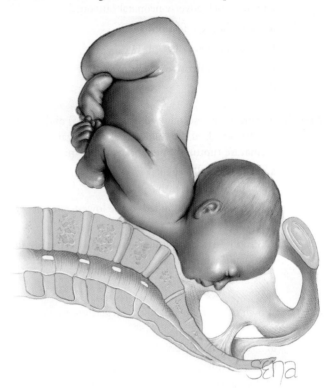

Reproduced with permission from Cunningham FG, Leveno KJ, Bloom SL, et al (eds): Abnormal labor. In Williams Obstetrics, 24th ed. New York, McGraw-Hill, 2014, Figure 23-6.

a. Brow presentation

b. Face presentation

c. Occiput presentation

d. Synciput presentation

23–28. Which of the following is a risk factor for face presentation?

a. Prematurity

b. Multiparity

c. Anencephaly

d. All of the above

23–29. This image illustrates which fetal presentation?

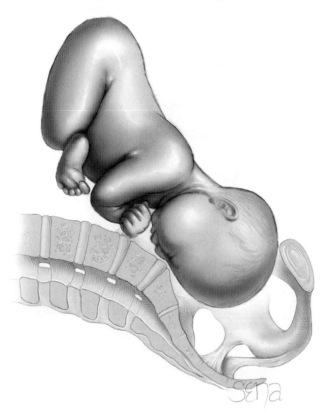

Reproduced with permission from Cunningham FG, Leveno KJ, Bloom SL, et al (eds): Abnormal labor. In Williams Obstetrics, 24th ed. New York, McGraw-Hill, 2014, Figure 23-8.

   a. Brow presentation
   b. Face presentation
   c. Occiput presentation
   d. Synciput presentation

23–30. This vigorous newborn most likely presented how during labor?

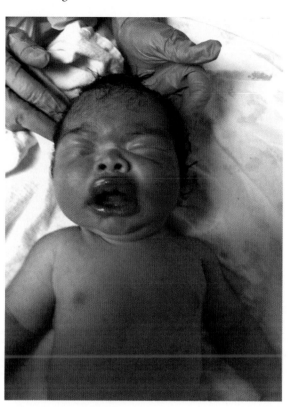

   a. Brow presentation
   b. Face presentation
   c. Occiput presentation
   d. Synciput presentation

23–31. Which of the following describes the position of the fetus in this drawing?

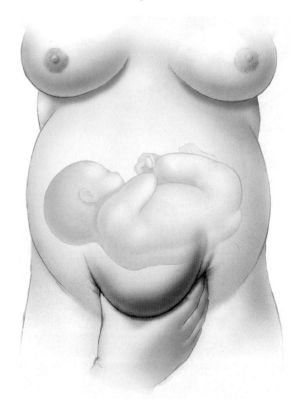

Reproduced with permission from Cunningham FG, Leveno KJ, Bloom SL, et al (eds): Abnormal labor. In Williams Obstetrics, 24th ed. New York, McGraw-Hill, 2014, Figure 23-9C.

    a. Left acromidorsoanterior

    b. Left acromidorsoposterior

    c. Right acromidorsoanterior

    d. Right acromidorsoposterior

23–32. Common causes of transverse lie include which of the following?

    a. Nulliparity

    b. Prolonged labor

    c. Placenta previa

    d. Oligohydramnios

23–33. Which of the following complications may follow vaginal delivery with the presentation shown here?

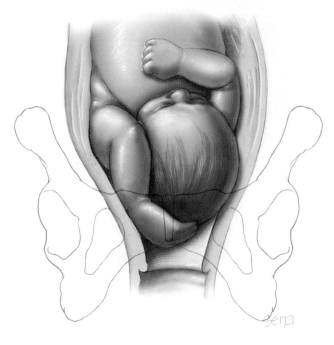

Reproduced with permission from Cunningham FG, Leveno KJ, Bloom SL, et al (eds): Abnormal labor. In Williams Obstetrics, 24th ed. New York, McGraw-Hill, 2014, Figure 23-11.

    a. Klumpke palsy

    b. Cookie-cutter scalp laceration

    c. Significant brachial plexus injury

    d. Ischemic necrosis of the presenting forearm

23–34. The following adverse outcomes are associated with dystocia?

    a. Chorioamnionitis

    b. Retained placenta

    c. Puerperal endometritis

    d. A and C

23–35. In which of the following clinical scenarios is prolonged labor associated with uterine rupture?

    a. High parity

    b. Previous cesarean delivery

    c. 32-week fetus in a transverse lie

    d. All of the above

23–36. Prolonged labor can result in which of the following maternal complications?

    a. Uterine rupture

    b. Fistula formation

    c. Symphyseal necrosis

    d. A and B

23–37. Which of the following nerves is more commonly injured during vaginal delivery due to poor patient positioning?

   a. Femoral nerve

   b. Ilioinguinal nerve

   c. Genitofemoral nerve

   d. Common fibular nerve (formerly common peroneal nerve)

References

Hannah M, Ohlsson A, Farine D, et al: International Term PROM Trial: a RCT of induction of labor for prelabor rupture of membranes at term. Am J Obstet Gynecol 174:303, 1996

Menticoglou SM, Manning F, Harman C, et al: Perinatal outcomes in relation to second-stage duration. Am J Obstet Gynecol 173:906, 1995a

Menticoglou SM, Perlman M, Manning FA: High cervical spinal cord injury in neonates delivered with forceps: report of 15 cases. Obstet Gynecol 86:589, 1995b

Peleg D, Hannah ME, Hodnett ED, et al: Predictors of cesarean delivery after prelabor rupture of membranes at term. Obstet Gynecol 93:1031, 1999

CHAPTER 23 ANSWER KEY

Question number	Letter answer	Page cited	Header cited
23–1	d	p. 455	Dystocia
23–2	c	p. 455	Dystocia Descriptors
23–3	b	p. 456	Mechanisms of Dystocia
23–4	d	p. 457	Table 23-3
23–5	c	p. 459	Table 23-5
23–6	d	p. 458	Abnormalities of the Expulsive Forces
23–7	a	p. 458	Types of Uterine Dysfunction
23–8	a	p. 458	Types of Uterine Dysfunction
23–9	d	p. 459	Active-Phase Disorders
23–10	b	p. 459	Active-Phase Disorders
23–11	c	p. 459	Second-Stage Disorders
23–12	c	p. 461	Maternal Pushing Efforts
23–13	c	p. 461	Fetal Station at Onset of Labor
23–14	d	p. 461	Epidural Anesthesia
23–15	b	p. 461	Chorioamnionitis
23–16	a	p. 461	Maternal Position During Labor
23–17	d	p. 462	Birthing Position in Second-Stage Labor
23–18	d	p. 462	Water Immersion
23–19	b	p. 462	Premature Ruptured Membranes at Term
23–20	d	p. 462	Precipitous Labor and Delivery
23–21	a	p. 462	Maternal Effects
23–22	d	p. 463	Contracted Inlet
23–23	c	p. 463	Contracted Midpelvis
23–24	b	p. 463	Contracted Outlet
23–25	c	p. 464	Pelvic Fractures
23–26	c	p. 464	Fetal Dimensions in Fetopelvic Disproportion
23–27	b	p. 466	Face Presentation
23–28	d	p. 466	Etiology
23–29	a	p. 467	Brow Presentation
23–30	b	p. 466	Face Presentation
23–31	c	p. 468	Transverse Lie
23–32	c	p. 468	Etiology
23–33	d	p. 469	Management and Prognosis
23–34	d	p. 470	Maternal Complications
23–35	d	p. 470	Uterine Rupture
23–36	d	p. 471	Fistula Formation
23–37	d	p. 471	Postpartum Lower Extremity Nerve Injury

CHAPTER 24

Intrapartum Assessment

24–1. Which of the following is currently the most prevalent obstetrical procedure performed in the United States?

  a. Episiotomy

  b. Fetal monitoring

  c. Cesarean delivery

  d. Operative vaginal delivery

24–2. Continuous R-to-R wave fetal heart rate computation is reflected clinically as which of the following?

  a. Periodic change

  b. Episodic change

  c. Beat-to-beat variability

  d. Shift in the heart rate baseline

24–3. Which of the following are scaling factors for fetal heart rate monitoring recommended by a 1997 National Institute of Child Health and Human Development (NICHD) workshop?

  a. 3 cm/min chart recorder paper speed

  b. 1 cm/min chart recorder paper speed

  c. 60 beats per minute per vertical centimeter

  d. None of the above

24–4. In cases of fetal demise, external Doppler ultrasound will most likely detect signals from which of the following?

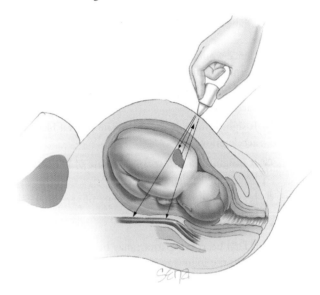

Reproduced with permission from Cunningham FG, Leveno KJ, Bloom SL, et al (eds): Intrapartum assessment. In Williams Obstetrics, 24th ed. New York, McGraw-Hill, 2014, Figure 24-5.

  a. Placenta

  b. Maternal heart

  c. Maternal aorta

  d. None of the above

24–5. According to the National Institute of Child Health and Human Development (NICHD), a fetal heart rate acceleration is defined by which of the following?

  a. Accelerations lasting > 5 minutes are considered a baseline change.

  b. It is considered prolonged, if it lasts ≥ 2 minutes and < 10 minutes.

  c. For all gestational ages, an acceleration lasts ≥ 15 seconds and rises ≥ 15 beats above the heart rate baseline.

  d. None of the above

24–6. Decreased fetal heart rate variability most closely reflects which of the following?

   a. Fetal hypoxia

   b. Fetal acidemia

   c. Fetal hyperglycemia

   d. None of the above

24–7. Which of the following would not be expected to decrease fetal heart rate variability?

   a. Meperidine

   b. Butorphanol

   c. Diphenhydramine

   d. Diabetic ketoacidosis

24–8. Evidence would suggest which of the following concerning magnesium sulfate?

   a. It insignificantly decreases fetal heart rate variability.

   b. It significantly increases the rate of fetal heart rate accelerations.

   c. It insignificantly increases the rate of late fetal heart rate decelerations.

   d. It significantly increases the rate of variable fetal heart rate decelerations.

24–9. This fetal heart rate pattern may be associated with which of the following conditions?

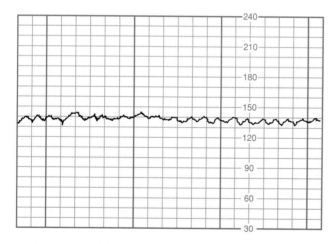

Reproduced with permission from Cunningham FG, Leveno KJ, Bloom SL, et al (eds): Intrapartum assessment. In Williams Obstetrics, 24th ed. New York, McGraw-Hill, 2014, Figure 24-13.

   a. Alloimmunization

   b. Intracranial hemorrhage

   c. Meperidine administration

   d. All of the above

24–10. Which of the following is the most common fetal heart rate deceleration?

   a. Late deceleration

   b. Early deceleration

   c. Variable deceleration

   d. Prolonged deceleration

24–11. This deceleration most likely reflects which of the following?

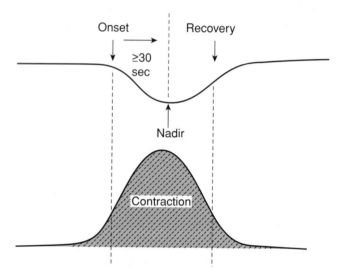

Reproduced with permission from Cunningham FG, Leveno KJ, Bloom SL, et al (eds): Intrapartum assessment. In Williams Obstetrics, 24th ed. New York, McGraw-Hill, 2014, Figure 24-14.

   a. Head compression

   b. Cord compression

   c. Maternal chronic anemia

   d. Uteroplacental insufficiency

24–12. This deceleration most likely reflects which of the following?

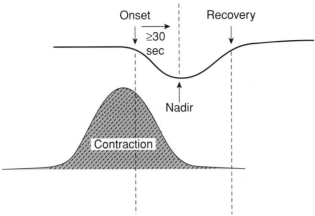

Reproduced with permission from Cunningham FG, Leveno KJ, Bloom SL, et al (eds): Intrapartum assessment. In Williams Obstetrics, 24th ed. New York, McGraw-Hill, 2014, Figure 24-16.

   a. Head compression

   b. Cord compression

   c. Maternal chronic anemia

   d. Uteroplacental insufficiency

24–13. The acceleration seen prior to the fetal heart deceleration characterized here is most likely due to which of the following?

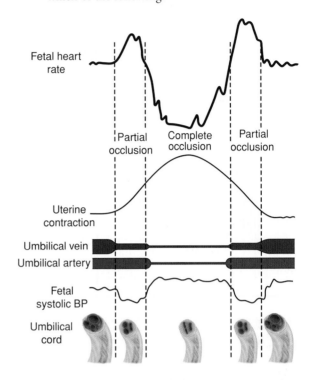

Reproduced with permission from Cunningham FG, Leveno KJ, Bloom SL, et al (eds): Intrapartum assessment. In Williams Obstetrics, 24th ed. New York, McGraw-Hill, 2014, Figure 24-22.

   a. Venous compression induces a baroreceptor-mediated acceleration.

   b. Venous compression induces a chemoreceptor-mediated acceleration.

   c. Arterial compression induces a baroreceptor-mediated acceleration.

   d. Partial placenta separation induces a chemoreceptor-mediated acceleration.

CHAPTER 24

24–14. Which of the following is true of this fetal heart rate pattern?

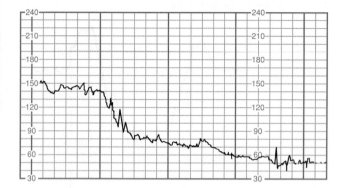

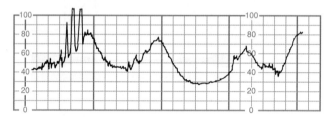

Reproduced with permission from Cunningham FG, Leveno KJ, Bloom SL, et al (eds): Intrapartum assessment. In Williams Obstetrics, 24th ed. New York, McGraw-Hill, 2014, Figure 24-24.

    a. This variable deceleration will resolve spontaneously.

    b. This late deceleration should prompt emergent delivery.

    c. This prolonged deceleration should prompt immediate intervention.

    d. This fetal bradycardia will be followed by compensatory fetal tachycardia.

24–15. Which of the following approximates the percentage of deliveries that have decelerations in the second stage of labor?

    a. 33%

    b. 50%

    c. 66%

    d. 90%

24–16. For low-risk pregnancies, continuous fetal monitoring at admission has which of the following affects on obstetrical outcome?

    a. Increases cesarean delivery rates

    b. Decreases perinatal mortality rates

    c. Decreases perinatal morbidity rates

    d. All of the above

24–17. Centralized monitoring has which of the following affects on obstetrical care?

    a. Increases cesarean delivery rates

    b. Decreases perinatal morbidity rates

    c. Decreases detection of critical fetal heart rate signals as the number of video display screens increases

    d. All of the above

24–18. Which of the following intrapartum stimulation tests are useful to exclude fetal acidemia?

    a. Vibroacoustic stimulation

    b. Digital stroking of the fetal scalp

    c. Allis clamp grasping of the fetal scalp

    d. All of the above

24–19. Which of the following is true of the diagnosis of fetal distress and asphyxia?

    a. Labor is ultimately an asphyxiating event.

    b. High degrees of interobserver agreement are found with fetal heart rate pattern interpretation.

    c. Attention should focus only on intrapartum events as these are the major contributors to poor fetal outcome.

    d. All of the above

24–20. In 2008, the National Institute of Child Health and Human Development (NICHD) convened a conference and constructed a three-tiered system for fetal heart rate pattern classification. Which of the following accurately characterizes the different tiers?

    a. Category I: absence of early decelerations and presence of normal baseline variability

    b. Category II: presence of recurrent late decelerations and absent baseline variability

    c. Category III: presence of recurrent variable decelerations and normal baseline variability

    d. None of the above

24–21. Since the introduction of the new National Institute of Child Health and Human Development (NICHD) classification of fetal heart rate patterns, which of the following is true regarding its effect on perinatal and maternal morbidity?

    a. Cesarean delivery rates have declined.

    b. Neonatal morbidity rates have declined.

    c. Identification of fetal acidosis is easier.

    d. There is not a consensus on interpretation and management recommendations for fetal heart rate patterns.

24–22. Growing evidence suggests which of the following regarding meconium aspiration syndrome (MAS) is true?

   a. Antepartum chronic hypoxia rarely leads to MAS.

   b. Most cases are secondary to acute intrapartum events.

   c. More than ½ of infants with MAS have cord pH values > 7.20.

   d. All of the above

24–23. Current guidelines from the American Academy of Pediatricians and the American College of Obstetricians and Gynecologists recommend which of following regarding intrapartum neonatal suctioning in the presence of meconium?

   a. Routine intrapartum suctioning decreases the incidence of meconium aspiration syndrome.

   b. For vigorous neonates, intubation and suctioning below the cords should not be performed.

   c. The neonate should immediately be handed to the pediatrician for suctioning below the vocal cords.

   d. None of the above

24–24. In the presence of a critical fetal heart rate change, what should the obstetrician do to resuscitate the fetus?

   a. Halt an oxytocin infusion

   b. Examine the cervix to exclude umbilical cord prolapse

   c. Move the patient to a left lateral decubitus position and correct epidural-related hypotension

   d. All of the above

24–25. Which of the following is true concerning tocolysis for treatment of nonreassuring fetal heart rate patterns during labor?

   a. Subcutaneous terbutaline lowers cesarean delivery rates.

   b. Small doses of intravenous nitroglycerine are not beneficial.

   c. The American College of Obstetricians and Gynecologists does not recommend tocolysis for nonreassuring fetal heart rate patterns due to insufficient evidence regarding its efficacy.

   d. None of the above

24–26. Regarding amnioinfusion, which of the following statements is true?

   a. It improves neonatal outcomes when used prophylactically for variable decelerations.

   b. It reduces cesarean delivery rates when used prophylactically for variable decelerations.

   c. According to the American College of Obstetricians and Gynecologists, it may be used to treat persistent variable decelerations.

   d. All of the above

24–27. Regarding prophylactic amnioinfusion for thick meconium, which of the following statements is true?

   a. It improves neonatal outcomes.

   b. It decreases the incidence of meconium aspiration syndrome.

   c. It can be completed in only a few cases that have thick meconium-stained fluid.

   d. It is not recommended by the American College of Obstetricians and Gynecologists for meconium-stained fluid.

24–28. The American College of Obstetricians and Gynecologists recommends obtaining umbilical cord blood gases in which of the following circumstances?

   a. Routinely

   b. 5-minute Apgar score ≤ 7

   c. Fetal-growth restriction

   d. None of the above

24–29. Regarding the mode of fetal heart rate monitoring during labor, the American Academy of Pediatricians and the American College of Obstetricians and Gynecologists recommend which of the following?

   a. In high-risk pregnancies, intermittent auscultation is acceptable.

   b. In low-risk pregnancies, continuous external monitoring is preferred.

   c. In high-risk pregnancies, intermittent auscultation should be preformed every 15 minutes during the second stage of labor.

   d. None of the above

24–30. Uterine contractions are typically associated with pain after they reach what intrauterine pressure threshold?

   a. 5 mm Hg

   b. 15 mm Hg

   c. 25 mm Hg

   d. 35 mm Hg

24–31. Your patient, a 34-year-old nullipara, is undergoing oxytocin induction of labor, and her cervix is dilated 6 to 7 cm. Her fetus has a cephalic presentation. She has been having six contractions per 10 minutes for the past 45 minutes. What term correctly describes this contraction pattern?

   a. Normal

   b. Hypersystole

   c. Tachysystole

   d. Hyperstimulation

24–32. During monitoring of the patient in Question 24–31, a prolonged fetal heart rate deceleration is noted during external monitoring. What is an acceptable response?

   a. Prepare for cesarean delivery

   b. Administer a 0.25-mg dose of terbutaline subcutaneously

   c. Halt oxytocin, move patient to a left lateral decubitus position, and provide oxygen by mask

   d. Clinical judgment should guide your actions, and all of the responses may be acceptable

24–33. For the patient in Question 24–31, the fetal heart rate pattern responds to conservative measures, and a scalp electrode is applied for direct monitoring. During the next 2 hours, she progresses to complete cervical dilatation. Fetal station is +1 to +2, and fetal head position is left occiput transverse. The fetal heart rate has lost all variability, and recurrent late decelerations are present. The patient has now developed chorioamnionitis, and you begin antibiotic therapy. Your appropriate next response is which of the following?

   a. Prepare for cesarean delivery

   b. Perform midforceps rotation and delivery

   c. Begin maternal pushing, and if prompt descent and internal rotation are noted, then complete a low forceps delivery from +2 station and occiput anterior position

   d. Clinical judgment should guide your actions, and all of the responses may be acceptable

CHAPTER 24 ANSWER KEY

Question number	Letter answer	Page cited	Header cited
24–1	b	p. 473	Introduction
24–2	c	p. 473	Electronic Fetal Monitoring
24–3	a	p. 475	Fetal Heart Rate Patterns
24–4	c	p. 474	External (Indirect) Electronic Monitoring
24–5	b	p. 477	Table 24-1
24–6	b	p. 479	Decreased Variability
24–7	c	p. 479	Decreased Variability
24–8	a	p. 479	Decreased Variability
24–9	d	p. 482	Sinusoidal Heart Rate Pattern
24–10	c	p. 484	Variable Deceleration
24–11	a	p. 483	Early Deceleration
24–12	d	p. 483	Late Deceleration
24–13	a	p. 484	Variable Deceleration
24–14	c	p. 487	Prolonged Deceleration
24–15	d	p. 487	Fetal Heart Rate Patterns During Second-Stage Labor
24–16	a	p. 487	Admission Fetal Monitoring in Low-Risk Pregnancies
24–17	c	p. 488	Centralized Monitoring
24–18	d	p. 489	Vibroacoustic Stimulation
24–19	a	p. 491	Pathophysiology and Diagnosis
24–20	a	p. 492	National Institutes of Health Workshops on Three-Tier Classification System
24–21	d	p. 492	National Institutes of Health Workshops on Three-Tier Classification System
24–22	c	p. 493	Meconium in the Amnionic Fluid
24–23	b	p. 493	Meconium in the Amnionic Fluid
24–24	d	p. 494	Management Options
24–25	c	p. 494	Tocolysis
24–26	d	p. 495	Prophylactic Amnioinfusion for Variable Decelerations
24–27	d	p. 495	Amnioinfusion for Meconium-Stained Amnionic Fluid
24–28	c	p. 496	Human Evidence
24–29	a	p. 497	Current Recommendations
24–30	b	p. 498	Patterns of Uterine Activity
24–31	c	p. 499	New Terminology for Uterine Contractions
24–32	d	p. 487	Clinical Correlation
24–33	d	p. 483	Clinical Correlation

CHAPTER 25

Obstetrical Analgesia and Anesthesia

25–1. Approximately what percentage of maternal deaths are attributable to anesthetic complications?

a. 1.2%

b. 2.4%

c. 3.6%

d. 4.8%

25–2. Which of the following statements is true regarding the American College of Obstetricians and Gynecologists opinion on which patients should receive anesthesia in labor?

a. All patients with heart disease

b. All patients with severe preeclampsia

c. All patients with gestational diabetes

d. Any woman who requests it and has no contraindication to its administration

25–3. Which parenteral anesthetic agent has the shortest neonatal half-life?

a. Morphine

b. Nalbuphine

c. Meperidine

d. Butorphanol

25–4. What is the half-life of meperidine in the newborn?

a. 4 hr

b. 9 hr

c. 13 hr

d. 21 hr

25–5. What percentage of newborns will need naloxone treatment in the delivery room if their mother has received meperidine in labor?

a. 1%

b. 3%

c. 5%

d. 10%

25–6. Which patient should not receive naloxone while in labor?

a. A patient with severe preeclampsia

b. A patient with respiratory depression

c. A newborn of a narcotic-addicted mother

d. A patient who has just received intravenous morphine

25–7. What is the direct cause of most maternal deaths involving regional anesthesia?

a. Drug reaction

b. Cardiac arrhythmia

c. High spinal blockade

d. Central nervous system infection

25–8. In the figure below, blockade at which sensory level would provide the best analgesia during early labor?

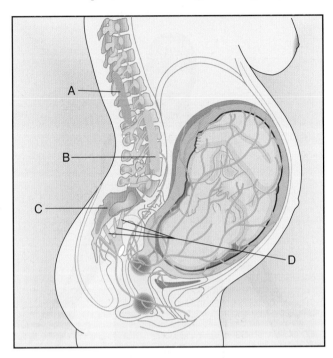

Modified with permission from Eltzschig HK, Lieberman ES, Camann WR: Medical progress: regional anesthesia and analgesia for labor and delivery. N Engl J Med 348: 319-332, 2003, Figure 1.

a. A

b. B

c. C

d. D

25–9. Which nerve is primarily involved with the pain associated with perineal stretching?

a. Ischial nerve

b. Pudendal nerve

c. Hypogastric nerve

d. Frankenhäuser ganglion

25–10. In the image shown below, which ligament is the needle passing through to reach the pudendal nerve?

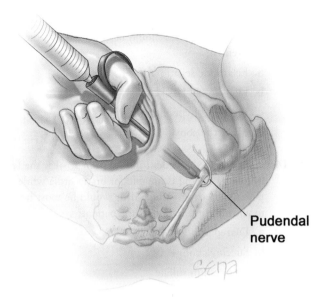

Modified with permission from Cunningham FG, Leveno KJ, Bloom SL, et al (eds): Obstetrical analgesia and anesthesia. In Williams Obstetrics, 24th ed. New York, McGraw-Hill, 2014, Figure 25-2.

a. Pudendal ligament

b. Sacroiliac ligament

c. Sacrospinous ligament

d. Sacrotuberous ligament

25–11. Which of the following statements is true regarding butorphanol in labor?

a. Neonatal depression is greater than with meperidine.

b. It can be administered contiguously with meperidine.

c. It can be associated with a transient sinusoidal fetal heart rate.

d. All of the above

25–12. A patient in early labor is sitting up for her epidural. An anesthetic test dose is given. The patient's heart rate and blood pressure rise immediately after administration of the test dose. What has most likely caused her change in vital signs?

a. The patient just had a contraction.

b. The test dose was given intravenously.

c. The text dose created high spinal blockade.

d. None of the above

25–13. A diabetic, preeclamptic patient requires cesarean delivery for breech presentation and is sitting up for a spinal anesthetic block. After administration of her spinal block, she has a seizure. Which of the following diagnoses should be considered in the differential?

a. Eclamptic seizure

b. High spinal blockade

c. Profound hypoglycemia

d. All of the above

25–14. Referring to the patient in Question 25–13, the fetal heart rate tracing is notable for bradycardia while the patient is seizing. Which drug would be most helpful in allowing intubation of the patient?

a. Diazepam

b. Succinylcholine

c. Magnesium sulfate

d. All of the above

25–15. Which anesthetic is associated with neurotoxicity and cardiotoxicity at virtually identical serum drug levels?

a. Lidocaine

b. Tetracaine

c. Bupivacaine

d. Ropivacaine

25–16. All **EXCEPT** which of the following are true for the quality of regional anesthesia that reaches the dermatome level marked by the X in this figure?

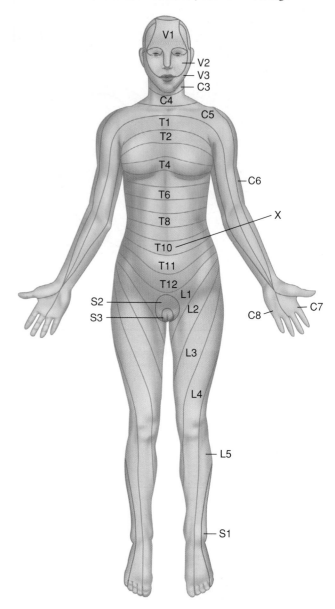

Modified with permission from Cunningham FG, Leveno KJ, Bloom SL, et al (eds): Obstetrical analgesia and anesthesia. In Williams Obstetrics, 24th ed. New York, McGraw-Hill, 2014, Figure 25-4A.

a. It is adequate for forceps delivery.

b. It is adequate for a cesarean delivery.

c. It is adequate for spontaneous vaginal delivery.

d. All of the above

25–17. Using the same image in Question 25–16, regional anesthesia that reaches which dermatome level is required for cesarean delivery?

a. T_4

b. T_6

c. T_8

d. T_{10}

25–18. Which complication occurs with approximately 15% of paracervical blocks?

    a. Infection

    b. Fetal bradycardia

    c. Hematoma formation

    d. Intravascular injection

25–19. What is the main reason for the addition of glucose to the anesthetic agents chosen for a spinal blockade?

    a. To make the solution hyperbaric

    b. To make the solution hypertonic

    c. To provide glucose to the patient, who should be NPO

    d. To minimize hypotension associated with spinal blockade

25–20. When used prophylactically in the obstetrical anesthesia setting, which vasopressor has been associated with fetal acidemia?

    a. Ephedrine

    b. Ergonovine

    c. Phenylephrine

    d. Methylergonovine

25–21. Which of the following interventions has been shown to reduce the incidence of postdural puncture headache?

    a. Vigorous prehydration

    b. Prophylactic blood patch

    c. Use of a smaller-gauge needle

    d. Keeping the patient supine during labor

25–22. Absolute contraindications to regional anesthesia include all **EXCEPT** which of the following?

    a. Scoliosis

    b. Maternal coagulopathy

    c. Skin infection over the site of needle placement

    d. Use of low-molecular-weight heparin in the prior 6 hours

25–23. Which structure in the image here is identified by the letter X?

    a. Dura mater

    b. Epidural space

    c. Ligamentum flavum

    d. Internal venous plexus

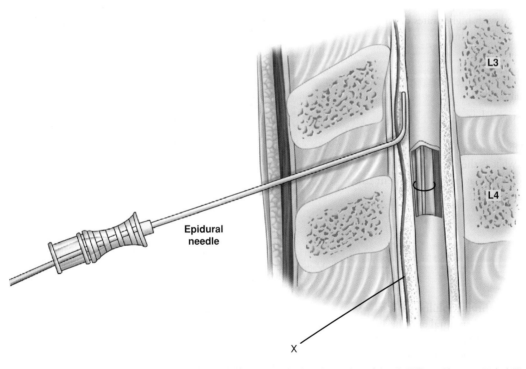

Modified with permission from Cunningham FG, Leveno KJ, Bloom SL, et al (eds): Obstetrical anesthesia. In Williams Obstetrics, 23rd ed. New York, McGraw-Hill, 2010, Figure 19-4.

25–24. The spread of anesthesia after epidural placement can be influenced by all **EXCEPT** which of the following?

a. Maternal position

b. Dose of anesthetic

c. Type of catheter used

d. Location of catheter tip

25–25. Which is the most common complication encountered during epidural anesthesia?

a. Fever

b. Hypotension

c. Total spinal blockade

d. Ineffective analgesia

25–26. All **EXCEPT** which of the following are associated with breakthrough pain after epidural anesthesia is initially established?

a. Nulliparity

b. Heavier fetal weight

c. Lower maternal body mass index (BMI)

d. Catheter placed at earlier cervical dilation

25–27. Compared with intravenous meperidine, epidural anesthesia is associated with higher rates of all **EXCEPT** which of the following?

a. Cesarean delivery

b. Oxytocin stimulation

c. Operative vaginal delivery

d. Prolonged first-stage labor

25–28. According to the American College of Obstetricians and Gynecologists, what is the threshold below which thrombocytopenia may prevent a patient from receiving epidural anesthesia?

a. 50,000

b. 75,000

c. 100,000

d. 150,000

25–29. A patient with a known thrombophilia has just had a vaginal delivery under epidural anesthesia. She had discontinued her low-dose low-molecular-weight anticoagulant prior to induction of labor. When would it be safe to restart her anticoagulant postpartum?

a. Prior to removal of her epidural catheter

b. As soon as her epidural catheter is removed

c. At least two hours after epidural catheter removal

d. When her partial thromboplastin time (PTT) is normal

25–30. An opiate was used for epidural analgesia in a patient's cesarean delivery, and now she is complaining of itching and being unable to empty her bladder. Which drug will eliminate her symptoms without affecting the analgesic action of the opiate?

a. Naloxone

b. Cetirizine

c. Bupivacaine

d. Diphenhydramine

25–31. A patient requiring emergent cesarean delivery has a patchy epidural block and needs local infiltration of anesthesia to augment the blockade. In the image here, which nerve is identified by the letter X?

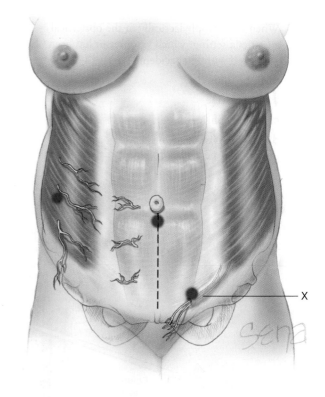

Modified with permission from Cunningham FG, Leveno KJ, Bloom SL, et al (eds): Obstetrical analgesia and anesthesia. In Williams Obstetrics, 24th ed. New York, McGraw-Hill, 2014, Figure 25-6.

a. Ischial nerve

b. Intercostal nerve

c. Hypogastric nerve

d. Ilioinguinal nerve

25–32. Of the following steps taken prior to the induction of general anesthesia, which has been the key factor in decreasing maternal mortality rates from general anesthesia?

   a. Antacids

   b. Preoxygenation

   c. Uterine displacement

   d. Aggressive intravenous hydration

25–33. What is the rate of failed intubation for general anesthesia in pregnancy?

   a. 1 in 100

   b. 1 in 250

   c. 1 in 400

   d. 1 in 550

25–34. Of agents used for induction of general anesthesia, which is associated with delirium and hallucinations?

   a. Ketamine

   b. Propofol

   c. Thiopental

   d. Succinylcholine

25–35. Which pulmonary lobe is most often involved in aspiration as a complication of general anesthesia?

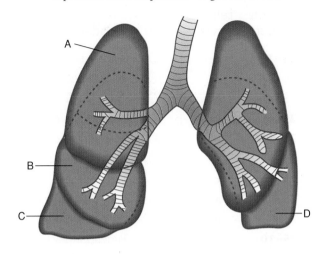

   a. Right upper lobe

   b. Right middle lobe

   c. Right lower lobe

   d. Left lower lobe

25–36. If a patient has emesis of gastric contents during induction of general anesthesia, which of the following steps is indicated to limit the complications of aspiration?

   a. Saline lavage

   b. Initiation of prophylactic antibiotics

   c. Administration of corticosteroid therapy

   d. Suctioning of inhaled fluid from pharynx and trachea

CHAPTER 25 ANSWER KEY

Question number	Letter answer	Page cited	Header cited
25–1	a	p. 504	Introduction
25–2	d	p. 504	Obstetrical Anesthesia Services
25–3	b	p. 507	Table 25-3
25–4	c	p. 506	Meperidine and Promethazine
25–5	b	p. 506	Meperidine and Promethazine
25–6	c	p. 507	Efficacy and Safety of Parenteral Agents
25–7	c	p. 504	Introduction
25–8	a	p. 505	Principles of Pain Relief
25–9	b	p. 505	Principles of Pain Relief
25–10	c	p. 508	Pudendal Block, Figure 25-2
25–11	c	p. 506	Butorphanol (Stadol)
25–12	b	p. 507	Anesthetic Agents
25–13	d	p. 507	Central Nervous System Toxicity
25–14	b	p. 507	Central Nervous System Toxicity
25–15	c	p. 508	Cardiovascular Toxicity
25–16	b	p. 510	Vaginal Delivery
25–17	a	p. 511	Cesarean Delivery
25–18	b	p. 509	Paracervical Block
25–19	a	p. 510	Vaginal Delivery
25–20	a	p. 511	Hypotension
25–21	c	p. 512	Postdural Puncture Headache
25–22	a	p. 512	Contraindications to Spinal Analgesia, Table 25-6
25–23	d	p. 510	Figure 25-3
25–24	c	p. 513	Continuous Lumbar Epidural Block
25–25	b	p. 511	Hypotension, Table 25-5
25–26	c	p. 514	Ineffective Analgesia
25–27	a	p. 515	Effect on Labor, Table 25-8
25–28	a	p. 516	Thrombocytopenia
25–29	c	p. 516	Anticoagulation
25–30	a	p. 517	Epidural Opiate Analgesia
25–31	d	p. 517	Local Infiltration for Cesarean Delivery, Figure 25-6
25–32	a	p. 518	Patient Preparation
25–33	b	p. 517	General Anesthesia
25–34	a	p. 518	Induction of Anesthesia
25–35	c	p. 519	Pathophysiology
25–36	d	p. 520	Treatment

CHAPTER 26

Induction and Augmentation of Labor

26–1. Compared with the *induction* of labor, the *augmentation* of labor differs in what regard?

a. The fetal membranes are intact.

b. Oxytocin is titrated to effect.

c. Contractions are pharmacologically stimulated.

d. Previously commenced labor fails to effect cervical change.

26–2. All **EXCEPT** which of the following are contraindications to labor induction?

a. Twin gestation

b. Breech presentation

c. Fetal-growth restriction

d. Prior vertical hysterotomy cesarean delivery

26–3. The risk for cesarean delivery is increased in women undergoing induction of labor in which of the following situations?

a. Low Bishop score

b. Engaged fetal head

c. Multiparous parturient

d. All of the above

26–4. Women whose labors are managed with amniotomy are at increased risk for which complication?

a. Uterine atony

b. Chorioamnionitis

c. Cervical lacerations

d. All of the above

26–5. A 30-year-old G2P1 at 37 weeks' gestation with one prior cesarean delivery presents with contractions and premature rupture of the fetal membranes. Her cervix is 3 cm dilated. She requests a trial of labor and is deemed an appropriate candidate. An oxytocin infusion is initiated, and 2 hours later, you are called to the room to evaluate the fetal heart rate tracing, which is shown below. According to a large study conducted by the Maternal-Fetal Medicine Units Network, the use of oxytocin increases the risk for uterine rupture by what magnitude in women with a prior cesarean delivery?

a. Threefold

b. Sixfold

c. Tenfold

d. No change from background risk in women undergoing trial of labor after cesarean

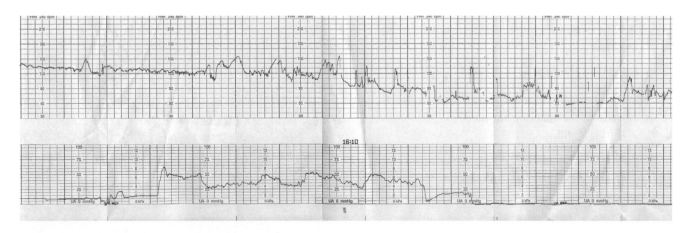

26–6. The patient presented in Question 26–5 is taken emergently for cesarean delivery due to uterine rupture. If misoprostol had been considered as an induction agent rather than oxytocin, what is the safest prostaglandin route and dose to use in a patient with a uterine cesarean scar?

a. Oral administration only

b. Low-dose preparation only

c. Vaginal administration only

d. They should be avoided completely.

26–7. Labor induction or augmentation increases the likelihood of which of the following peripartum complications?

a. Hysterectomy

b. Uterine atony

c. Postpartum hemorrhage

d. All of the above

26–8. Which of the following women would be most likely to have a successful induction of labor?

a. G2P1 with a body mass index of 34 and a neonatal birthweight of 3250 g

b. G1P0 with a body mass index of 25 and a neonatal birthweight of 3800 g

c. G2P1 with a body mass index of 27 and a neonatal birthweight of 3150 g

d. G1P0 with a body mass index of 31 and a neonatal birthweight of 2900 g

26–9. Which of the following administration routes is acceptable for preinduction cervical ripening with prostaglandin E_2 (dinoprostone)?

a. Intravenous

b. Intravaginal

c. Intramuscular

d. All of the above

26–10. Use of cervical ripening agents is associated with which of the following outcomes?

a. Labor initiation

b. Decreased cesarean delivery rate

c. Decreased maternal morbidity rate

d. All of the above

26–11. A 22-year-old primigravida is diagnosed with severe preeclampsia at 39 weeks' gestation. A magnesium sulfate infusion is initiated for seizure prophylaxis, and plans are made for induction of labor. Her cervix is 3 cm dilated, 50-percent effaced, slightly soft, and located anteriorly. The fetal head is at –1 station. What is her Bishop score?

a. 6

b. 7

c. 8

d. 9

26–12. Of the five elements that comprise the Bishop scoring system, only three are significantly associated with predicting successful vaginal delivery. This simplified Bishop scoring system includes all **EXCEPT** which of the following?

a. Fetal station

b. Cervical dilation

c. Cervical effacement

d. Cervical consistency

26–13. Intracervical administration of dinoprostone (Prepidil) for the purpose of cervical ripening may be repeated every 6 hours with a maximum of how many doses?

a. 2

b. 3

c. 4

d. 5

26–14. When administering dinoprostone using the device shown here, which of the following should be avoided?

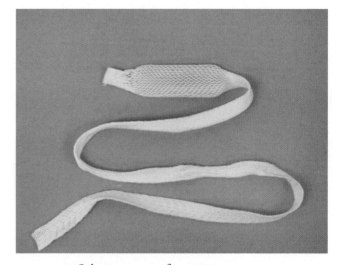

a. Subsequent use of oxytocin

b. Use of lubricants during insertion

c. Removal of the device with labor onset

d. Recumbent positioning for the first 2 hours after insertion

26–15. Based on the available literature, the use of dinoprostone appears to have what effect on the cesarean delivery rate?

  a. Unchanged

  b. Decreased

  c. Increased for fetal distress

  d. Increased for labor dystocia

26–16. A 16-year-old primigravida is admitted to the hospital for preterm, premature rupture of the fetal membranes at 32 weeks' gestation. Two days later, she complains of contractions and vaginal bleeding, and the following fetal heart rate tracing is noted to be associated with frequent uterine contractions. According to the definitions established by the American College of Obstetricians and Gynecologists, what is the appropriate term for this condition?

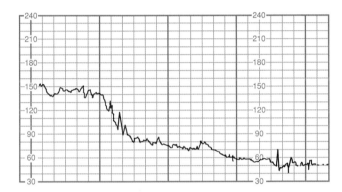

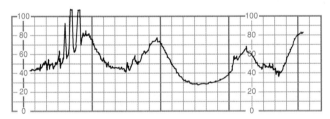

Reproduced with permission from Cunningham FG, Leveno KJ, Bloom SL, et al (eds): Intrapartum assessment. In Williams Obstetrics, 24th ed. New York, McGraw-Hill, 2014, Figure 24-24.

  a. Uterine hypertonus

  b. Uterine tachysystole

  c. Uterine hyperstimulation

  d. Uterine hypercontractility

26–17. A 25-year-old G2P1 at 41 weeks' gestation presents for preinduction cervical ripening, and a 10-mg dinoprostone insert (Cervidil) is placed in the posterior vaginal fornix. Thirty minutes later, she is noted to have 6 contractions every 10 minutes. What is the most appropriate next step in management?

  a. Remove the insert

  b. Irrigate the vagina

  c. Administer supplemental oxygen

  d. Increase intravenous fluid administration rate

26–18. Misoprostol (prostaglandin E_1) is approved by the U.S. Food and Drug Administration for what indication?

  a. Labor induction

  b. Cervical ripening

  c. Cholelithiasis pain

  d. Peptic ulcer prevention

26–19. When administered vaginally for labor induction, what is the recommended dose of misoprostol (prostaglandin E_1)?

  a. 25 μg

  b. 25 mg

  c. 100 μg

  d. 100 mg

26–20. Which of the following observations prompted investigators to search for clinical agents that stimulate nitric oxide (NO) production?

  a. NO is a mediator of cervical ripening.

  b. NO metabolite levels are increased in early labor.

  c. NO production prior to labor is low in postterm pregnancies.

  d. All of the above

26–21. For cervical ripening, the addition of nitric oxide donors to prostaglandins has been demonstrated to have which of the following outcomes compared with prostaglandins alone?

  a. Shortened time to vaginal delivery

  b. Enhanced cervical ripening in term pregnancies

  c. Enhanced cervical ripening in preterm pregnancies

  d. None of the above

26–22. When using a transcervical catheter to mechanically promote cervical ripening, concurrent extraamnionic saline infusion through the catheter reduces what complication compared with catheter placement without infusion?

    a. Tachysystole

    b. Uterine rupture

    c. Chorioamnionitis

    d. Placental abruption

26–23. Compared with prostaglandins for cervical ripening, transcervical catheters have what benefit?

    a. Lower cesarean delivery rate

    b. Lower rates of supplemental oxytocin use

    c. Fewer cases of cardiotocographic changes

    d. All of the above

26–24. For cervical ripening, use of the mechanical dilating device shown here has which of the following benefits compared with prostaglandins?

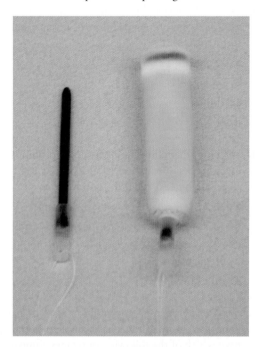

Reproduced with permission from Cunningham FG, Leveno KJ, Bloom SL, et al (eds): Abortion. In Williams Obstetrics, 24th ed. New York, McGraw-Hill, 2014, Figure 18-8B.

    a. Low cost

    b. Patient comfort

    c. Lower chorioamnionitis rate

    d. Shorter induction-to-delivery intervals

26–25. All **EXCEPT** which of the following statements regarding oxytocin are accurate?

    a. It was the first polypeptide hormone synthesized.

    b. It may be used for labor induction or augmentation.

    c. It can be administered by intravenous or intravaginal routes.

    d. It is one of the most frequently used medications in the United States.

26–26. In general, oxytocin infusions should be discontinued if the number of contractions per 10 minutes consistently exceeds what value?

    a. 3

    b. 5

    c. 7

    d. 10

26–27. What is the mean half-life of oxytocin?

    a. 1 minute

    b. 5 minutes

    c. 10 minutes

    d. 20 minutes

26–28. Potential benefits of a high-dose oxytocin regimen (4.5 to 6 mU/mL) compared with a low-dose regimen (0.5–1.5 mU/mL) include which of the following?

    a. Fewer failed inductions

    b. Decreased admission-to-delivery intervals

    c. Lower rates of intrapartum chorioamnionitis

    d. All of the above

26–29. At what oxytocin infusion dose does free-water clearance begin to decrease markedly?

    a. 10 mIU/mL

    b. 20 mIU/mL

    c. 36 mIU/mL

    d. 48 mIU/mL

26–30. On average, epidural analgesia prolongs the active phase of labor how many minutes?

    a. 60 minutes

    b. 90 minutes

    c. 120 minutes

    d. 180 minutes

26–31. Which of the following can follow amniotomy?

    a. Cord prolapse

    b. Placental abruption

    c. Variable fetal heart rate decelerations

    d. All of the above

26–32. Membrane stripping has been associated with which of the following untoward outcomes?

    a. Chorioamnionitis

    b. Precipitous labor

    c. Patient discomfort

    d. Premature rupture of the fetal membranes

CHAPTER 26 ANSWER KEY

Question number	Letter answer	Page cited	Header cited
26–1	d	p. 523	Introduction
26–2	c	p. 523	Labor Induction—Contraindications
26–3	a	p. 524	Cesarean Delivery Rate
26–4	b	p. 524	Chorioamnionitis
26–5	a	p. 524	Rupture of a Prior Uterine Incision
26–6	d	p. 524	Rupture of a Prior Uterine Incision
26–7	d	p. 524	Uterine Atony
26–8	c	p. 524	Factors Affecting Successful Induction
26–9	b	p. 525	Table 26-1
26–10	a	p. 525	Preinduction Cervical Ripening
26–11	c	p. 525	Cervical Favorability
26–12	d	p. 525	Cervical Favorability
26–13	b	p. 526	Prostaglandin E_2
26–14	b	p. 526	Prostaglandin E_2
26–15	a	p. 526	Prostaglandin E_2
26–16	b	p. 527	Side Effects
26–17	a	p. 527	Side Effects
26–18	d	p. 527	Prostaglandin E_1
26–19	a	p. 527	Prostaglandin E_1
26–20	d	p. 527	Nitric Oxide Donors
26–21	d	p. 527	Nitric Oxide Donors
26–22	c	p. 528	Transcervical Catheter
26–23	c	p. 528	Transcervical Catheter
26–24	a	p. 528	Hygroscopic Cervical Dilators
26–25	c	p. 529	Oxytocin
26–26	b	p. 529	Intravenous Oxytocin Administration
26–27	b	p. 529	Intravenous Oxytocin Administration
26–28	d	p. 529	Oxytocin Regimens
26–29	b	p. 530	Risks versus Benefits
26–30	a	p. 531	Active Phase Arrest
26–31	d	p. 531	Amniotomy for Induction and Augmentation; Elective Amniotomy
26–32	c	p. 532	Membrane Stripping for Labor Induction

DELIVERY

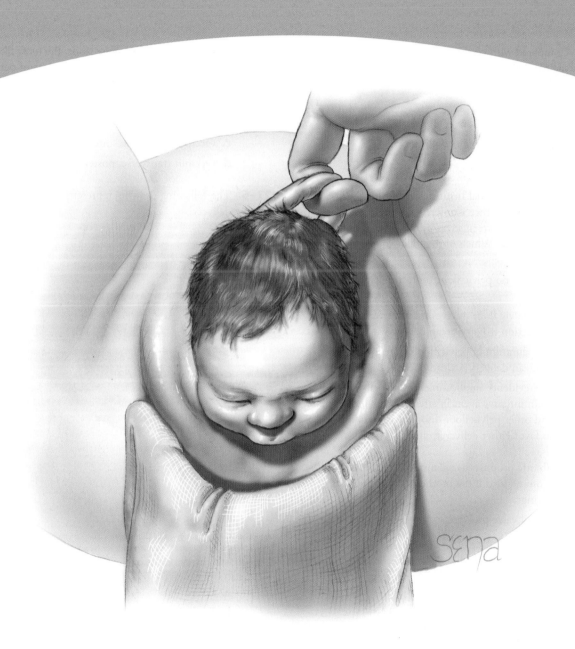

CHAPTER 27

Vaginal Delivery

27–1. Compared with cesarean delivery, spontaneous vaginal delivery has lower associated rates of which of the following?

    a. Hemorrhage

    b. Maternal infection

    c. Anesthesia-related complications

    d. All of the above

27–2. In 2006, a National Institutes of Health (NIH) State-of-the-Science Conference summarized the associations between stress urinary incontinence and delivery route. Which of the following reflects their findings?

    a. There is no pelvic floor protection from cesarean delivery.

    b. The pelvic floor receives substantive durable protection from cesarean delivery.

    c. The duration of pelvic floor protection from cesarean delivery is clearly defined.

    d. The evidence implicating vaginal delivery as the main putative agent in stress urinary incontinence and other pelvic floor disorders is weak and fails to favor either delivery route.

27–3. Antibiotic prophylaxis against infective endocarditis is recommended if the mother has which of the following?

    a. Mitral valve prolapse

    b. Cyanotic heart disease

    c. Prosthetic heart valve

    d. B and C

27–4. Regarding patient positioning during second-stage labor, which of the following is true?

    a. Dorsal lithotomy position is the most widely used.

    b. The legs should not be strapped, and this allows quick flexion of the thighs should shoulder dystocia develop.

    c. Within the leg holder, the popliteal region should rest comfortably in the proximal portion and the heel in the distal portion.

    d. All of the above

27–5. At the end of second-stage labor, the most likely position of the fetal occiput at the time of perineal distention is which of the following?

    a. Occiput anterior

    b. Occiput posterior

    c. Occiput transverse, anterior asynclitic

    d. Occiput transverse, posterior asynclitic

27–6. The following drawing represents which event in delivery?

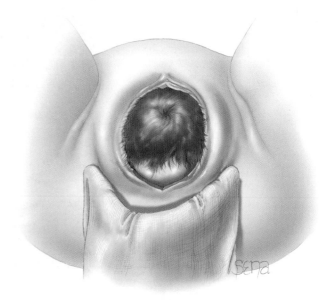

Reproduced with permission from Cunningham FG, Leveno KJ, Bloom SL, et al (eds): Vaginal delivery. In Williams Obstetrics, 24th ed. New York, McGraw-Hill, 2014, Figure 27-1.

    a. Crowning

    b. Extension

    c. Expulsion

    d. Perineal massage

27–7. If expulsive efforts of the parturient are inadequate for delivery when the fetal head is on the perineum, which of the following may be done to aid delivery?

    a. Low forceps

    b. Ritgen maneuver

    c. Rectal misoprostol

    d. A and B

27–8. Which of the following is true of routine episiotomy during vaginal delivery?

   a. Leads to anterior tears involving the urethra and labia

   b. Is preferred instead of individualized use of episiotomy

   c. Increases the risk of third- and fourth-degree lacerations

   d. B and C

27–9. During the cardinal movements of labor, when the bisacromial diameter rotates at the introitus after extension, which of the following is true?

   a. This rotation is termed external rotation.

   b. The shoulders rotate to a transverse position.

   c. Most often, the shoulders require extraction after external rotation.

   d. B and C

27–10. Regarding nasopharyngeal suctioning following the birth of a neonate, the American Heart Association recommends which of the following?

   a. Nasal bulb suctioning should be performed if thick meconium is present.

   b. Nasal bulb suctioning is performed only if the initial Apgar score is < 4.

   c. The need for nasal bulb suctioning should be determined by the resuscitating team.

   d. A and C

27–11. Which of the following is true regarding delayed umbilical cord clamping after birth of the neonate?

   a. It is recommended for preterm fetuses.

   b. It delays resuscitation of the depressed infant.

   c. There is currently insufficient evidence to support its use in term neonates in the United States.

   d. All of the above

27–12. In the early 20th century, when cesarean delivery was still associated with excessive maternal mortality rates, a persistent occiput posterior presentation was an important problem during second-stage labor. Which of the following statements is true regarding this figure of a study cohort?

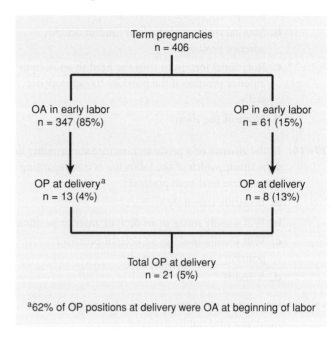

Reproduced with permission from Cunningham FG, Leveno KJ, Bloom SL, et al (eds): Vaginal delivery. In Williams Obstetrics, 24th ed. New York, McGraw-Hill, 2014, Figure 27-6.

   a. Most occiput anterior presentations at delivery were initially occiput posterior in early labor.

   b. Most persistent occiput posterior presentations were initially occiput anterior in early labor.

   c. Approximately 50% of persistent occiput posterior presentations were originally occiput posterior in early labor.

   d. Approximately 75% of persistent occiput posterior presentations were originally occiput posterior in early labor.

27–13. During evaluation of a persistent occiput posterior presentation, the fetal scalp is noted at the introitus, and the fetal head is palpated above the pubic symphysis. Which of the following is appropriate action?

　　a. Vacuum-assisted delivery if appropriate anesthesia is in place

　　b. Manual rotation of the fetal head to occiput anterior position

　　c. Rotational forceps to turn the head to an occiput anterior position if the provider has appropriate skills

　　d. None of the above

27–14. In the absence of a pelvic architecture abnormality or asynclitism, which of the following is true regarding a transverse fetal head position?

　　a. Is usually transitory

　　b. Will usually rotate to an occiput anterior position

　　c. Will usually rotate to an occiput posterior position

　　d. A and B

27–15. Which of the following is true regarding the incidence of shoulder dystocia?

　　a. Approximates 1%

　　b. Varies depending on the definition used

　　c. Has increased likelihood because of increasing fetal birthweights

　　d. All of the above

27–16. Which of the following is the most common neonatal injury with shoulder dystocia?

　　a. Fractured clavicle

　　b. Brachial plexus injury

　　c. Hypoxic ischemic encephalopathy

　　d. B and C

27–17. Regarding shoulder dystocia, which of the following is true?

　　a. It is now relatively predictable.

　　b. Elective inductions in women with suspected macrosomia may help to reduce maternal and neonatal morbidity.

　　c. Elective cesarean delivery may be considered for the diabetic mother whose fetus has an estimated weight $\geq$ 4500 g.

　　d. B and C

27–18. Rouse and Owen (1999) predicted that how many prophylactic cesarean deliveries for macrosomia would need to be performed to prevent one case of permanent brachial plexus injury?

　　a. 100

　　b. 500

　　c. 1000

　　d. 2000

27–19. Which maneuver(s) is illustrated in the following graphic?

    a. Rubin maneuver

    b. McRoberts maneuver

    c. Suprapubic pressure

    d. B and C

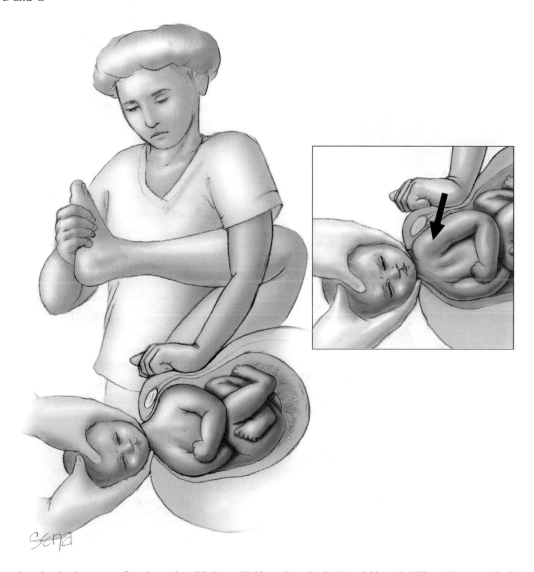

Reproduced with permission from Cunningham FG, Leveno KJ, Bloom SL, et al (eds): Vaginal delivery. In Williams Obstetrics, 24th ed. New York, McGraw-Hill, 2014, Figure 27-7.

27–20. Rubin recommended two maneuvers, one of which is depicted here. His maneuvers involve which of the following steps?

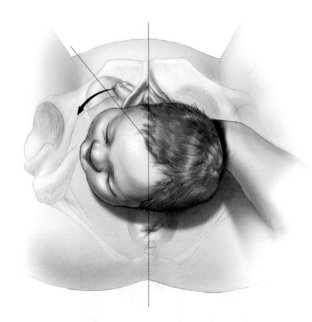

Reproduced with permission from Cunningham FG, Leveno KJ, Bloom SL, et al (eds): Vaginal delivery. In Williams Obstetrics, 24th ed. New York, McGraw-Hill, 2014, Figure 27-10B.

   a. The posterior shoulder is progressively rotated 180 degrees in a corkscrew fashion.

   b. The fetal shoulders are rocked side-to-side by applying force to the maternal abdomen.

   c. The most easily accessible fetal shoulder is pushed toward the anterior surface of the fetal chest.

   d. B and C

27–21. Which of the following is the initial step in performing a Zavanelli maneuver?

   a. Perform laparotomy

   b. Flex the head and push it back into the vagina

   c. Administer subcutaneous terbutaline to relax the uterus

   d. Restore the fetal head to an occiput anterior or occiput posterior position

27–22. Which of the following is true regarding shoulder dystocia drills?

   a. A McRoberts maneuver involves at least two assistants.

   b. Suprapubic pressure is the initial approach recommended by the American College of Obstetricians and Gynecologists.

   c. Traction and fundal pressure should be tried first followed by a call for anesthesia, additional provider help, and pediatric resuscitation.

   d. A and B

27–23. Regarding women with prior pelvic reconstructive surgery and delivery route, which of the following is true?

   a. Vaginal delivery is prohibited in this population.

   b. Cesarean delivery is always protective against symptom recurrence.

   c. Most women with prior antiincontinence surgery can be delivered vaginally without symptom recurrence.

   d. A and B

27–24. Regarding a hydrocephalic fetus with macrocephaly, which of the following is true concerning delivery route?

   a. The fetus may not deliver vaginally if the biparietal diameter is < 10 cm.

   b. At the time of cesarean delivery, a long classical incision should be performed.

   c. Cephalocentesis performed suprapubically on the breech fetus may allow a vaginal delivery.

   d. B and C

27–25. Goals of a successful third stage of labor include which of the following?

   a. Prevention of uterine inversion

   b. Prevention of shoulder dystocia

   c. Completion of episiotomy repair

   d. All of the above

27–26. What important points of placenta delivery are shown in this drawing?

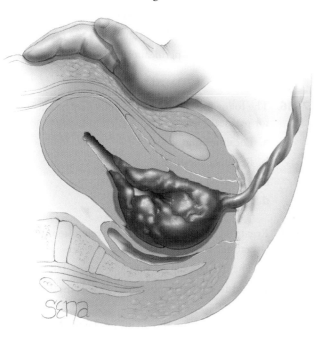

a. The fundus is being elevated.

b. The placenta remains in the uterus.

c. The umbilical cord is being pulled taut.

d. The hand is pushing the fundus toward the vagina.

27–27. Which of the following is most effective to decrease postpartum hemorrhage in third-stage labor?

a. Uterotonics

b. Fundal massage

c. Early cord clamping

d. Manual placenta removal

27–28. Which of the following is the mean half-life of oxytocin?

a. 1 minute

b. 5 minutes

c. 10 minutes

d. 15 minutes

27–29. Intravenous bolus doses of oxytocin may be particularly dangerous for which of the following parturients?

a. Morbidly obese women

b. Women with cardiovascular disease

c. Women suffering significant postpartum hemorrhage

d. B and C

27–30. High-dose oxytocin for extended periods with large volumes of electrolyte-free, dextrose-containing solutions can have which of the following effects?

a. Can have a profound diuretic action

b. Can lead to seizures in mothers and newborns

c. Can concentrate electrolytes such as sodium and lead to water intoxication

d. A and C

27–31. The ergot alkaloid methergine may be given by which of the following routes?

a. Orally

b. Intravenously

c. Intramuscularly

d. All of the above

27–32. Which of the following is true regarding misoprostol?

a. It is an E_2 prostaglandin.

b. It is more effective than oxytocin in preventing postpartum hemorrhage.

c. It can be given as a single, oral 600-μg dose to prevent postpartum hemorrhage.

d. It is best administered intramuscularly directly into the uterus at the time of hemorrhage.

27–33. This image represents which of the following perineal lacerations?

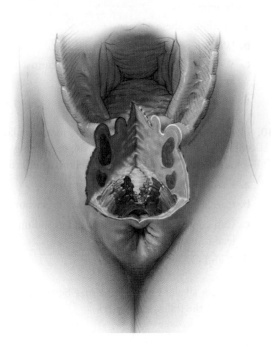

Reproduced with permission from Cunningham FG, Leveno KJ, Bloom SL, et al (eds): Vaginal delivery. In Williams Obstetrics, 24th ed. New York, McGraw-Hill, 2014, Figure 27-15C.

    a. First-degree laceration

    b. Second-degree laceration

    c. Third-degree laceration

    d. Fourth-degree laceration

27–34. Which of the following is true regarding midline episiotomies?

    a. They increase the incidence of anal sphincter tears.

    b. They should never be used in lieu of spontaneous laceration.

    c. They should be routinely cut during the delivery of nulliparous patients.

    d. A and C

27–35. The restrictive use of episiotomy is associated with which of the following?

    a. More healing complications

    b. Less anterior perineal trauma

    c. Less posterior perineal trauma

    d. A and C

27–36. The following anesthesia methods may be adequate for perineal repair?

    a. Local infiltration

    b. Regional anesthesia

    c. Pudendal nerve block

    d. All of the above

27–37. Regarding repair of a fourth-degree episiotomy or laceration, which of the following is true?

    a. The overlapping technique is acceptable.

    b. End-to-end anal sphincter repair is the superior method.

    c. Chromic suture should always be used due to less tissue inflammation.

    d. Prophylactic antibiotic administration has strong evidence to support its use with fourth-degree laceration repair.

References

Rouse DJ, Owen J: Prophylactic cesarean delivery for fetal macrosomia diagnosed by means of ultrasonography—a Faustian bargain? Am J Obstet Gynecol 181:332, 1999

CHAPTER 27 ANSWER KEY

Question number	Letter answer	Page cited	Header cited
27–1	d	p. 536	Route of Delivery
27–2	d	p. 536	Route of Delivery
27–3	d	p. 536	Preparation for Delivery
27–4	d	p. 536	Preparation for Delivery
27–5	a	p. 537	Occiput Anterior Position
27–6	a	p. 537	Delivery of the Head
27–7	b	p. 537	Delivery of the Head
27–8	c	p. 537	Delivery of the Head
27–9	a	p. 538	Delivery of the Shoulders
27–10	c	p. 538	Delivery of the Shoulders
27–11	d	p. 539	Umbilical Cord Clamping
27–12	b	p. 539	Persistent Occiput Posterior Position
27–13	d	p. 540	Delivery of Persistent Occiput Posterior Position
27–14	d	p. 540	Occiput Transverse Position
27–15	d	p. 541	Shoulder Dystocia
27–16	b	p. 541	Shoulder Dystocia
27–17	c	p. 541	Prediction and Prevention
27–18	c	p. 541	Birthweight
27–19	d	p. 542	Management
27–20	d	p. 542	Management
27–21	d	p. 542	Management
27–22	a	p. 542	Management
27–23	c	p. 545	Prior Pelvic Reconstructive Surgery
27–24	c	p. 546	Anomalous Fetuses
27–25	a	p. 546	Delivery of the Placenta
27–26	a	p. 546	Delivery of the Placenta
27–27	a	p. 547	Management of the Third Stage
27–28	b	p. 547	High-Dose Oxytocin
27–29	d	p. 547	High-Dose Oxytocin
27–30	b	p. 547	High-Dose Oxytocin
27–31	d	p. 548	Ergonovine and Methylergonovine
27–32	c	p. 548	Misoprostol
27–33	c	p. 548	Birth Canal Lacerations
27–34	a	p. 550	Episiotomy Indications and Consequences
27–35	c	p. 550	Episiotomy Indications and Consequences
27–36	d	p. 551	Repair of Episiotomy or Perineal Laceration
27–37	a	p. 552	Fourth-Degree Laceration Repair

Breech Delivery

28–1. What percentage of term singleton pregnancies present breech?

  a. 1–2%

  b. 3–4%

  c. 5–6%

  d. 7–8%

28–2. Regarding the prevalence of breech presentation, which of the following statements is true?

  a. It is stable throughout pregnancy.

  b. It approximates 80% at 24 weeks' gestation.

  c. Across pregnancy, it increases with gestational age.

  d. Across pregnancy, it decreases with gestational age.

28–3. The Term Breech Collaborative Group studied vaginal delivery of the breech fetus. Which of the following is a criticism of this study?

  a. Serious morbidity was defined too strictly.

  b. Only nulliparas were included in the trial.

  c. Most of the providers were unskilled at breech delivery.

  d. More than 10% of participants had radiological pelvimetry.

28–4. All **EXCEPT** which of the following are true regarding the "stargazer" breech fetus?

  a. The fetal head is hyperextended.

  b. Forceps are indicated for delivery.

  c. Cesarean delivery is the safest delivery route.

  d. The cervical spinal cord can be injured during vaginal delivery.

28–5. What is the risk that breech presentation will reoccur at term in a second pregnancy?

  a. 0.5%

  b. 2%

  c. 10%

  d. 12%

28–6. Which of the following is a known risk factor for breech presentation?

  a. Oligohydramnios

  b. Maternal diabetes

  c. Prior forceps delivery

  d. Anterior placental implantation

28–7. After reviewing all available studies, which of the following general statements can be made regarding vaginal delivery of the term breech fetus compared with cesarean delivery?

  a. Neonatal mortality rates are lower with cesarean delivery.

  b. Neonatal morbidity rates are lower with cesarean delivery.

  c. After vaginal breech birth, children at age 2 years have lower intelligence scores.

  d. None of the above

28–8. Which of the following statements is true regarding the preterm breech fetus?

  a. It is always best to deliver a preterm breech by cesarean.

  b. Neonatal survival rates are equal with vaginal or cesarean delivery.

  c. There are no randomized studies regarding optimal delivery route for the preterm breech fetus.

  d. None of the above

28–9. All **EXCEPT** which of the following statements are true regarding maternal morbidity and mortality in breech delivery?

  a. Hysterotomy extensions can occur with forceps use.

  b. Maternal genital tract lacerations can lead to infection.

  c. Maternal death is less likely if the breech is delivered by cesarean.

  d. Anesthesia needed for relaxation to deliver the breech can lead to postpartum hemorrhage.

28–10. Which of the following is the least common bone fractured in neonates who are delivered vaginally from a breech presentation?

   a. Femur

   b. Radius

   c. Humerus

   d. Clavicle

28–11. Which of the following outcomes that may be seen with breech presentation is not related to delivery mode?

   a. Erb palsy

   b. Hip dysplasia

   c. Spinal cord injury

   d. Sternocleidomastoid muscle hematoma

28–12. Based on imaging studies, which of the following biometric thresholds should be used to assess fetal suitability for vaginal breech delivery?

   a. BPD > 80 mm

   b. EFW < 2500 g

   c. EFW > 3500 g

   d. None of the above

28–13. What is the best indicator of pelvic adequacy for vaginal breech delivery?

   a. Fetal lie

   b. Pelvic radiograph

   c. Clinical pelvimetry

   d. Normal progression of labor

28–14. Which of the following statements is false regarding the cardinal movements of breech delivery?

   a. The fetal head is born by flexion.

   b. The back of the fetus is directed posteriorly.

   c. The anterior hip usually descends more rapidly than the posterior hip.

   d. Engagement and descent usually occur with the bitrochanteric diameter in an oblique plane.

28–15. Which of the following best describes a breech fetus that delivers spontaneously up to the umbilicus, but whose remaining body is delivered with operator traction?

   a. Breech decomposition

   b. Total breech extraction

   c. Partial breech extraction

   d. Spontaneous breech delivery

28–16. A 24-year-old G4P2 presents at term for a routine prenatal visit. She has had two prior vaginal deliveries of 6-pound neonates and one prior miscarriage. On examination, you suspect a breech-presenting fetus. Which of the following does not favor vaginal breech delivery?

   a. The fetal head is hyperflexed.

   b. Fetal weight approximates 7 lb.

   c. The patient requests cesarean delivery.

   d. The patient has had a prior pregnancy loss.

28–17. The patient in Question 28-16 is now in advanced labor and presents to Labor and Delivery. She wishes to attempt vaginal breech delivery. Sonographic evaluation shows that her fetus has both hips flexed and both knees extended. Which best describes fetal position?

   a. Frank breech

   b. Total breech

   c. Complete breech

   d. Incomplete breech

28–18. Following emergence of the fetal legs during vaginal or cesarean delivery of a breech fetus, this photograph demonstrates which next step?

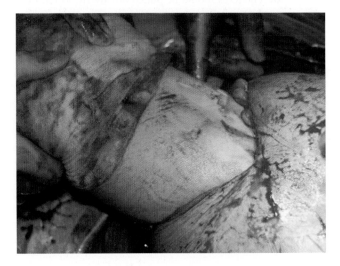

   a. Traction on the fetal waist

   b. Continued traction on the fetal legs

   c. Placement of thumbs on the fetal sacrum

   d. Placement of thumbs on the anterior superior iliac crests

28–19. To resolve the complication shown in this image, which of the following should be attempted?

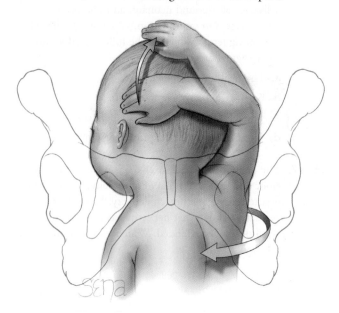

Reproduced with permission from Cunningham FG, Leveno KJ, Bloom SL, et al (eds): Breech delivery. In Williams Obstetrics, 24th ed. New York, McGraw-Hill, 2014, Figure 28-10.

a. The fetus should be rotated through a half circle.

b. The fetus should be pulled downward to release the arm.

c. The fetus should be rotated to bring its back directly posterior.

d. The humerus or clavicle should be fractured to reduce the bisacromial diameter.

28–20. What is the utility of the maneuver shown in this image?

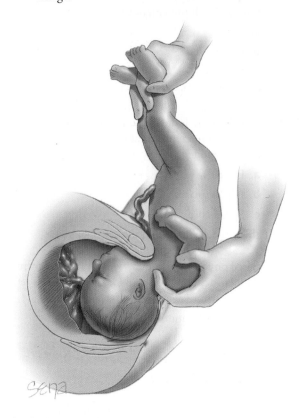

Reproduced with permission from Cunningham FG, Leveno KJ, Bloom SL, et al (eds): Breech delivery. In Williams Obstetrics, 24th ed. New York, McGraw-Hill, 2014, Figure 28-11.

a. Breech decomposition

b. Safest delivery method for the head of a preterm breech

c. Fetal head delivery when the back is oriented posteriorly

d. Release of the aftercoming head in an incompletely dilated cervix

28–21. Which of the following is true regarding the forceps used in this image?

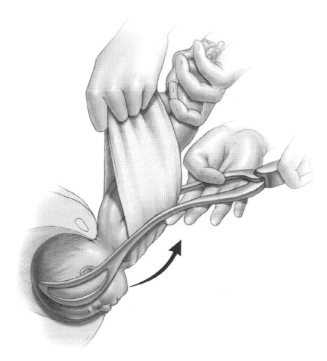

Reproduced with permission from Cunningham FG, Leveno KJ, Bloom SL, et al (eds): Breech delivery. In Williams Obstetrics, 24th ed. New York, McGraw-Hill, 2014, Figure 28-13C.

    a. They have a prominent pelvic curve.

    b. They have a downward arc in the shank.

    c. They must be rotated through a 45-degree angle.

    d. They must be disarticulated prior to fetal head delivery.

28–22. A patient presents in preterm labor at 30 weeks' gestation. Her cervix is completely dilated, and the fetus is breech. You are unable to deliver the fetal head. What procedure, used to resolve this complication, is demonstrated in this image?

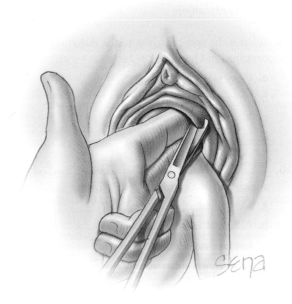

Reproduced with permission from Cunningham FG, Leveno KJ, Bloom SL, et al (eds): Breech delivery. In Williams Obstetrics, 24th ed. New York, McGraw-Hill, 2014, Figure 28-14.

    a. Symphysiotomy

    b. Zavanelli maneuver

    c. Dührssen incisions

    d. Mauriceau maneuver

28–23. If the procedure performed in Question 28–22 is not successful, which of the following may aid fetal delivery?

    a. Piper forceps

    b. Fundal pressure

    c. Zavanelli maneuver

    d. Intravenous nitroglycerin

28–24. What is the process called in which a frank breech presentation is converted to a footling breech presentation within the upper birth canal?

    a. Retraction

    b. Relaxation

    c. Displacement

    d. Decomposition

28–25. What is the eponym given to the maneuver described in Question 28–24?

    a. Piper maneuver

    b. Pinard maneuver

    c. Mauriceau maneuver

    d. Zavanelli maneuver

28–26. What is likely to be the most adequate method of anesthesia for a vaginal breech delivery?

    a. General anesthesia

    b. Pudendal anesthesia

    c. Epidural anesthesia

    d. Intravenous sedation

28–27. A 26-year-old G2P1 presents for a routine visit at 32 weeks' gestation. She is worried because her fetus was breech during her most recent sonographic examination. Which of the following are correct statements during your counseling regarding external cephalic version?

    a. The success rate is 80%.

    b. It can be performed when she presents in labor.

    c. It should be performed after 36 weeks' gestation.

    d. Amnionic fluid volume is unrelated to the success rate.

28–28. The patient in Question 28–27 chooses an external cephalic version attempt at 37 weeks' gestation. Sonographically, the fetus has a transverse lie, the amnionic fluid index is 18 cm, and the estimated fetal weight is 2800 g. The placenta is anterior. Which of the following does not aid successful version completion?

    a. Multiparity

    b. Anterior placenta

    c. Abundant amnionic fluid

    d. Fetal size of 2500–3000 g

28–29. Before proceeding with the requested version attempt, you counsel the patient in Question 28–27 regarding potential risks. Which of the following are complications of external cephalic version?

    a. Uterine rupture

    b. Placental abruption

    c. Emergency cesarean delivery

    d. All of the above

28–30. All **EXCEPT** which of the following are absolute contraindications for external cephalic version?

    a. Placenta previa

    b. Prior myomectomy

    c. Multifetal gestation

    d. Nonreassuring fetal status

28–31. Which of the following interventions has been shown most consistently to increase the success rate of external cephalic version attempts?

    a. Nifedipine

    b. Terbutaline

    c. Nitroglycerin

    d. Epidural analgesia

28–32. Internal podalic version is usually reserved for which of the following clinical situations?

    a. Frank breech deliveries

    b. Complete breech deliveries

    c. Delivery of an aftercoming twin

    d. Preterm breech deliveries, regardless of presentation

CHAPTER 28 ANSWER KEY

Question number	Letter answer	Page cited	Header cited
28–1	b	p. 558	Introduction
28–2	d	p. 559	Fig. 28-1
28–3	b	p. 558	Introduction
28–4	b	p. 559	Classification of Breech Presentations
28–5	c	p. 559	Risk Factors
28–6	a	p. 559	Risk Factors
28–7	d	p. 560	Term Breech Fetus
28–8	c	p. 561	Preterm Breech Fetus
28–9	c	p. 561	Maternal Morbidity and Mortality
28–10	b	p. 561	Perinatal Morbidity and Mortality
28–11	b	p. 561	Perinatal Morbidity and Mortality
28–12	b	p. 561	Imaging Techniques: Sonography
28–13	d	p. 562	Management of Labor and Delivery
28–14	b	p. 563	Cardinal Movements with Breech Delivery
28–15	c	p. 563	Partial Breech Extraction
28–16	c	p. 562	Table 28-1
28–17	a	p. 559	Fig. 28-2
28–18	c	p. 563	Partial Breech Extraction
28–19	a	p. 564	Nuchal Arm
28–20	c	p. 564	Modified Prague Maneuver
28–21	b	p. 567	Forceps to Aftercoming Head
28–22	c	p. 567	Entrapment of the Aftercoming Head
28–23	c	p. 567	Entrapment of the Aftercoming Head
28–24	d	p. 568	Frank Breech
28–25	b	p. 568	Frank Breech
28–26	c	p. 570	Analgesia and Anesthesia
28–27	c	p. 570	Indications
28–28	b	p. 570	Indications
28–29	d	p. 570	Complications
28–30	b	p. 570	Indications
28–31	b	p. 570	Tocolysis
28–32	c	p. 571	Internal Podalic Version

CHAPTER 29

Operative Vaginal Delivery

29–1. Accepted maternal indications for operative vaginal delivery include all **EXCEPT** which of the following?

 a. Mitral stenosis

 b. Spinal cord injury

 c. Pelvic floor protection

 d. Second-stage labor lasting > 2 hr in a multipara with epidural analgesia

29–2. Accepted fetal indications for forceps delivery include which of the following?

 a. Nonreassuring fetal heart rate pattern

 b. Prevention of intracranial hemorrhage from maternal pushing in the fragile preterm fetal head

 c. Prevention of intracranial hemorrhage from maternal pushing in the fetus with known coagulopathy

 d. All of the above

29–3. Which of the following is true of high forceps delivery?

 a. Indicated for fetal distress

 b. No role in modern obstetrics

 c. Forceps applied when the fetal head is engaged

 d. Indicated for those with prolonged second-stage labor

29–4. All **EXCEPT** which of the following criteria must be met prior to operative vaginal delivery?

 a. Membranes ruptured

 b. Cervix completely dilated

 c. Regional anesthesia placed

 d. Fetal head position determined

29–5. In all **EXCEPT** which of the following settings would forceps delivery be preferred to vacuum extraction?

 a. Maternal Marfan disease

 b. Delivery of a 33-week gestation

 c. Mentum anterior face presentation

 d. Rotation of the fetal head from occiput transverse to occiput anterior position

29–6. You are called to see your multigravid patient for prolonged fetal bradycardia. She is now 10 cm dilated, and membranes are ruptured. The head is at +2 station and shows poor descent with pushing. The fetal head is positioned left occiput posterior and is resistant to an attempt of manual rotation to an occiput anterior position. Forceps delivery of this patient would be classified as which of the following?

 a. Low

 b. High

 c. Outlet

 d. Low outlet

29–7. Which of the following describes forceps that are applied to the fetal head with the scalp visible at the introitus without manual separation of the labia?

 a. Low

 b. Mid

 c. High

 d. Outlet

29–8. Maternal morbidity with forceps delivery is most closely predicted by which of the following?

 a. Fetal station

 b. Maternal parity

 c. Degree of fetal distress

 d. Degree of fetal head molding

29–9. Third-degree laceration is more common with operative vaginal delivery compared with spontaneous vaginal delivery. Practices that may limit rates of this morbidity include which of the following?

 a. Early forceps disarticulation

 b. Selection of vacuum rather than forceps

 c. Selection of midline rather than mediolateral episiotomy

 d. Creation of episiotomy with each operative vaginal delivery

29–10. Compared with spontaneous vaginal delivery, operative vaginal delivery is confirmed to have higher long-term risks for which of the following?

  a. Anal incontinence

  b. Urinary incontinence

  c. Pelvic organ prolapse

  d. None of the above

29–11. Examples of subgaleal and cephalohematoma are shown here. Compared with forceps delivery, all **EXCEPT** which of the following have higher associated rates with vacuum extraction?

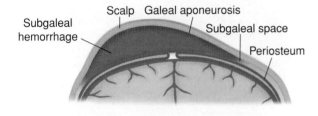

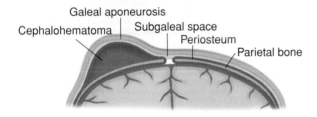

Modified with permission from Cunningham FG, Leveno KJ, Bloom SL, et al (eds): Diseases and injuries of the term newborn. In Williams Obstetrics, 24th ed. New York, McGraw-Hill, 2014, Figure 33-1.

  a. Cephalohematoma

  b. Shoulder dystocia

  c. Subgaleal hemorrhage

  d. Brachial plexus injury

29–12. The perinatal complication shown here is seen more frequently with which of the following delivery routes?

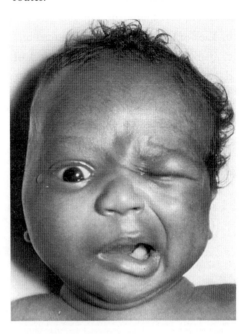

Reproduced with permission from Cunningham FG, Leveno KJ, Bloom SL, et al (eds): Diseases and injuries of the newborn. In Williams Obstetrics, 23rd ed. New York, McGraw-Hill, 2010, Figure 29-13A.

  a. Forceps delivery

  b. Vacuum extraction

  c. Cesarean delivery

  d. Spontaneous vaginal delivery

29–13. The rate of which neurodevelopmental disorder is increased by operative vaginal delivery?

  a. Epilepsy

  b. Cerebral palsy

  c. Cognitive delay

  d. None of the above

29–14. All **EXCEPT** which of the following are known factors associated with a failed trial of forceps and need for cesarean delivery?

  a. Birthweight > 4000 g

  b. Poor maternal pushing efforts

  c. Persistent occiput posterior position

  d. Absence of regional or general anesthesia

29–15. Which of the following findings should influence abandonment of operative vaginal delivery and election of cesarean delivery?

   a. Multiple vacuum cup "pop offs"

   b. Lack of fetal head descent with traction

   c. Inability to articulate the English lock of forceps

   d. All of the above

29–16. The opening in this forceps blade mainly serves which of the following functions?

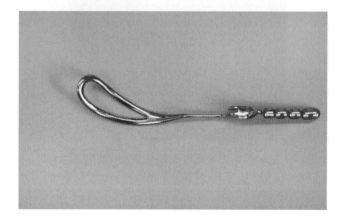

   a. Protects the fetal ears

   b. Allows blades to grip the fetal head firmly

   c. Offers a smaller metal surface area against the fetal skull

   d. Provides diminished traction forces against the maternal vaginal sidewall

29–17. This pair of forceps is ideally suited for which of the following obstetrical situations?

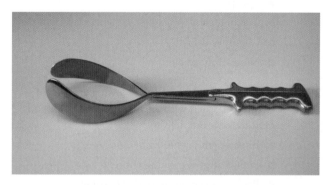

   a. Delivery of a fetus with a round head

   b. Delivery of a fetus with a molded head

   c. Delivery of a fetus with mentum posterior presentation

   d. Rotation of the fetal head from occiput transverse to occiput anterior position

29–18. Your primigravid patient had a forceps-assisted delivery of the newborn shown here after 3 hours of pushing with epidural analgesia. Prior to delivery, the fetal head position was noted to be left occiput anterior and the sagittal suture was aligned 45 degrees from the vertical axis. Which type of forceps would have been ideally suited for this delivery?

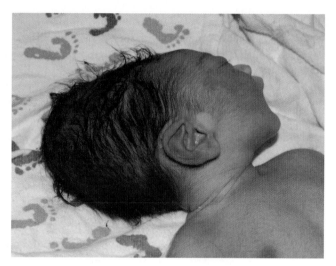

   a. Piper

   b. Simpson

   c. Kielland

   d. Tucker-McLane

29–19. Kielland forceps are ideally suited for which of the following obstetrical situations?

   a. Delivery of a fetus with a round head

   b. Delivery of a fetus with a molded head

   c. Delivery of a fetus with mentum posterior head position

   d. Rotation of the fetal head from occiput transverse to occiput anterior position

29–20. With delivery of a fetus whose head is in an occiput anterior position, correct blade application and positioning is reflected by all **EXCEPT** which of the following?

   a. The English lock can be articulated.

   b. One blade is positioned over the fetal brow and the other overlies the occiput.

   c. The long axis of the blades lies along the occipitomental diameter of the fetal head.

   d. The forceps blade edge on both the right and left is one fingerbreadth away from the adjacent fetal head lambdoidal suture.

29–21. During forceps placement, positioning of this operator's right hand deeper into the vagina serves what role?

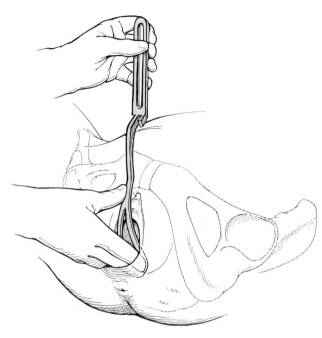

a. Protects the fetal ear

b. Identifies the ischial spines

c. Provides fetal scalp stimulation during the procedure

d. Guides the forceps into position and protects the vaginal sidewall

29–22. During operative delivery of a fetus from a +2 station and right occiput anterior position, movements of the forceps following lock articulation should most closely follow which sequence to effect delivery?

a. Outward traction, clockwise rotation, downward traction

b. Counterclockwise rotation, upward traction, outward traction

c. Clockwise rotation, downward and outward traction, upward traction

d. Downward and outward traction, counter clockwise rotation, upward traction

29–23. Which of the following pelvic types is generally
associated with persistent occiput posterior position?

    a. Android

    b. Gynecoid

    c. Anthropoid

    d. Platypelloid

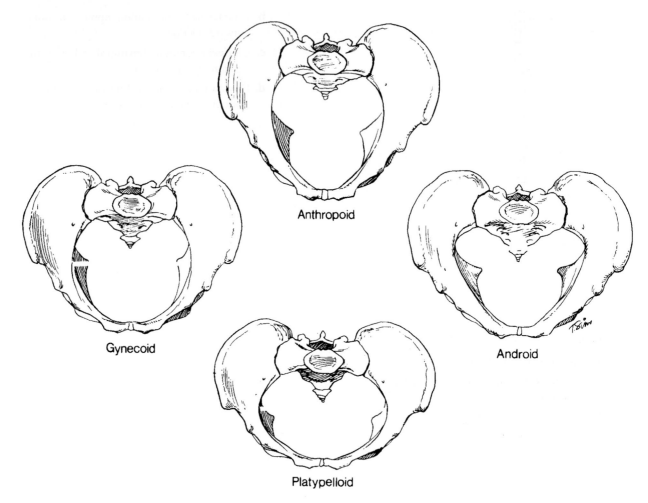

Anthropoid

Gynecoid

Android

Platypelloid

Modified with permission from Cunningham FG, Leveno KJ, Bloom SL, et al (eds): Maternal anatomy. In Williams Obstetrics, 24th ed. New York, McGraw-Hill, 2014, Figure 2-20.

29–24. Your primigravid patient at term has a completely dilated and effaced cervix, and the fetal head lies at +2 station. The fetal head position is right occiput posterior. The fetus begins to have severe variable decelerations with maternal pushing efforts. Her labor has not been augmented, her labor epidural is providing adequate analgesia, and her vital signs are normal. Despite attempts at maternal repositioning and oxygen supplementation, these variables persist and are deepening. All **EXCEPT** which of the following are suitable options?

　a. Perform vacuum extraction from occiput posterior position

　b. Manually rotate the head to occiput anterior position

　c. Perform vacuum rotation to occiput anterior position and then complete vacuum extraction

　d. Perform forceps rotation to occiput anterior position with Kielland forceps and then complete forceps delivery

29–25. Compared with forceps delivery from an occiput anterior position, which of the following is true of delivery from an occiput posterior position?

　a. Equal rates of episiotomy

　b. Lower rates of fetal Erb palsy

　c. Higher rates fetal facial palsy

　d. Equal rates of vaginal laceration

29–26. Which of the following describes the wandering technique of Kielland forceps blade placement for the left occiput transverse position?

　a. The anterior blade is swept up and around the fetal brow.

　b. The anterior blade is swept up and around the fetal occiput.

　c. The posterior blade is inserted under the symphysis and is swept down and around the fetal brow.

　d. The posterior blade is inserted under the symphysis and is swept down and around the fetal occiput.

29–27. Compared with soft cups for vacuum extraction, hard cups differ in which of the following regards?

　a. Lower scalp laceration rate

　b. Higher subgaleal hemorrhage rates

　c. Generation of greater traction force

　d. All of the above

29–28. Centering the vacuum cup over the flexion point provides which of the following advantages?

　a. Extends the fetal head

　b. Minimizes traction forces

　c. Delivers the smallest diameter through the pelvic outlet

　d. All of the above

29–29. Which of the following letters reflects the correct flexion point used for vacuum extraction? The color-coordinated larger circles reflect the actual cup placement for their respective flexion points.

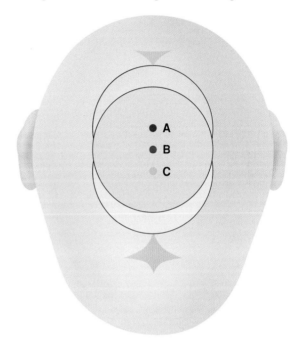

Modified with permission from Cunningham FG, Leveno KJ, Bloom SL, et al (eds): Operative vaginal delivery. In Williams Obstetrics, 24th ed. New York, McGraw-Hill, 2014, Figure 29-16.

　a. A

　b. B

　c. C

　d. None of the above

29–30. Which of the following is the preferred total negative pressure generated prior to initiation of traction during vacuum extraction?

　a. 0.2 kg/cm^2

　b. 0.8 kg/cm^2

　c. 1.2 kg/cm^2

　d. 1.6 kg/cm^2

29–31. With vacuum extraction, cup rotation, which generates torque, is avoided during traction to help avert all **EXCEPT** which of the following?

   a. Cephalohematoma

   b. Cup displacement

   c. Scalp laceration

   d. Retinal hemorrhage

29–32. Ideally, traction during vacuum extraction should be applied in which of the following manners?

   a. Continuously

   b. Intermittently and with contractions

   c. Intermittently and between contractions

   d. Intermittently with cycles of 20 seconds of traction followed by 1 minute of rest

CHAPTER 29 ANSWER KEY

Question number	Letter answer	Page cited	Header cited
29–1	c	p. 574	Indications
29–2	a	p. 574	Indications
29–3	b	p. 574	Classification and Prerequisites
29–4	c	p. 574	Classification and Prerequisites; Table 29-1
29–5	a	p. 574	Classification and Prerequisites; Table 29-1
29–6	a	p. 575	Table 29-1
29–7	d	p. 575	Table 29-1
29–8	a	p. 575	Morbidity
29–9	a	p. 575	Lacerations
29–10	d	p. 576	Pelvic Floor Disorders
29–11	d	p. 576	Acute Perinatal Injuries
29–12	a	p. 576	Acute Perinatal Injuries
29–13	d	p. 577	Long-Term Infant Morbidity
29–14	b	p. 577	Trial of Operative Vaginal Delivery
29–15	d	p. 577	Trial of Operative Vaginal Delivery; Technique
29–16	b	p. 578	Forceps Design
29–17	a	p. 578	Forceps Design
29–18	b	p. 578	Forceps Design
29–19	d	p. 582	Rotation from Occiput Transverse Positions
29–20	b	p. 578	Forceps Blade Application and Delivery
29–21	d	p. 578	Forceps Blade Application and Delivery
29–22	c	p. 578	Forceps Blade Application and Delivery
29–23	c	p. 580	Delivery of Occiput Posterior Positions
29–24	c	p. 580	Delivery of Occiput Posterior Positions
29–25	c	p. 580	Delivery of Occiput Posterior Positions
29–26	a	p. 582	Rotation from Occiput Transverse Positions
29–27	c	p. 583	Vacuum Extractor Design
29–28	c	p. 583	Technique
29–29	a	p. 583	Technique
29–30	b	p. 583	Technique
29–31	d	p. 583	Technique
29–32	b	p. 583	Technique

Cesarean Delivery and Peripartum Hysterectomy

30–1. By definition, the term *cesarean delivery* includes abdominal delivery of a fetus in all **EXCEPT** which of the following situations?

   a. Delivery of a stillborn infant

   b. Delivery of a previable infant

   c. Delivery of an abdominal pregnancy

   d. Delivery in a mother who has just died

30–2. The cesarean delivery rate has steadily increased during the past 30 years with the exception of what epoch. During this epoch, the vaginal birth after cesarean (VBAC) rate was increasing commensurate with a decreasing cesarean delivery rate?

   a. 1970–1978

   b. 1980–1988

   c. 1989–1996

   d. 2000–2008

30–3. Reasons for increasing use of cesarean delivery include all **EXCEPT** which of the following?

   a. Rising average maternal age

   b. Greater percentage of births to multiparas

   c. Declining use of operative vaginal delivery

   d. Increased use of electronic fetal monitoring

30–4. *Elective* cesarean deliveries are increasingly being performed for what indication?

   a. Maternal request

   b. Medically indicated preterm birth

   c. Concerns regarding pelvic floor injury

   d. All of the above

30–5. Although the indications for cesarean delivery are manifold, 85 percent are performed for four reasons. These principle indications include all **EXCEPT** which of the following?

   a. Labor dystocia

   b. Placenta previa

   c. Previous cesarean delivery

   d. Abnormal fetal presentation

30–6. Compared with planned primary vaginal delivery, the maternal risks associated with planned primary cesarean include which of the following?

   a. Higher morbidity and mortality rates

   b. Equivalent morbidity and mortality rates

   c. Higher morbidity but decreased mortality rates

   d. Higher morbidity but equivalent mortality rates

30–7. Compared with planned primary vaginal birth, potential maternal benefits of elective primary cesarean delivery include which of the following?

   a. Decreased risk for hemorrhage

   b. Decreased rehospitalization rate

   c. Decreased risk for thromboembolism

   d. Decreased rate of hysterectomy

30–8. A 21-year-old primigravida at 41 weeks' gestation is undergoing labor induction for oligohydramnios. She progresses to the second stage of labor, but the fetal head does not descend below 0 station despite 3 hours of pushing efforts. Cesarean delivery is undertaken but extraction is difficult and requires upward pressure from the vagina. A radiograph of the newborn head is shown here and reveals a depressed skull fracture (*white arrow*). Approximately what percentage of cesarean deliveries are complicated by some type of fetal injury?

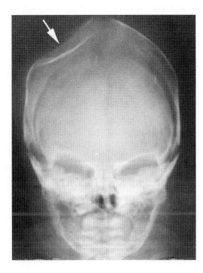

Reproduced with permission from Cunningham FG, Leveno KJ, Bloom SL, et al (eds): Diseases and injuries of the term newborn. In Williams Obstetrics, 24th ed. New York, McGraw-Hill, 2014, Figure 33-1.

a. 0.5%

b. 1%

c. 3%

d. 5%

30–9. Although controversial, cesarean delivery on maternal request should only be considered as an option when which of the following criteria have been met?

a. The mother plans to have three subsequent pregnancies.

b. There is a history of cerebral palsy in a previous child.

c. The pregnancy has reached at least 39 weeks' gestation.

d. The patient is concerned about inadequate pain control in labor.

30–10. Preoperative preparation for cesarean delivery should include all **EXCEPT** which of the following?

a. Administer an antacid

b. Place an indwelling bladder catheter

c. Place the supine woman in left lateral tilt

d. Shave pubic hair if it obstructs the operative field

30–11. Recommendations for antibiotic prophylaxis at cesarean delivery for women with a significant penicillin allergy include a single dose of which of the following agents?

a. Clindamycin

b. Levofloxacin

c. Clindamycin plus gentamicin

d. Clindamycin plus metronidazole

30–12. To reduce postoperative infectious morbidity, the American College of Obstetricians and Gynecologists recommends antibiotic prophylaxis be given within how many minutes prior to delivery?

a. 30

b. 60

c. 90

d. 120

30–13. When creating a Pfannenstiel incision, which vessels should be anticipated halfway between the skin and fascia, several centimeters from the midline?

a. External pudendal

b. Inferior epigastric

c. Superficial epigastric

d. Superficial circumflex iliac

30–14. Compared with a midline incision, a Pfannenstiel incision offers which of the following benefits?

a. Less postoperative pain

b. Improved cosmetic result

c. Decreased rates of fascial wound dehiscence

d. All of the above

30–15. When performing dissection through a Pfannenstiel incision, the two fascial layers are incised individually as is illustrated in this image. The first layer encountered, which is incised already in this image, is the aponeurosis of what muscle?

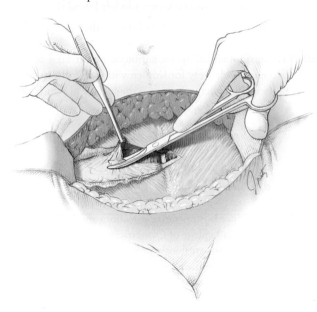

Reproduced with permission from Word L, Hoffman BL: Surgeries for benign gynecologic conditions. In Hoffman BL, Schorge JO, Schaffer JI, et al (eds): Williams Gynecology, 2nd ed. New York, McGraw-Hill, 2012, Figure 41-2.1.

   a. Transversalis

   b. External oblique

   c. Internal oblique

   d. Transversus abdominis

30–16. Transverse uterine incisions are generally preferred to vertical incisions for all **EXCEPT** which of the following reasons?

   a. Ease of closure

   b. Decreased rates of postpartum metritis

   c. Less likely to rupture in subsequent pregnancy

   d. Lower risk of incisional adhesions to bowel or omentum

30–17. Failure to recognize dextrorotation of the uterus prior to hysterotomy increases the risk of damage to what structure?

   a. Left ureter

   b. Right ureter

   c. Left uterine artery

   d. Right uterine artery

30–18. Caudad separation of the bladder from the lower uterine segment, as shown in the figure below, usually does not exceed 5 cm in depth. In what clinical situation, however, may extended dissection be recommended?

   a. Placenta previa

   b. Planned cesarean hysterectomy

   c. Second-stage cesarean delivery

   d. All of the above

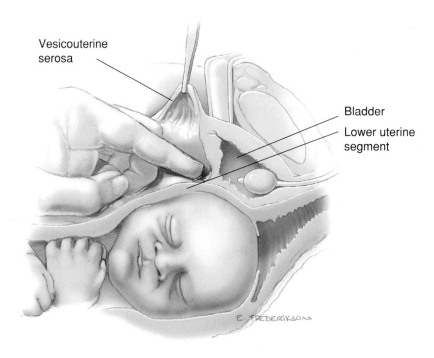

Reproduced with permission from Cunningham FG, Leveno KJ, Bloom SL, et al (eds): Cesarean delivery and peripartum hysterectomy. In Williams Obstetrics, 24th ed. New York, McGraw-Hill, 2014, Figure 30-3.

30–19. During cesarean delivery, a hysterotomy incision is made in the lower uterine segment, as shown here. In which of the following settings is it imperative to incise relatively higher on the uterus to avoid uterine vessel laceration or unintended entry into the vagina?

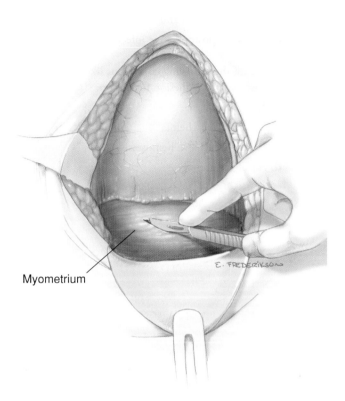

Myometrium

Reproduced with permission from Cunningham FG, Leveno KJ, Bloom SL, et al (eds): Cesarean delivery and peripartum hysterectomy. In Williams Obstetrics, 24th ed. New York, McGraw-Hill, 2014, Figure 30-4.

   a. An anemic mother
   b. A completely dilated cervix
   c. A breech-presenting fetus
   d. Cesarean performed prior to labor onset

30–20. Shown in the image below are two methods of extending the hysterotomy once the endometrial cavity has been entered. Compared with blunt extension, the use of bandage scissors for sharp extension has been associated with an increase in which of the following?

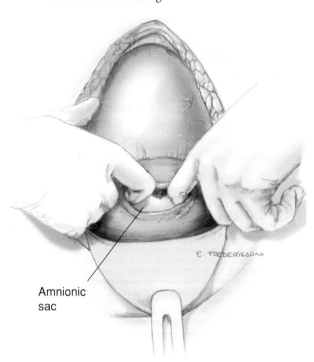

Amnionic sac

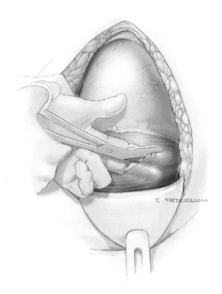

Reproduced with permission from Cunningham FG, Leveno KJ, Bloom SL, et al (eds): Cesarean delivery and peripartum hysterectomy. In Williams Obstetrics, 24th ed. New York, McGraw-Hill, 2014, Figure 30-5.

   a. Estimated blood loss
   b. Blood transfusion rate
   c. Postoperative infection rate
   d. None of the above

30–21. A 22-year-old primigravida undergoes a cesarean delivery for breech presentation. As the hysterotomy is being closed, her blood pressure is noted to be 82/40. The estimated blood loss is normal. Concentrated administration of which of the following could explain this finding?

a. Oxytocin

b. Methergine

c. Misoprostol

d. Tranexamic acid

30–22. Compared with manual extraction, spontaneous delivery of the placenta with fundal massage, as shown in the figure, has been shown to reduce the risk of which complication?

a. Retained placenta

b. Postpartum infection

c. Deep-vein thrombosis

d. Amnionic fluid embolism

30–23. Which of the following is a disadvantage of uterine exteriorization to repair the hysterotomy during cesarean delivery?

a. Increased blood loss

b. Increased operative injury rate

c. Increased nausea and vomiting rate

d. Increased postoperative infection rate

30–24. Which of the following conditions likely contributes to postoperative adhesion formation?

a. Infection

b. Local tissue ischemia

c. Failure to achieve hemostasis

d. All of the above

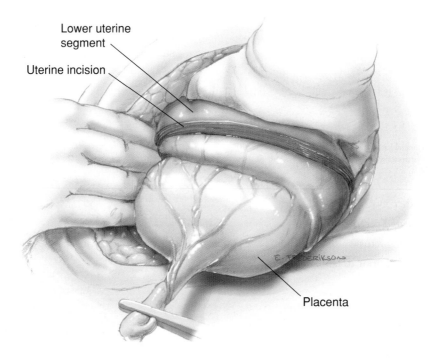

Reproduced with permission from Cunningham FG, Leveno KJ, Bloom SL, et al (eds): Cesarean delivery and peripartum hysterectomy. In Williams Obstetrics, 24th ed. New York, McGraw-Hill, 2014, Figure 30-9.

30–25. What is a potential advantage of closure of the parietal peritoneum prior to closure of the fascia?

   a. Less adhesion formation

   b. Shorter operative times

   c. Avoidance of distended bowel

   d. Decreased postoperative pain

30–26. Subcutaneous tissue greater than what depth should be closed with suture to avoid postoperative wound disruption?

   a. 2 cm

   b. 4 cm

   c. 6 cm

   d. 10 cm

30–27. All **EXCEPT** which of the following would be considered potential indications for a classical (vertical) hysterotomy?

   a. Cervical cancer

   b. Densely adhered bladder

   c. Back-up transverse fetal lie

   d. Significant maternal obesity

30–28. A 33-year-old G2P1 with one prior cesarean delivery presents at 35 weeks' gestation with active vaginal bleeding. She is taken emergently for repeat cesarean delivery and is found to have a placenta previa with accreta that requires cesarean hysterectomy. Compared with patients who have this procedure performed electively, this woman is at increased risk for which of the following complications?

   a. Bowel injury

   b. Urinary tract injury

   c. Venous thromboembolism

   d. All of the above

30–29. When performing the step shown in this image as a part of a peripartum hysterectomy, particular care must be taken to avoid injury to what structure?

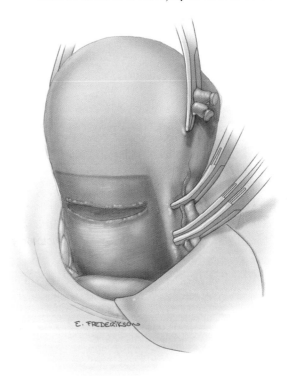

Reproduced with permission from Cunningham FG, Leveno KJ, Bloom SL, et al (eds): Cesarean delivery and peripartum hysterectomy. In Williams Obstetrics, 24th ed. New York, McGraw-Hill, 2014, Figure 30-18A.

   a. Ureter

   b. Bladder

   c. Urethra

   d. Sigmoid colon

30–30. When cystotomy complicates cesarean delivery, the bladder should be closed with a two- or three-layer running closure. Which layer is being closed in the image shown?

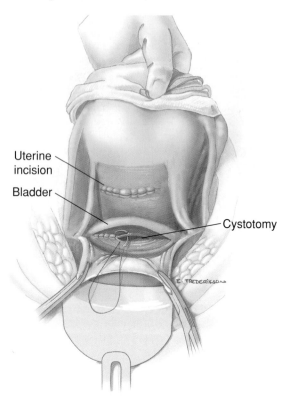

Reproduced with permission from Cunningham FG, Leveno KJ, Bloom SL, et al (eds): Cesarean delivery and peripartum hysterectomy. In Williams Obstetrics, 24th ed. New York, McGraw-Hill, 2014, Figure 30-23A.

    a. Mucosa

    b. Serosa

    c. Muscularis

    d. Visceral peritoneum

30–31. Women who have normal blood volume expansion and a hematocrit of at least 30 volume percent will usually tolerate blood loss up to what volume without hemodynamic compromise?

    a. 2000 mL

    b. 3000 mL

    c. 4000 mL

    d. 5000 mL

30–32. Although fluid sequestration in the "third space" is not typically seen in women who undergo cesarean delivery, this extracellular fluid sequestration can be problematic in women who have what pathological process?

    a. Sepsis

    b. Preeclampsia

    c. Excessive hemorrhage

    d. All of the above

CHAPTER 30 ANSWER KEY

Question number	Letter answer	Page cited	Header cited
30–1	c	p. 587	Introduction
30–2	c	p. 587	Cesarean Delivery in the United States
30–3	b	p. 587	Cesarean Delivery in the United States
30–4	d	p. 587	Cesarean Delivery in the United States
30–5	b	p. 587	Cesarean Delivery Indications and Risks
30–6	a	p. 588	Maternal Mortality and Morbidity
30–7	a	p. 588	Maternal Mortality and Morbidity
30–8	b	p. 589	Neonatal Morbidity
30–9	c	p. 589	Patient Choice in Cesarean Delivery
30–10	d	p. 590	Perioperative Care
30–11	c	p. 590	Infection Prevention
30–12	b	p. 590	Infection Prevention
30–13	c	p. 591	Abdominal Incision
30–14	d	p. 591	Abdominal Incision
30–15	b	p. 591	Transverse Incisions
30–16	b	p. 592	Hysterotomy
30–17	c	p. 592	Low Transverse Cesarean Section
30–18	b	p. 592	Low Transverse Cesarean Section
30–19	b	p. 592	Low Transverse Cesarean Section
30–20	a	p. 593	Uterine Incision
30–21	a	p. 594	Delivery of the Fetus
30–22	b	p. 596	Placental Delivery
30–23	c	p. 596	Uterine Repair
30–24	d	p. 597	Adhesions
30–25	c	p. 597	Abdominal Closure
30–26	a	p. 597	Abdominal Closure
30–27	c	p. 598	Classical Cesarean Incision—Indications
30–28	b	p. 599	Peripartum Hysterectomy—Indications
30–29	a	p. 600	Peripartum Hysterectomy—Technique
30–30	a	p. 604	Cystotomy
30–31	a	p. 604	Peripartum Management—Intravenous Fluids
30–32	d	p. 604	Analgesia, Vital Signs, Intravenous Fluids

CHAPTER 31

Prior Cesarean Delivery

31–1. What is the least common neonatal morbidity seen with elective repeat cesarean delivery?

a. Sepsis

b. Respiratory distress syndrome

c. Transient tachypnea of the newborn

d. None of the above

31–2. What is most the most common maternal complication seen with repeat cesarean delivery?

a. Transfusion

b. Hysterectomy

c. Wound infection

d. Deep-vein thrombosis

31–3. Which of the following contributes to a rising rate of primary cesarean delivery?

a. Maternal request

b. Reduced use of oxytocin

c. Increased rate of breech presentation

d. All of the above

31–4. A patient underwent a primary cesarean in her first pregnancy for a frank breech presentation at term. In general, what is the rate of successful vaginal delivery in a subsequent pregnancy in patients with this original indication?

a. 30%

b. 50%

c. 75%

d. 90%

31–5. The patient in Question 31–4 had this type of uterine incision at her first delivery. Which of the following statements is most accurate in planning the timing of her second pregnancy?

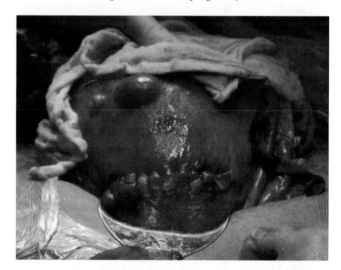

a. The risk of uterine rupture is unrelated to the interdelivery interval.

b. Lowest uterine rupture rates are seen in women who wait at least 24 months to become pregnant.

c. Interdelivery periods < 18 months are associated with a tripling of the uterine rupture risk.

d. None of the above

31–6. The patient in Question 31–5 returns for an initial prenatal care visit 12 months after her last delivery and is interested in vaginal birth with this pregnancy. When is the most appropriate time to begin discussion on this topic?

a. At the first prenatal visit

b. When the hospital consent is signed

c. When she is admitted to Labor and Delivery

d. None of the above

31–7. For the patient in Question 31–5, what is her absolute risk for uterine rupture if she chooses a trial of labor with a future pregnancy?

    a. 1/1000

    b. 7/1000

    c. 1/100

    d. 5/100

31–8. The patient in Question 31–5 also wants more information about neonatal risks. Which of the following statements regarding neonatal outcomes is most accurate?

    a. The perinatal death rate associated with a trial of labor is 1.3%.

    b. The perinatal mortality rate is 11 times greater if she chooses a trial of labor.

    c. Trial of labor is associated with a reduced risk for hypoxic ischemic encephalopathy.

    d. There is no difference in perinatal mortality rates if she chooses planned repeat cesarean section or trial of labor.

31–9. Sonographic examination of this pregnancy is done in the office with the following finding. Now, how should the patient be counseled regarding her risk of complications associated with vaginal birth after cesarean (VBAC)?

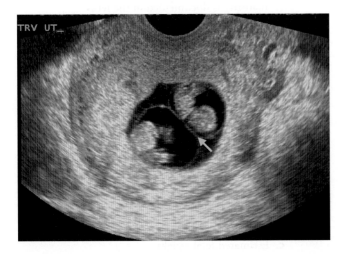

Reproduced with permission from Cunningham FG, Leveno KJ, Bloom SL, et al (eds): Multifetal gestation. In Williams Obstetrics, 23rd ed. New York, McGraw-Hill, 2010, Figure 39-7B.

    a. The risk for uterine rupture is not increased with this finding.

    b. A repeat cesarean section should be planned because of low rates of successful VBAC.

    c. Permitting an attempt at vaginal birth will depend on the gestational age at delivery.

    d. None of the above

31–10. What was the rate of cesarean delivery in the United States in 2011?

    a. 20%

    b. 26%

    c. 33%

    d. 38%

31–11. How does the risk of hysterectomy, uterine rupture, or operative injury change if a patient's attempt at vaginal delivery is unsuccessful and she undergoes a repeat cesarean delivery?

    a. Twofold higher

    b. Fivefold higher

    c. Tenfold higher

    d. No risk difference

31–12. Which of the following neonatal complications is more frequently seen in newborns following elective repeat cesarean delivery?

    a. 5-minute Apgar score < 7

    b. Hypoxic ischemic encephalopathy

    c. Transient tachypnea of the newborn

    d. Neonatal intensive care unit admission

31–13. The rate of which of the following is significantly increased in newborns of women attempting trial of labor compared with those delivered by repeat cesarean?

    a. Term neonatal death

    b. Intrapartum stillbirth

    c. Term hypoxic ischemic encephalopathy

    d. All of the above

31–14. The American College of Obstetricians and Gynecologists considers which of the following factors the most important in selecting a suitable candidate for trial of labor?

    a. Prior uterine incision type

    b. Infection at the time of the original surgery

    c. Gestational age at the time of the original surgery

    d. Degree of uterine distention during the current pregnancy

SECTION 8

31–15. How does the type of uterine closure seen in this image affect the risk of complications in a subsequent pregnancy?

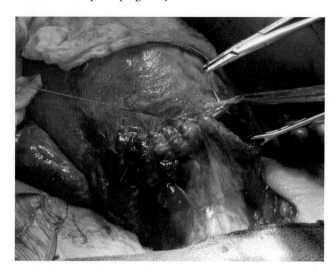

Used with permission from Dr. Donald Anderson.

    a. The risk of uterine rupture is reduced.

    b. The risk of uterine rupture is increased.

    c. The risk of uterine dehiscence is reduced.

    d. Data are unclear regarding the role that closure type plays in subsequent uterine rupture.

31–16. A nonpregnant patient presents with vaginal bleeding 7 months after having a primary cesarean delivery for arrest of descent during the second stage of labor. Transvaginal sonography reveals the finding below in this sagittal image of the uterus. Which of the following statements is accurate?

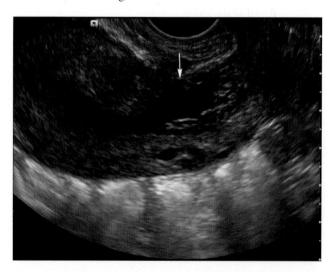

    a. Future pregnancies should be discouraged.

    b. She should undergo an exploratory laparotomy.

    c. Her risk for uterine rupture in a future pregnancy is increased.

    d. All of the above

31–17. Two years previously, your patient had the type of cesarean delivery depicted in the image below for a preterm twin gestation. She is currently pregnant with a singleton gestation. What do the authors feel is the optimal management plan for delivery in this scenario?

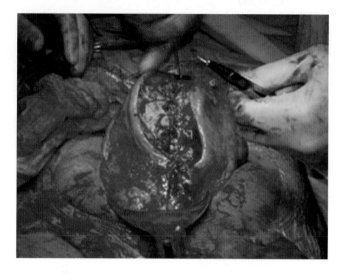

    a. Schedule a repeat cesarean delivery at 39 weeks' gestation

    b. Perform a repeat cesarean delivery when she presents in early labor

    c. Schedule a cesarean delivery as soon as pulmonary maturity is documented in the fetus

    d. Allow a trial of labor only if there is immediate availability of obstetrical and anesthesia staff in the hospital where she plans to deliver

31–18. A 28-year-old G3P2 underwent a primary low transverse cesarean delivery for a prolapsed cord at term in her last pregnancy. She is currently at 38 weeks' gestation, and her obstetrician estimates the fetal size to be 6½ lb. Her cervix is 2-cm dilated. What is the most favorable prognostic indicator that this patient will have a vaginal delivery?

    a. Cervical examination

    b. Obstetrical history

    c. Estimated fetal weight

    d. Indication for her prior cesarean delivery

31–19. What does the graph below suggest about the effect of maternal obesity on a successful vaginal birth after cesarean (VBAC) attempt?

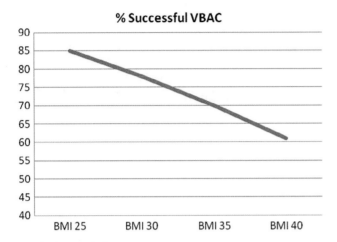

% Successful VBAC

BMI = Body mass index

a. Obesity has no effect on VBAC success rates.

b. The overall success rate for all women is 85%.

c. The success rate in women with a BMI of 35 is 70%.

d. The overall success rate for obese parturients is 60%.

31–20. Use of which of the following methods of labor induction is contraindicated in a patient with a prior cesarean delivery?

a. Oxytocin

b. Amniotomy

c. Misoprostol

d. None of the above

31–21. What is the most common sign of uterine rupture?

a. Abdominal pain

b. Vaginal bleeding

c. Loss of fetal station

d. Fetal heart rate decelerations

31–22. Which of the following is a valid reason to avoid epidural analgesia during labor in patients with prior cesarean delivery?

a. It may mask the signs of uterine scar dehiscence.

b. Higher doses of medication are required in women undergoing trial of labor.

c. It is associated with decreased success rates for vaginal birth after cesarean.

d. None of the above

31–23. During routine exploration of the lower uterine segment following a vaginal delivery in a patient with a previous cesarean delivery, the obstetrician discovers a defect in the myometrium. The patient's vital signs are stable, and she has a normal amount of vaginal bleeding. What is the most appropriate next step in the management of this patient?

a. Immediate exploratory laparotomy

b. Diagnostic laparoscopy 6 weeks postpartum

c. Abdominal computed tomography (CT) scan to assess the defect size

d. None of the above

31–24. What is the greatest risk factor for uterine dehiscence or incomplete uterine rupture?

a. Grand multiparity

b. Multifetal gestation

c. Prior cesarean delivery

d. Use of uterotonic agents

31–25. During uterine rupture, which of the following improves the chances of a neonate surviving and retaining normal neurological function?

a. Cephalic presentation

b. Intact fetal membranes prior to rupture

c. Location of placenta away from the rupture site

d. Reassuring fetal heart rate tracing prior to rupture

31–26. According to investigators from Utah, delivery within how many minutes following uterine rupture is associated with normal neonatal neurological outcomes?

a. 18 minutes

b. 30 minutes

c. 40 minutes

d. None of the above

31–27. When uterine rupture occurs, what is the risk for neonatal death?

a. 0.5%

b. 1%

c. 5%

d. 25%

31–28. While undergoing labor induction at 41 weeks' gestation, a primigravida has spontaneous uterine rupture that is repaired. How should she be counseled about the recurrence risk in future pregnancies?

 a. 2–3%

 b. 25–30%

 c. 50%

 d. No increase in risk

31–29. Which of the following obstetrical complications is **NOT** increased with the diagnosis shown in the following images?

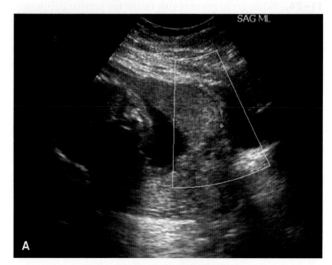

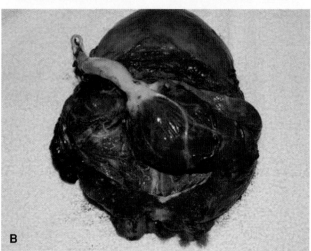

 a. Hemorrhage

 b. Hysterectomy

 c. Maternal mortality

 d. None of the above

31–30. Which of the following statements regarding the figure below is accurate?

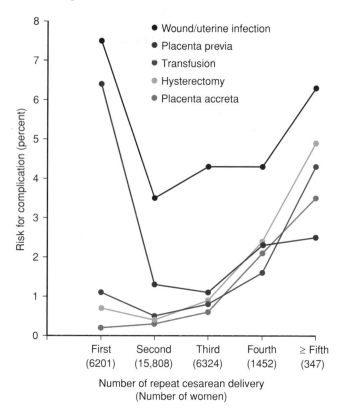

Reproduced with permission from Cunningham FG, Leveno KJ, Bloom SL, et al (eds): Prior cesarean delivery. In Williams Obstetrics, 24th ed. New York, McGraw-Hill, 2014, Figure 31-5.

 a. The risk for wound infection is halved with the second repeat cesarean delivery.

 b. Placenta previa complicates approximately 6% of first repeat cesarean deliveries.

 c. The risk of placenta accreta continues to increase as the number of repeat cesarean deliveries increases.

 d. All of the above

31–31. In this figure, the trend from 1989 to 1995 may be explained by which of the following?

  a. Increased demand for cesarean delivery by patients

  b. Increased numbers of pregnancies secondary to fertility treatments

  c. Increased awareness of risks of vaginal birth after cesarean delivery

  d. A recommendation from American College of Obstetricians and Gynecologists that most women with a previous low transverse cesarean section should attempt vaginal birth in a subsequent pregnancy

31–32. Which of the following statements regarding maternal deaths from uterine rupture is most accurate?

  a. Worldwide mortality rate from uterine rupture is < 1%.

  b. Individual maternal mortality risk can be predicted based on comorbidities.

  c. Rates for maternal mortality vary widely depending on availability of medical services.

  d. None of the above

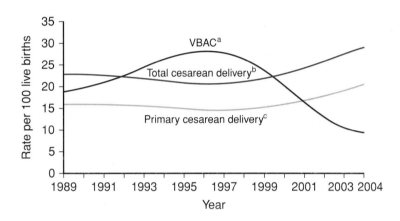

Reproduced with permission from Cunningham FG, Leveno KJ, Bloom SL, et al (eds): Prior cesarean delivery. In Williams Obstetrics, 23rd ed. New York, McGraw-Hill, 2010, Figure 26-1.

CHAPTER 31 ANSWER KEY

Question number	Letter answer	Page cited	Header cited
31–1	a	p. 615	Figure 31-3
31–2	c	p. 618	Figure 31-5
31–3	a	p. 609	100 Years of Controversy
31–4	d	p. 614	Indication for Prior Cesarean Delivery
31–5	c	p. 614	Interdelivery Intervals
31–6	a	p. 610	Factors That Influence a Trial of Labor
31–7	b	p. 610	Maternal Risks
31–8	b	p. 610	Maternal Risks
31–9	a	p. 614	Multifetal Gestations
31–10	c	p. 609	100 Years of Controversy
31–11	b	p. 610	Maternal Risks
31–12	c	p. 612	Fetal and Neonatal Risks
31–13	c	p. 611	Table 31-2
31–14	a	p. 612	Prior Incision Type
31–15	d	p. 612	Prior Incision Type
31–16	c	p. 614	Imaging of Prior Incision
31–17	c	p. 614	Prior Uterine Rupture
31–18	b	p. 614	Prior Vaginal Delivery
31–19	c	p. 615	Maternal Obesity
31–20	c	p. 615	Cervical Ripening and Labor Stimulation
31–21	d	p. 616	Epidural Analgesia
31–22	d	p. 616	Epidural Analgesia
31–23	d	p. 616	Uterine Scar Exploration
31–24	c	p. 617	Classification
31–25	c	p. 617	Decision-to-Delivery Time
31–26	a	p. 617	Decision-to-Delivery Time
31–27	c	p. 617	Decision-to-Delivery Time
31–28	b	p. 618	Hysterectomy versus Repair
31–29	d	p. 618	Complications with Multiple Repeat Cesarean Deliveries
31–30	d	p. 618	Figure 31-5
31–31	d	p. 609	100 Years of Controversy
31–32	c	p. 617	Decision-to-Delivery Time

THE NEWBORN

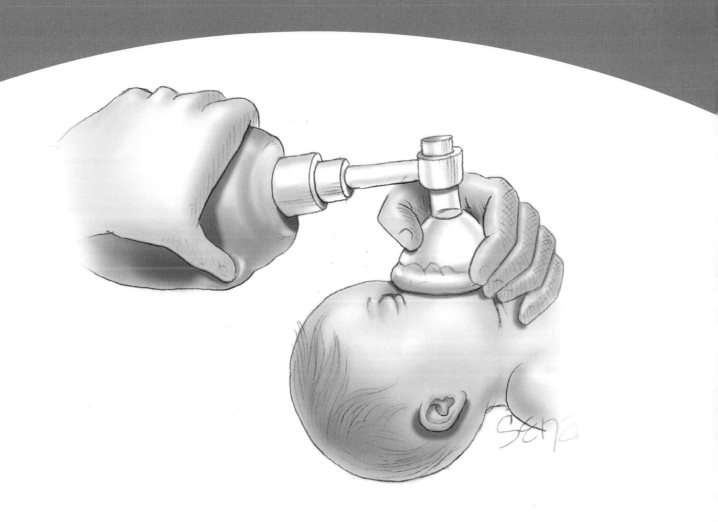

CHAPTER 32

The Newborn

32–1. Removal of fluid from the newborn respiratory tract occurs through which of the following mechanisms?

   a. Physical compression of the thorax

   b. Absorption of fluid into the pulmonary circulation

   c. Absorption of fluid into the pulmonary lymphatic system

   d. All of the above

32–2. Which of the following events aids in closure of the ductus arteriosus in the newborn?

   a. Fall in pulmonary arterial pressure

   b. Thoracic compression during delivery

   c. Postnatal accumulation of carbon dioxide

   d. Increased compression of pulmonary vasculature

32–3. Delayed removal or absorption of amnionic fluid from the pulmonary system results in which of the following conditions?

   a. Respiratory distress syndrome

   b. Persistent pulmonary hypertension

   c. Transient tachypnea of the newborn

   d. Premature closure of the ductus arteriosus

32–4. What type of cell produces surfactant in the fetal lung?

   a. Type I pneumocytes

   b. Type II pneumocytes

   c. Smooth muscle cells

   d. Squamous epithelial cells

32–5. A 25-year-old primigravida explains to her obstetrician that she is considering a home delivery with a local midwife. Which of the following is an accurate statement regarding home births?

   a. Neonatal death rates are doubled for infants born at home.

   b. One in 10 neonates born at home needs extensive resuscitation.

   c. When patients are properly selected, neonatal complication rates are not increased.

   d. None of the above

32–6. What differentiates secondary apnea from primary apnea in the newborn?

   a. It is resolved with simple stimulation.

   b. It is accompanied by a fall in heart rate.

   c. Clinical signs are markedly different for the two conditions.

   d. Respiratory efforts will not spontaneously resume without intervention.

32–7. A multiparous patient with rapid labor has moderate staining of her amnionic fluid with meconium. She received a single 50-mg dose of meperidine intravenously for pain relief. Following variable decelerations to 90 beats per minute (bpm) with pushing, she delivers the neonate. What is the first step in newborn resuscitation?

   a. Administer naloxone (Narcan)

   b. Bulb suction the oropharynx

   c. Warm, dry, and stimulate the newborn

   d. Prophylactically intubate and suction

32–8. The newborn in Question 32–7 has a heart rate of 80 bpm and gasping respirations. Which of the following should be the next step of resuscitation?

   a. Intubation and room air administration

   b. Positive pressure ventilation with room air

   c. Positive pressure ventilation with 50% oxygen

   d. Nasal continuous airway pressure with 28% oxygen

32–9. Which of the following scenarios is an indication for endotracheal intubation?

   a. Gestational age < 28 weeks

   b. Heart rate < 100 bpm for > 60 seconds

   c. Heart rate < 100 bpm for > 30 seconds

   d. Meperidine administration 1 hour prior to delivery

32–10. Which of the following demonstrates correct placement of the endotracheal tube in the neonate?

   a. Symmetric chest wall motion

   b. Equal breath sounds bilaterally

   c. Absence of gurgling sounds in epigastrium

   d. All of the above

32–11. Where is the correct location of fingers during chest compressions in the neonate?

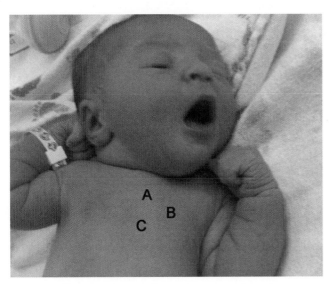

Used with permission from Stephanie Raynish.

    a. A

    b. B

    c. C

    d. None of the above

32–12. What is the correct ratio of chest compressions to breaths per minute in the term neonate?

    a. 30 compressions: 90 breaths

    b. 45 compressions: 15 breaths

    c. 90 compressions: 30 breaths

    d. 60 compressions: 30 breaths

32–13. Despite ventilatory support and chest compressions, the neonatal heart rate is 45 bpm. What is the appropriate management?

    a. Increase respiratory rate

    b. Administer intramuscular naloxone

    c. Administer intravenous fluid bolus

    d. Administer endotracheal epinephrine

32–14. Which of the following is **NOT** an element of the Apgar score?

    a. Cry

    b. Color

    c. Muscle tone

    d. Respiratory effort

32–15. Which of the following is **NOT** an appropriate use of the 1- and 5-minute Apgar scores?

    a. Prognostic indicator of neonatal survival

    b. Prognostic indicator of long-term neurologic outcome

    c. Measure of effectiveness of neonatal resuscitation effort

    d. All of the above are appropriate uses

32–16. Which of the following conditions may influence the Apgar score?

    a. Immaturity

    b. Maternal infection

    c. Medication administration

    d. All of the above

32–17. A 25-year-old primigravida with gestational hypertension has new-onset vaginal bleeding that is accompanied by fetal decelerations. She undergoes an emergency cesarean delivery, and the placental findings below are noted. According to the American College of Obstetricians and Gynecologists and the American Academy of Pediatrics, which of the following would support the diagnosis of hypoxia-induced metabolic acidemia?

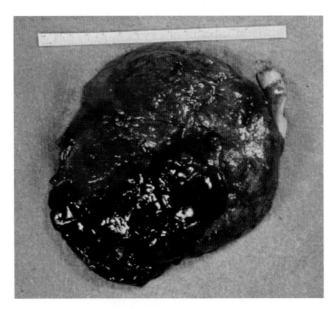

Reproduced with permission from Cunningham FG, Leveno KJ, Bloom SL, et al (eds): Obstetrical hemorrhage. In Williams Obstetrics, 23rd ed. New York, McGraw-Hill, 2010, Figure 35-5.

    a. 5-minute Apgar score of 2

    b. Umbilical artery pH of 7.05

    c. Transient tachypnea of the newborn

    d. Neonatal seizure in the first 24 hours of life

32–18. Which of the following actions is critical in obtaining an appropriate umbilical blood sample for acid-base analysis?

   a. The specimen is collected in a heparinized syringe.

   b. The specimen must be immediately placed on ice until testing is performed.

   c. The specimen is best obtained from sampling of the arteries on the fetal surface of the placenta.

   d. The cord segment used for the sample is isolated immediately following delivery of the placenta.

32–19. How does the normal result of an umbilical venous sample of cord blood differ from that of an umbilical arterial sample?

   a. The pH is higher.

   b. The P_{CO_2} is higher.

   c. The base excess is higher.

   d. None of the above.

32–20. Metabolic acidemia at birth is most closely linked to long-term neurological outcome in which of the following circumstance?

   a. When the birthweight is < 1000 g

   b. When infant has a 5-minute Apgar < 7

   c. When the gestational age at delivery is < 36 weeks

   d. When the mother is a known group B *Streptococcus* carrier

32–21. According to the American College of Obstetricians and Gynecologists, which of following is **NOT** an indication for cord blood gas determination?

   a. Twin gestation

   b. Maternal thyroid disease

   c. Vaginal bleeding before delivery

   d. Abnormal fetal heart rate tracing during labor

32–22. Which of the following regimens is **NOT** recommended prophylaxis for the condition shown here?

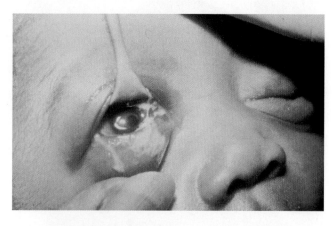

Reproduced with permission from Levsky ME, DeFlorio P: Ophthalmologic conditions. In Knoop KJ, Stack LB, Storrow AB, et al (eds): The Atlas of Emergency Medicine, 3rd ed. New York, McGraw-Hill, 2010, Figure 2-1.

   a. 1% tetracycline ophthalmic ointment

   b. 1% silver nitrate ophthalmic solution

   c. 0.5% erythromycin ophthalmic ointment

   d. 300-mg ceftriaxone intramuscular injection

32–23. Neonatal conjunctivitis can follow vaginal delivery in a mother with an active chlamydial infection. Which of the following is a true statement regarding chlamydial conjunctivitis?

   a. 1% of newborns born to women with active chlamydial infections will develop conjunctivitis.

   b. Prophylaxis for gonorrheal conjunctivitis adequately conveys protection against chlamydial infection.

   c. Prophylactic ophthalmic treatment for chlamydial conjunctivitis does not reliably reduce the incidence of the disease.

   d. Treatment of newborn chlamydial infection consists of a single dose of ceftriaxone 100 mg/kg given intravenously or intramuscularly.

32–24. During her prenatal course, a patient is discovered to be positive for both the hepatitis B surface antigen and the e antigen. Which of the following is the appropriate evaluation and management for her newborn?

   a. Administer hepatitis B immune globulin immediately after delivery

   b. Test for neonatal hepatitis B antigen status to determine appropriate therapy

   c. Administer hepatitis B immune globulin and immunize against hepatitis B during hospital stay

   d. None of the above

32–25. What is the reason that vitamin K is administered to newborns within 1 hour of birth?

a. To enhance newborn bone development

b. To prevent vitamin K–dependent hemorrhagic disease of the newborn

c. To reduce the incidence of necrotizing enterocolitis in premature infants

d. To augment the lower vitamin K levels found in breast milk compared with those in commercial infant formulas

32–26. Which of the following is the most accurate statement regarding newborn screening?

a. The United States federal government mandates newborn screening.

b. Some newborn screening tests do not rely on hematologic testing.

c. All newborn screening tests are performed within the first 24 hours after delivery.

d. None of the above

32–27. A patient whose labor was complicated by chorioamnionitis and gestational hypertension returns to your office on postpartum day 5 to have her blood pressure checked. She brings her newborn and is concerned about the appearance of the umbilical cord stump, which is shown below. What is the appropriate response to her concern?

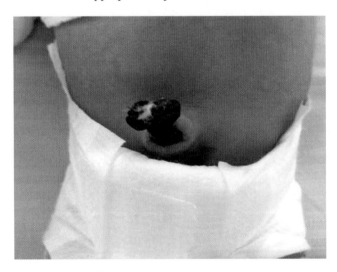

Used with permission from Kelly Buruca.

a. This is a normal finding, and no treatment is required.

b. There is concern for cord necrosis and a need for local resection.

c. This likely represents an infection of the cord, and antibiotics are indicated.

d. The patient should hasten the process by covering the remaining umbilical cord with petroleum jelly and gauze.

32–28. A patient who is exclusively breast feeding her infant is concerned because her child has lost 6 oz in the first 3 days of life. What advice should you give this patient?

a. Switch feedings entirely to a high-caloric infant formula

b. Expect the infant to regain its weight over the next week

c. Supplement the breast feedings with formula until the infant's weight stabilizes

d. None of the above

32–29. Meconium stooling in the delivery room suggests which of the following?

a. An imperforate anus

b. Intrapartum fetal distress

c. Gastrointestinal tract patency

d. Concurrent intrauterine infection

32–30. A reduced risk of which of the following is **NOT** a benefit of neonatal male circumcision?

a. Phimosis

b. Penile cancer

c. Endometrial cancer in female partner

d. Human immunodeficiency virus infection

32–31. Which of the following is **NOT** a recommended method of anesthesia for neonatal circumcision?

a. Local infiltration with lidocaine

b. Topical lidocaine-prilocaine cream

c. Dorsal penile block with lidocaine

d. Ring block with lidocaine and epinephrine

32–32. Which of the following are associated with reduced maternal postpartum lengths of stay?

a. Decreased neonatal mortality rates

b. Decreased neonatal infection rates

c. Increased neonatal readmission rates

d. Increased rates of exclusive breast feeding

CHAPTER 32 ANSWER KEY

Question number	Letter answer	Page cited	Header cited
32–1	d	p. 624	Initiation of Air Breathing
32–2	a	p. 624	Initiation of Air Breathing
32–3	c	p. 624	Initiation of Air Breathing
32–4	b	p. 624	Initiation of Air Breathing
32–5	a	p. 625	Newborn Resuscitation
32–6	d	p. 625	Newborn Resuscitation
32–7	c	p. 626	Figure 32-2
32–8	b	p. 625	Assessment at 30 Seconds of Life
32–9	b	p. 625	Assessment at 60 Seconds of Life
32–10	d	p. 626	Tracheal Intubation
32–11	c	p. 626	Chest Compressions
32–12	c	p. 626	Chest Compressions
32–13	d	p. 626	Epinephrine and Volume Expansion
32–14	a	p. 627	Table 32-1
32–15	b	p. 627	Apgar Score
32–16	d	p. 627	Apgar Score
32–17	d	p. 630	Metabolic Acidemia
32–18	a	p. 628	Umbilical Cord Blood Acid-Base Studies
32–19	a	p. 630	Table 32-2
32–20	a	p. 630	Metabolic Acidemia
32–21	c	p. 630	Recommendations for Cord Blood Gas Determinations
32–22	d	p. 631	Gonococcal Infection
32–23	c	p. 631	Chlamydial Infection
32–24	c	p. 631	Hepatitis B Immunization
32–25	b	p. 631	Vitamin K
32–26	b	p. 631	Newborn Screening
32–27	a	p. 632	Care of Skin and Umbilical Cord
32–28	b	p. 633	Feeding and Weight Loss
32–29	c	p. 633	Stools and Urine
32–30	c	p. 633	Newborn Male Circumcision
32–31	d	p. 633	Anesthesia for Circumcision
32–32	c	p. 634	Hospital Discharge

CHAPTER 33

Diseases and Injuries of the Term Newborn

33–1. Of the following, which is the most common cause of respiratory distress syndrome in a term infant?

  a. Severe asphyxia

  b. Meconium aspiration

  c. Elective cesarean delivery

  d. Perinatal infection with sepsis syndrome

33–2. Which of the following statements regarding intrapartum amnioinfusion is true?

  a. It improves the perinatal death rate.

  b. It decreases cesarean delivery rates.

  c. It prevents meconium aspiration syndrome.

  d. It has been used successfully in women with variable fetal heart rate decelerations.

33–3. Hyperalertness, irritability, and hyper/hypotonia define which level of hypoxic-ischemic encephalopathy?

  a. Mild

  b. Severe

  c. Moderate

  d. None of the above

33–4. Which form(s) of cerebral palsy result(s) from acute peripartum ischemia?

  a. Ataxia

  b. Spastic diplegia

  c. Spastic quadriplegia

  d. All of the above

33–5. Which of the following is **NOT** a risk factor for neonatal acidosis?

  a. Thick meconium

  b. General anesthesia

  c. Prior cesarean delivery

  d. Maternal age < 35 years

33–6. Which of the following is **NOT** strongly predictive of cerebral palsy?

  a. Perinatal infection

  b. Birthweight < 2000 g

  c. Obstetrical complication

  d. Birth earlier than 32 weeks' gestation

33–7. Which of the following statements regarding intrapartum fetal heart rate monitoring is true?

  a. There are no specific fetal heart rate patterns predictive of cerebral palsy.

  b. Evidence does not support its ability to predict or reduce cerebral palsy risk.

  c. An abnormal fetal heart rate pattern in fetuses that ultimately develop cerebral palsy may reflect a preexisting neurological abnormality.

  d. All are true.

33–8. Which of the following statements regarding Apgar scores and cerebral palsy is true?

  a. Survivors with Apgar scores of 0 at 10 minutes have surprisingly good outcomes.

  b. 1- and 5-minute Apgar scores are generally good predictors of long-term neurological impairment.

  c. With a 20-minute Apgar score of ≤ 2, there is a 60-percent mortality rate and a 57-percent cerebral palsy rate.

  d. All are true.

33–9. The threshold for clinically significant cord blood acidemia is which of the following?

  a. < 6.9

  b. < 7.0

  c. < 7.1

  d. < 7.2

33–10. Encephalopathy develops in 40 percent of newborns with a base deficit of which of the following?

  a. 8 to 10 mmol/L

  b. 10 to 12 mmol/L

  c. 12 to 16 mmol/L

  d. > 16 mmol/L

33–11. Regarding neuroimaging in the neonatal period, which of the following statements is true?

  a. Imaging precisely determines the timing of a brain injury.

  b. Sonographic studies are generally normal on the day of birth.

  c. Magnetic resonance imaging is most helpful at 2 weeks of life.

  d. Computed-tomography scans will detect abnormalities on the first day of life in term infants.

33–12. Which of the following is **LEAST** likely to cause isolated intellectual disability?

  a. Gene mutation

  b. Perinatal hypoxia

  c. Chromosomal abnormality

  d. Congenital malformation

33–13. According to the Centers for Disease Control and Prevention (2012), what is the frequency of autism in the United States?

  a. 0.1%

  b. 0.5%

  c. 1%

  d. 5%

33–14. According to the Centers for Disease Control and Prevention (2012), what is the frequency of attention deficit hyperactivity disorders in the United States?

  a. 1%

  b. 5%

  c. 7%

  d. 10%

33–15. After 35 weeks' gestation, what is the expected mean cord hemoglobin concentration?

  a. Less than 10 g/dL

  b. Less than 14 g/dL

  c. Approximately 17 g/dL

  d. Approximately 27 g/dL

33–16. Which of the following is **NOT** a cause of neonatal polycythemia?

  a. Chronic hypoxia

  b. Fetal liver trauma

  c. Fetal-growth restriction

  d. Twin-twin transfusion syndrome

33–17. Which of the following statements regarding serum bilirubin levels in newborns is true?

  a. Even in the mature newborn, serum bilirubin levels usually increase for 3 to 4 days.

  b. In preterm infants, the bilirubin level does not increase to the same extent as in term infants.

  c. In 25 percent of term newborns, bilirubin levels cause clinically visible skin color changes.

  d. Ten to 20 percent of neonates delivered at ≥ 35 weeks' gestation have a maximum serum bilirubin level > 20 mg/dL.

33–18. Which of the following is **NOT** a characteristic of acute bilirubin encephalopathy?

  a. Lethargy

  b. Hypotonia

  c. Spasticity

  d. Poor feeding

33–19. The mainstay of prevention and treatment of neonatal hyperbilirubinemia is which of the following?

  a. Ursodiol

  b. Hydration

  c. Phototherapy

  d. Exchange transfusions

33–20. Which of the following is **NOT** a vitamin K–dependent clotting factor?

    a. Factor III

    b. Factor V

    c. Factor VII

    d. Factor IX

33–21. What is recommended by the American Academy of Pediatrics and the American College of Obstetricians and Gynecologists for routine prophylaxis against hemorrhagic disease of the newborn?

    a. Vitamin K_1 1 mg intramuscularly

    b. Phytonadione 5 mg intravenously

    c. Phytonadione 25 mg by mouth once daily for two doses

    d. 2 mg elemental iron/kg/day by mouth divided into 1 to 3 doses

33–22. Which of the following statements regarding hemorrhagic disease of the newborn is true?

    a. It becomes apparent 4 to 6 months after birth.

    b. Mothers who took anticonvulsant drugs are at lower risk.

    c. It results from abnormally high levels of proteins C and S.

    d. The disorder is characterized by spontaneous internal or external bleeding beginning any time after birth.

33–23. Which of the following is associated with severe fetal thrombocytopenia?

    a. Preeclampsia

    b. Systemic lupus erythematosus

    c. Immunological thrombocytopenia

    d. Neonatal autoimmune thrombocytopenia

33–24. Which of the following types of neonatal intracranial hemorrhage is common and almost always benign?

    a. Subdural

    b. Intracerebellar

    c. Intraventricular

    d. Primary subarachnoid

33–25. Which of the following statements regarding the condition depicted in the figure below is true?

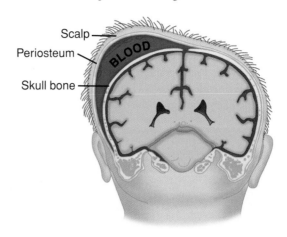

Reproduced with permission from Cunningham FG, Leveno KJ, Bloom SL, et al (eds): Diseases and injuries of the fetus and newborn. In Williams Obstetrics, 23rd ed. New York, McGraw-Hill, 2010, Figure 29-12.

    a. It enlarges rapidly.

    b. It resolves in hours.

    c. It is identified immediately at delivery.

    d. It results from laceration of the emissary or diploic veins.

33–26. Which of the following statements regarding the condition depicted in the figure below is true?

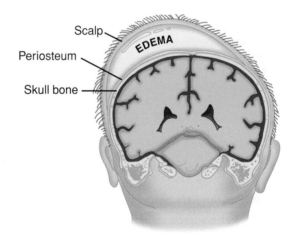

Reproduced with permission from Cunningham FG, Leveno KJ, Bloom SL, et al (eds): Diseases and injuries of the fetus and newborn. In Williams Obstetrics, 23rd ed. New York, McGraw-Hill, 2010, Figure 29-12.

    a. It is rare.

    b. It reaches maximum size at birth.

    c. It may persist for weeks to months.

    d. It becomes apparent hours after delivery.

33–27. A 33-year-old G1P0 at 42 weeks' gestation is delivered by cesarean for arrest of descent. The patient pushed for 3 hours without progressing past +1 station. At the time of cesarean, difficulty in delivering the head is encountered. Several different maneuvers are required to disimpact the head. After delivery, a radiograph is performed of the fetal head. It is provided below. Which of the following is **NOT** the likely etiology of the depressed skull fracture?

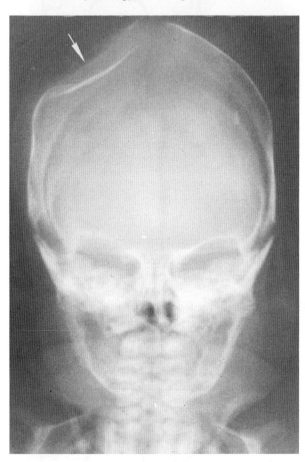

Reproduced with permission from Cunningham FG, Leveno KJ, Bloom SL, et al (eds): Diseases and injuries of the fetus and newborn. In Williams Obstetrics, 23rd ed. New York, McGraw-Hill, 2010, Figure 29-14.

a. Forceful retraction of the bladder blade

b. Skull compression against the sacral promontory

c. Upward transvaginal hand pressure by an assistant

d. Pressure from the surgeon's hand as the head is lifted upward

33–28. Which of the following statements regarding birth injury of the brachial plexus is **NOT** true?

a. Nerve roots at C_{3-7} and T_1 are injured.

b. The incidence is 1.5/1000 vaginal deliveries.

c. Chances of recovery are good if there is no avulsion.

d. Risk factors include breech delivery and shoulder dystocia.

33–29. A 25-year-old G4P3 presents in active labor at 10 cm dilation. The fetal presentation is breech. She proceeds to deliver vaginally. After delivery, the right arm of the newborn is noted to be straight and internally rotated with the elbow extended and the wrists and fingers flexed. The affected nerve root is likely:

a. C_{2-3}

b. C_{3-4}

c. C_{5-6}

d. C_8-T_1

33–30. A 20-year-old G2P1 undergoes a forceps-assisted vaginal delivery for a nonreassuring fetal heart tracing. After delivery, the newborn is noted to have an asymmetric grimace. A photograph is provided below. Which nerve is most likely injured?

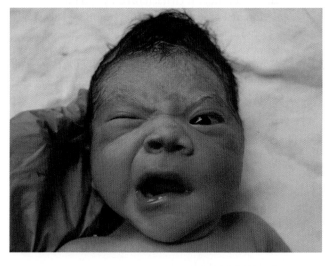

Reproduced with permission from Cunningham FG, Leveno KJ, Bloom SL, et al (eds): Diseases and injuries of the term newborn. In Williams Obstetrics, 24th ed. New York, McGraw-Hill, 2014, Figure 33-3.

a. Cranial nerve V

b. Cranial nerve VII

c. Cranial nerve IX

d. Cranial nerve XI

33–31. Which of the following birth fractures is the most
common?

  a. Femoral fracture

  b. Humeral fracture

  c. Clavicular fracture

  d. Mandibular fracture

33–32. The image below represents the most common
type of humeral fracture seen, frequently after an
uneventful birth. What is this type of fracture called?

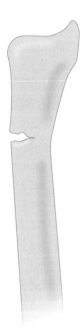

Reproduced with permission from Menkes JS: Initial evaluation and management of
orthopedic injuries. In Tintinalli JE, Stapczynski JS, Cline DM, et al (eds): Tintinalli's
Emergency Medicine: A Comprehensive Study Guide, 7th ed. New York, McGraw-Hill,
2011, Figure 264-2G.

  a. Torus

  b. Spiral

  c. Segmental

  d. Greenstick

References:

Centers for Disease Control and Prevention: Key findings: trends
in the prevalence of developmental disabilities in U.S. children
1997–2008. 2012. Available at: http://www.cdc.gov/ncbddd/features/
birthdefects-dd-keyfindings. html. Accessed June 6, 2013

CHAPTER 33 ANSWER KEY

Question number	Letter answer	Page cited	Header cited
33–1	d	p. 637	Respiratory Distress Syndrome
33–2	d	p. 638	Prevention
33–3	a	p. 639	Neonatal Encephalopathy
33–4	c	p. 639	Neonatal Encephalopathy
33–5	d	p. 640	Sentinel Event
33–6	c	p. 640	Incidence and Epidemiological Correlates
33–7	d	p. 641	Intrapartum Fetal Heart Rate Monitoring
33–8	c	p. 642	Apgar Scores
33–9	b	p. 642	Umbilical Cord Blood Gas Studies
33–10	d	p. 642	Umbilical Cord Blood Gas Studies
33–11	b	p. 642	Neuroimaging in Neonatal Period
33–12	b	p. 643	Intellectual Disability and Seizure Disorders
33–13	b	p. 643	Autism Spectrum Disorders
33–14	c	p. 643	Autism Spectrum Disorders
33–15	c	p. 643	Anemia
33–16	b	p. 643	Polycythemia and Hyperviscosity
33–17	a	p. 644	Hyperbilirubinemia
33–18	c	p. 644	Acute Bilirubin Encephalopathy and Kernicterus
33–19	c	p. 644	Prevention and Treatment
33–20	a	p. 644	Hemorrhagic Disease of the Newborn
33–21	a	p. 644	Hemorrhagic Disease of the Newborn
33–22	d	p. 644	Hemorrhagic Disease of the Newborn
33–23	d	p. 644	Thrombocytopenia
33–24	d	p. 646	Table 33-5
33–25	d	p. 646	Extracranial Hematomas
33–26	b	p. 646	Extracranial Hematomas
33–27	a	p. 647	Skull Fractures
33–28	a	p. 648	Brachial Plexopathy
33–29	c	p. 648	Brachial Plexopathy
33–30	b	p. 648	Facial Paralysis
33–31	c	p. 648	Facial Paralysis
33–32	d	p. 648	Fractures

CHAPTER 34

The Preterm Newborn

34–1. Neonates born prematurely compared with term newborns have higher associated rates of which of the following?

   a. Congenital malformations

   b. Necrotizing enterocolitis

   c. Bronchopulmonary dysplasia

   d. All of the above

34–2. Following birth, neonatal alveoli must rapidly clear amnionic fluid and remain expanded to permit gas exchange. All **EXCEPT** which of the following assist this transition?

   a. Lymphatic absorption of amnionic fluid

   b. Pulmonary vasculature absorption of amnionic fluid

   c. Chest compression by the vaginal walls during delivery

   d. Surfactant-related increases in alveolar surface tension

34–3. Clinical signs of respiratory distress syndrome include all **EXCEPT** which of the following?

   a. Grunting

   b. Hypertension

   c. Respiratory acidosis

   d. Chest wall retraction during inspiration

34–4. A 30-week newborn displays grunting, nasal flaring, chest retractions, and diminished oxygen saturation. Chest radiography shows a moderate left pneumothorax, seen here. In general, all **EXCEPT** which of the following should be included in the initial differential diagnosis of respiratory distress in a preterm neonate?

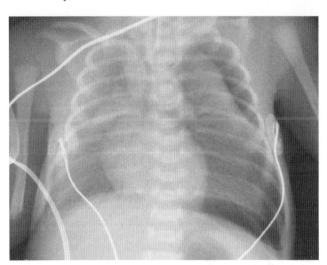

   a. Sepsis

   b. Diaphragmatic hernia

   c. Bronchopulmonary dysplasia

   d. Persistent fetal circulation

34–5. With respiratory distress syndrome, as shown here, a chest radiograph will most likely display which of the following?

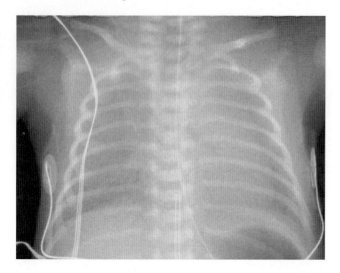

a. Perihilar infiltrate
b. Diffuse reticulogranular infiltrate
c. Increased central bronchovascular markings
d. Honeycomb pattern with or without air-fluid levels

34–6. Once diagnosed, respiratory distress syndrome is preferably treated with which of the following?

a. Intravenous corticosteroids
b. High inspired-oxygen concentration
c. High-frequency oscillatory ventilation
d. All the above

34–7. All **EXCEPT** which of the following are available surfactant products for use in humans?

a. Exosurf (synthetic)
b. Infasurf (calf-derived)
c. Survanta (bovine-derived)
d. Surfamet (murine-derived)

34–8. Your patient delivers her son prematurely at 27 weeks' gestation. He develops respiratory distress syndrome, and his neonatologist plans treatment with surfactant. You counsel her that among its benefits, prophylactic surfactant lowers subsequent rates of all **EXCEPT** which of the following?

a. Pneumonitis
b. Pneumothorax
c. Neonatal death
d. Bronchopulmonary dysplasia

34–9. To lower rates of respiratory distress syndrome, the American College of Obstetricians and Gynecologists (ACOG) recommends antenatal corticosteroid therapy for women at risk of preterm delivery at what gestational ages?

a. 20–30 weeks
b. 22–32 weeks
c. 24–34 weeks
d. 26–36 weeks

34–10. After 34 weeks' gestation, approximately what percentage of newborns develops respiratory distress syndrome?

a. 0.5%
b. 4%
c. 9%
d. 16%

34–11. Complications of hyperoxia used to treat respiratory distress syndrome typically include all **EXCEPT** which of the following?

a. Pulmonary hypertension
b. Necrotizing enterocolitis
c. Retinopathy of prematurity
d. Bronchopulmonary dysplasia

34–12. A 35-year-old G3P2 with two prior cesarean deliveries presented for her initial prenatal visit at 28 weeks' gestation. Her fundal height measured 30 cm, and a sonographic evaluation performed at that time yielded measurements that were concurrent with her last menstrual period. She desires repeat cesarean delivery and has now reached 40 weeks' gestation without spontaneous labor onset. Suitable measures for fetal lung maturity include all **EXCEPT** which of the following?

a. Lamellar body count
b. Surfactant – albumin ratio
c. Lecithin – sphingomyelin ratio
d. Mature type II pneumocyte – type I pneumocyte ratio

34–13. Clinical settings that may alter lecithin – sphingomyelin assessment of fetal lung maturity include all **EXCEPT** which of the following?

a. Blood-stained amnionic fluid
b. Meconium-stained amnionic fluid
c. Maternal corticosteroid administration
d. Elevated fetal fibronectin concentrations in amnionic fluid

34–14. Values greater than what lecithin – sphingomyelin ratio threshold indicate fetal lung maturity?

a. 2

b. 4

c. 6

d. 10

34–15. This diagram shows the normal rise in the concentration of lecithin relative to that of sphingomyelin. At what gestational age does this begin?

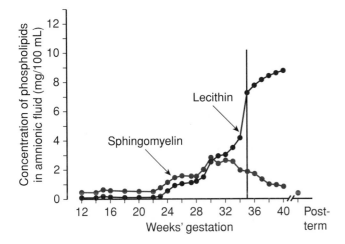

Reproduced with permission from Cunningham FG, Leveno KJ, Bloom SL, et al (eds): The preterm newborn. In Williams Obstetrics, 24th ed. New York, McGraw-Hill, 2014, Figure 34-1.

a. 24 weeks

b. 28 weeks

c. 30 weeks

d. 34 weeks

34–16. Lamellar bodies are counted in amnionic fluid samples to assess fetal lung maturity. These phospholipid storage organelles are derived from which of the following?

a. Amniocytes

b. Type II pneumocytes

c. Syncytiotrophoblast

d. Pulmonary endothelium

34–17. Which of the following are common clinical findings in a preterm neonate with necrotizing enterocolitis?

a. Bloody stools

b. Scaphoid abdomen

c. Hyperperistalic colon

d. None of the above

34–18. With retinopathy of prematurity, which of the following is the ultimate step leading to blindness?

a. Retinal detachment

b. Vitreous humor hemorrhage

c. Retinal neovascularization

d. Retinal vessel vasoconstriction

34–19. Which of the following modalities is initially preferred to identify brain abnormalities in the newborn?

a. Sonography

b. Computed tomography

c. Magnetic resonance imaging

d. Positron emission tomography

34–20. In addition to subdural hemorrhage, the other main neonatal intracranial hemorrhage categories include all **EXCEPT** which of the following?

a. Cephalohematoma

b. Subarachnoid hemorrhage

c. Intracerebellar hemorrhage

d. Peri- or intraventricular hemorrhage

34–21. This coronal sonographic image is from a neonate born at 26 weeks' gestation. In preterm newborns, which cerebral lesion, shown here (*asterisk*), is strongly associated with adverse neurodevelopmental outcomes?

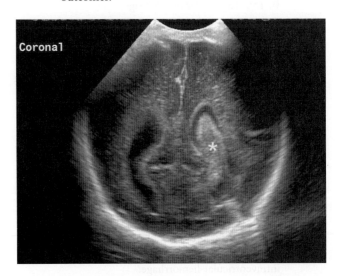

a. Subdural hemorrhage

b. Subgaleal hemorrhage

c. Intraventricular hemorrhage

d. None of the above

34–22. Because of the ventricular dilatation shown in the image from Question 34–21, which grade best describes this hemorrhage?

a. I

b. II

c. III

d. IV

34–23. Which of the following is the most grave sequela in those who survive intraventricular hemorrhage?

a. Proliferative gliosis

b. Ependymal cell atrophy

c. Periventricular leukomalacia

d. Choroidal neovascularization

34–24. Approximately what percentage of all neonates born before 34 weeks' gestation will have evidence of intraventricular hemorrhage?

a. 0.5

b. 10

c. 30

d. 50

34–25. Several organizations recommend antenatal corticosteroid therapy for women at risk for preterm delivery to prevent which of the following?

a. Neonatal death

b. Intraventricular hemorrhage

c. Respiratory distress syndrome

d. All of the above

34–26. In addition to corticosteroids, which of the following has the greatest evidence supporting its efficacy antenatally to reduce the sequelae of periventricular hemorrhage?

a. Vitamin K

b. Vitamin E

c. Indomethacin

d. Magnesium sulfate

34–27. Which of the following obstetrical practices has been shown to be superior to lower the rate of intraventricular hemorrhage?

a. Forceps delivery

b. Cesarean delivery

c. Spontaneous vaginal delivery

d. None is superior

34–28. Which of the following statements about periventricular leukomalacia is true?

a. It is associated with cerebral palsy.

b. Cyst size does not correlate with risk of cerebral palsy.

c. Cysts seen on neuroimaging studies require approximately 2 days to develop.

d. All of the above

34–29. Which of the following types of cerebral palsy is the least common?

a. Diplegia

b. Hemiplegia

c. Spastic quadriplegia

d. Choreoathetoid types

34–30. Preterm neonates are most susceptible to brain ischemia and periventricular leukomalacia. This stems from which of the following vascular limitations of prematurity?

a. A fine cortical capillary network that limits blood flow

b. Poor anastomoses between cortical and ventricular vascular systems

c. Vessels with underdeveloped tunica media and poor autoregulation

d. Vessels with a low density of receptors specific for adrenergic vasodilators

34–31. Which of the following are underlying risks for periventricular leukomalacia?

a. Ischemia

b. Perinatal infection

c. Intraventricular hemorrhage

d. All of the above

CHAPTER 34 ANSWER KEY

Question number	Letter answer	Page cited	Header cited
34–1	d	p. 653	Introduction
34–2	d	p. 653	Respiratory Distress Syndrome
34–3	b	p. 653	Clinical Course
34–4	c	p. 653	Clinical Course
34–5	b	p. 653	Clinical Course
34–6	c	p. 654	Treatment
34–7	d	p. 654	Surfactant Prophylaxis
34–8	a	p. 654	Surfactant Prophylaxis
34–9	c	p. 654	Antenatal Corticosteroids
34–10	b	p. 654	Antenatal Corticosteroids
34–11	b	p. 654	Complications
34–12	d	p. 655	Amniocentesis for Fetal Lung Maturity
34–13	d	p. 655	Lecithin-Sphingomyelin Ratio
34–14	a	p. 655	Lecithin-Sphingomyelin Ratio
34–15	d	p. 655	Lecithin-Sphingomyelin Ratio
34–16	b	p. 655	Other Tests
34–17	a	p. 655	Necrotizing Enterocolitis
34–18	a	p. 656	Retinopathy of Prematurity
34–19	a	p. 656	Brain Disorders
34–20	a	p. 656	Intracranial Hemorrhage
34–21	c	p. 656	Periventricular-Intraventricular Hemorrhage
34–22	c	p. 657	Incidence and Severity
34–23	c	p. 656	Pathology
34–24	d	p. 657	Incidence and Severity
34–25	d	p. 657	Prevention with Antenatal Corticosteroids
34–26	d	p. 657	Other Preventative Methods
34–27	d	p. 657	Other Preventative Methods
34–28	a	p. 656	Periventricular-Intraventricular Hemorrhage; Periventricular Leukomalacia
34–29	d	p. 657	Cerebral Palsy
34–30	b	p. 658	Ischemia
34–31	d	p. 657	Cerebral Palsy

CHAPTER 35

Stillbirth

35–1. In the United States, which of the following gestational ages has the lowest associated fetal mortality rate per 1000 births?

    a. 20 weeks

    b. 30 weeks

    c. 39 weeks

    d. 42 weeks

35–2. In the United States, the definition of a fetal death includes all **EXCEPT** which of the following characteristics?

    a. Death occurs prior to fetal expulsion.

    b. No signs of life are apparent at birth.

    c. Induced terminations of pregnancy are excluded.

    d. It applies only to gestational ages greater than 14 weeks.

35–3. Reporting requirements for fetal deaths are determined by which level of government?

    a. Local

    b. State

    c. County

    d. Federal

35–4. The fetal mortality rate has declined since 1990 for which of the following gestational age ranges?

    a. < 20 weeks

    b. 20–27 weeks

    c. > 28 weeks

    d. None of the above

35–5. A 41-year-old G6P5 presents for fetal sonographic evaluation at 19 weeks' gestation. The following image is obtained, which demonstrates an absent calvarium (an arrow indicates the chin and asterisks mark the eyes). Her medical history is significant for poorly controlled hypertension and diabetes. Her obstetrical history is significant for having a previous child with Down syndrome and a major cardiac defect. Which of the following conditions likely contributed to this particular fetal anomaly?

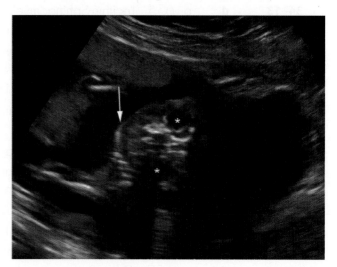

    a. Diabetes mellitus

    b. Advanced maternal age

    c. History of an anomalous infant in a prior pregnancy

    d. History of an aneuploid infant in a prior pregnancy

35–6. The patient from Question 35–5 declines intervention. She represents at 35 weeks' gestation for a prenatal care visit and is found to have a stillbirth. Induction is undertaken, and she delivers the infant pictured below. Based on the Stillbirth Collaborative Research Writing Group's categories, how would this stillbirth be classified with regard to the underlying cause?

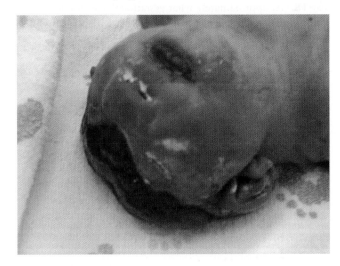

Used with permission from Dr. Tiffany Woodus.

    a. Unknown

    b. Possible

    c. Probable

    d. None of the above

35–7. After a systematic evaluation, approximately what percentage of stillbirths could be assigned a cause in the Stillbirth Collaborative Research Network study (2011)?

    a. 25%

    b. 50%

    c. 75%

    d. 90%

35–8. Referencing the study from Question 35–7, what was the categorical leading cause of fetal death?

    a. Infection

    b. Fetal malformations

    c. Placental abnormalities

    d. Obstetrical complications

35–9. All **EXCEPT** which of the following are recognized risk factors for antepartum stillbirth?

    a. Smoking

    b. Multiparity

    c. African American race

    d. Advanced maternal age

35–10. Determining the cause of a stillbirth via systematic evaluation can be important for which of the following reasons?

    a. Helps parents cope with the loss

    b. May prompt a specific therapy

    c. Allows for more accurate counseling regarding recurrence risk

    d. All of the above

35–11. A 40-year-old G5P4 presents at 28 weeks' gestation with complaints of contractions and vaginal bleeding. Her blood pressure is 166/98, and heavy proteinuria is found on urinalysis. Her cervix is 8 cm dilated, and there is active vaginal bleeding. No fetal heart tones can be found, and a stillbirth is confirmed by sonographic examination. She is stabilized, has a vaginal delivery, and the placenta is noted to have the following appearance. What is the most common associated risk factor for this condition?

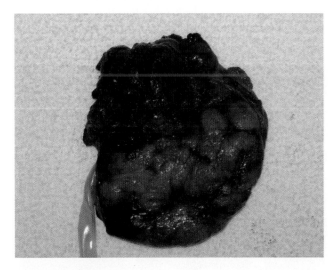

    a. High parity

    b. Hypertension

    c. Family history

    d. Advanced maternal age

35–12. For the patient presented in Question 35–11, what additional testing is recommended?

    a. Autopsy

    b. Karyotyping

    c. Examination of the fetus

    d. All of the above

35–13. For the patient presented in Question 35–11, what additional maternal blood test might be useful in this particular clinical situation?

    a. Kleihauer-Betke staining

    b. Serum glucose measurement

    c. Lupus anticoagulant testing

    d. Anticardiolipin antibody testing

35–14. The American College of Obstetricians and Gynecologists recommends karyotyping of stillborns with which of the following characteristics?

a. Those with morphologic anomalies

b. Those born to women of advanced maternal age

c. Those whose serum screening tests indicated an increased risk for aneuploidy

d. All stillborns

35–15. Acceptable specimens for cytogenetic analysis from a stillborn include all **EXCEPT** which of the following?

a. A placental block

b. A fetal skin specimen

c. A fetal patella specimen

d. An umbilical cord segment

35–16. If parents decline an autopsy, in addition to a fetogram shown here, other tests that can aid determination of the cause of death include all **EXCEPT** which of the following?

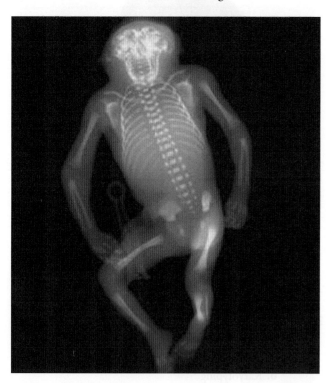

a. Photography

b. Viral culture

c. Chromosomal studies

d. Magnetic resonance imaging

35–17. Almost half of all fetal deaths are associated with what pregnancy complication?

a. Preeclampsia

b. Oligohydramnios

c. Fetal malformations

d. Fetal-growth restriction

35–18. At approximately what gestational age should antenatal testing begin in women with a history of a stillbirth in a prior pregnancy?

a. 26 weeks

b. 28 weeks

c. 30 weeks

d. 32 weeks

35–19. For women with an unexplained stillbirth in a previous pregnancy, recommendations for delivery planning would include an induction of labor at what gestational age in a well-dated pregnancy?

a. 37 weeks

b. 38 weeks

c. 39 weeks

d. 40 weeks

References:

Stillbirth Collaborative Research Network Writing Group: Causes of death among stillbirths. JAMA 306(22):2459, 2011

CHAPTER 35 ANSWER KEY

Question number	Letter answer	Page cited	Header cited
35–1	b	p. 661	Introduction
35–2	d	p. 661	Definition of Fetal Mortality
35–3	b	p. 661	Definition of Fetal Mortality
35–4	c	p. 661	Definition of Fetal Mortality; Figure 35-3
35–5	a	p. 662	Causes of Fetal Death
35–6	c	p. 662	Causes of Fetal Death
35–7	c	p. 662	Causes of Fetal Death
35–8	d	p. 662	Causes of Fetal Death; Table 35-1
35–9	b	p. 662	Risk Factors for Fetal Death
35–10	d	p. 664	Evaluation of the Stillborn
35–11	b	p. 663	Table 35-1
35–12	d	p. 664	Clinical Examination
35–13	a	p. 664	Laboratory Evaluation
35–14	d	p. 664	Laboratory Evaluation
35–15	b	p. 664	Laboratory Evaluation
35–16	b	p. 665	Autopsy
35–17	d	p. 665	Management of Women with a Prior Stillbirth
35–18	d	p. 665	Management of Women with a Prior Stillbirth
35–19	c	p. 665	Management of Women with a Prior Stillbirth

THE PUERPERIUM

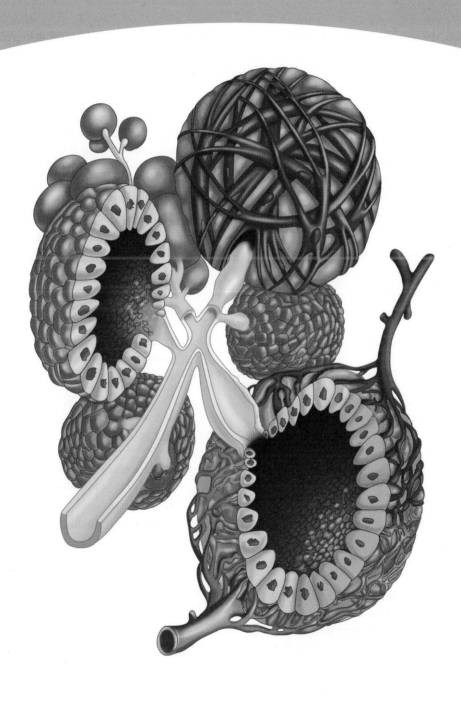

CHAPTER 36

The Puerperium

36–1. By definition, the puerperium lasts what time interval following delivery?

a. 3 weeks

b. 6 weeks

c. 9 weeks

d. 12 weeks

36–2. According to data from the Pregnancy Risk Assessment Surveillance System, which of the following concerns is most frequently expressed by women in the first 2 to 9 months postpartum?

a. Altered libido

b. Altered body image

c. Breast-feeding issues

d. Ability to return to work

36–3. Typically, one finger can easily be inserted through the internal cervical os for up to what time interval postpartum?

a. 3 days

b. 10 days

c. 21 days

d. 42 days

36–4. What interval following delivery is required for the typical uterus to complete involution?

a. 1 week

b. 4 weeks

c. 10 weeks

d. 16 weeks

36–5. Sonographically, approximately what percentage of women will have demonstrable uterine tissue or fluid in their endometrial cavity 2 weeks postpartum?

a. 20%

b. 40%

c. 60%

d. 80%

36–6. Your multigravid patient delivered 12 hours ago in a delivery with an estimated blood loss of 500 mL and without perineal laceration. Her epidural catheter has been removed, and she now complains of strong uterine contractions that accompany initial attempts at nursing. Her temperature is 37.0°C; pulse, 84 bpm; and blood pressure, 98/66 mm Hg. She has voided twice for a total of 800 mL. Her fundus is firm and minimal bright red blood is noted on her perineal pad. This clinical picture should prompt which of the following management plans?

a. Transvaginal sonography

b. Analgesia administration and reassurance

c. Hematocrit assessment and initiation of uterotonics

d. Hematocrit assessment and initiation of prophylactic broad-spectrum antibiotics

36–7. Lochia, in its various forms, typically resolves after how many weeks postpartum?

a. 1 week

b. 5 weeks

c. 9 weeks

d. 13 weeks

36–8. Which organism has been implicated in late postpartum hemorrhage?

a. *Escherichia coli*

b. *Neisseria gonorrhoeae*

c. *Mycoplasma genitalium*

d. *Chlamydia trachomatis*

36–9. Your patient is now 14 days postpartum following an uncomplicated vaginal delivery. She notes heavy vaginal bleeding and passage of clots. Her temperature is 37.1°C; pulse, 88 bpm; and blood pressure, 112/72 mm Hg. Physical findings reveal approximately 60 mL of clot in the vaginal vault, a closed cervical os, and a 12-week-size boggy nontender uterus. Her hematocrit has declined 2 volume percent from that measured following delivery and is 30 volume percent. A sagittal sonographic image of her uterus is shown here, and calipers measure the endometrial cavity. The most appropriate management for this patient includes which of the following?

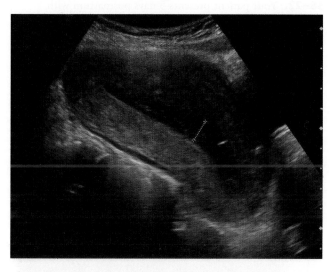

   a. Dilatation and curettage

   b. Methergine administration

   c. Uterine artery embolization

   d. Intravenous broad-spectrum antibiotics

36–10. Secondary postpartum hemorrhage is defined as bleeding from 24 hours to 12 weeks postpartum. It may be caused by all **EXCEPT** which of the following?

   a. Endomyometritis

   b. Placental abruption

   c. Abnormal involution

   d. Retained placental tissue

36–11. Your patient had a vaginal delivery yesterday complicated by a first-degree perineal laceration after a 12-hour labor. She is asymptomatic, afebrile, and has normal vital signs. Her uterus is firm and nontender. Her remaining physical examination is unremarkable. She has voided several times, and total urine output for the past 12 hours is 1400 mL. Her complete blood count from this morning reveals the following: hemoglobin, 9.8 g/dL; hematocrit, 31 volume percent; white blood cell count, 16,000/mm³; platelet count 118,000/mm³. Which of the following is the next best management step?

   a. Chest radiograph

   b. Urinalysis and urine culture

   c. Continue routine postpartum care

   d. Blood culture and intravenous broad-spectrum antibiotics

36–12. You counsel your puerperal patient that most women first approach their prepregnancy weight by which time interval following delivery?

   a. 2 months

   b. 6 months

   c. 12 months

   d. 24 months

36–13. Compared with colostrum, mature milk typically has greater amounts of which of the following per volume weight?

   a. Fat

   b. Protein

   c. Minerals

   d. All of the above

36–14. Concentrations of which two vitamins are reduced or absent from mature breast milk and require supplementation?

   a. Vitamins C and D

   b. Vitamins D and K

   c. Vitamins B₆ and K

   d. None of the above

36–15. Benefits of breast feeding include lower rates of all **EXCEPT** which of the following?

   a. Puerperal mastitis

   b. Maternal breast cancer

   c. Infant respiratory infections

   d. Maternal postpartum weight retention

36–16. All **EXCEPT** which of the following are included in the World Health Organization steps to successful breast feeding?

   a. Discourage breast feeding on demand by infants

   b. Initiate breast feeding within an hour of birth

   c. Inform all pregnant women about breast-feeding advantages

   d. Under no circumstances provide free-of-charge breast milk substitutes

36–17. Contraindications to breast feeding include maternal infection caused by which of the following viruses?

   a. Hepatitis C virus

   b. Genital herpes simplex virus

   c. Human immunodeficiency virus

   d. All of the above

36–18. To minimize neonatal drug exposure from maternal medications, which drug quality is preferred during selection?

   a. Long half-life

   b. Poor lipid solubility

   c. Superior oral absorption

   d. None of the above

36–19. All **EXCEPT** which of the following therapies are absolutely contraindicated during breast feeding?

   a. Methotrexate

   b. Thyroid radioablation

   c. Radionuclide imaging with technetium

   d. Selective serotonin-reuptake inhibitors

36–20. In a woman who chooses not to breast feed, treatment of bilateral breast engorgement that is associated with fever in the first few postpartum days is managed best with which of the following?

   a. Breast pumping

   b. Antibiotics with gram-positive coverage

   c. Antipyretic analgesia and breast binding

   d. All of the above

36–21. Your patient who is breast feeding presents 8 weeks postpartum with complaints of breast pain and associated mass that has enlarged during the last 2 weeks. A significantly tender, fluctuant nonerythematous mass is present. She is afebrile and has normal vital signs. Management of this patient should primarily include which of the following?

   a. Diagnostic excision

   b. Therapeutic needle aspiration

   c. Broad-spectrum antibiotic therapy

   d. Incision and drainage and antibiotics with primarily gram-positive coverage

36–22. Your patient presents 5 days postpartum with an axillary mass. She noted it during pregnancy, although it was much smaller. It became significantly larger and tender yesterday. Her face is shielded, and a sagittal photograph of her breast, axilla, and arm is shown below. She denies fever or other complaints. Management of this patient should primarily include which of the following?

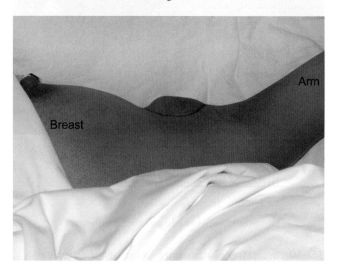

Used with permission from Dr. William Griffith.

   a. Needle aspiration

   b. Observation and reassurance

   c. Axillary lymph node excision

   d. Antibiotic therapy with primarily gram-positive coverage

36–23. All **EXCEPT** which of the following are typical components of in-hospital puerperal care?

   a. Encourage bed rest

   b. Monitor voiding frequency and volume

   c. Assess uterus regularly to confirm contracted tone

   d. Advance diet as tolerated for all puerperal patients

36–24. Your patient had a 3-hour second-stage labor and vaginal delivery without laceration. As her epidural analgesia subsides, she complains of perineal pain. Her temperature is 37.2°C; pulse, 84 bpm; and blood pressure, 120/68 mm Hg. Her first void yielded 300 mL of urine. Management of this patient should primarily include which of the following?

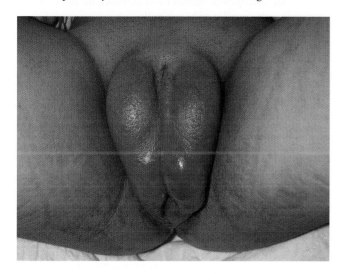

Used with permission from Dr. Marlene Corton.

   a. Perineal cool pack

   b. Surgical evacuation

   c. Diagnostic needle aspiration

   d. Broad-spectrum intravenous antibiotic therapy

36–25. Your patient is a multipara who developed a swollen anterior cervical lip during her protracted first- and second-stage labor. Immediately postpartum, the anterior lip was seen prolapsed past the introitus as shown here. How is this condition best managed?

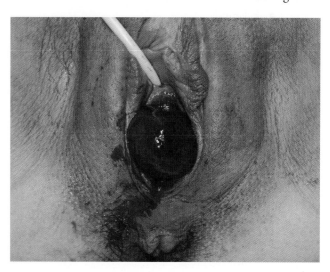

   a. Vaginal packing

   b. Strict bed rest and Foley catheter placement

   c. Digital replacement of the prolapse and observation for urinary retention

   d. All of the above

36–26. Which of the following is not associated with postpartum urinary retention?

   a. Prolonged labor

   b. Chorioamnionitis

   c. Oxytocin induction

   d. Perineal laceration

36–27. A depressed mood within the first week postpartum in a patient with no prior psychiatric history should prompt which of the following management plans?

   a. Observation

   b. Psychiatric admission

   c. Psychiatric consultation

   d. Initiation of antidepressant medications

36–28. Following spontaneous vaginal delivery, your patient complains of right leg weakness. Examination reveals an inability to flex the right hip and extend the leg. A common risk factor for this complication includes which of the following?

   a. Eclampsia

   b. Epidural anesthesia

   c. Prolonged second-stage labor

   d. Fourth-degree perineal laceration

36–29. Your multigravid patient delivered 5 hours ago in a precipitous delivery without perineal laceration. Her epidural catheter has been removed, and she now complains of pain with flexion or extension of either leg and with walking or weight bearing. She has normal lower extremity sensation and muscle strength. She is afebrile, vital signs are normal, and laboratory testing is unremarkable. Her pelvic radiograph is shown here. Management includes which of the following?

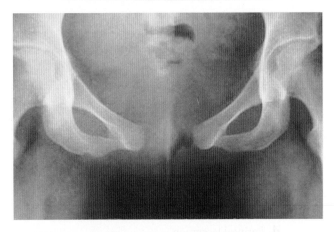

Reproduced with permission from Cunningham FG, Leveno KJ, Bloom SL, et al (eds): The puerperium. In Williams Obstetrics, 23rd ed. New York, McGraw-Hill, 2010, Figure 30-4.

   a. Supine bed rest

   b. Tightly fitted pelvic binder

   c. Surgery for all cases with separation > 3 cm

   d. All of the above

36–30. For women who are not breast feeding, menses will typically return during which time frame postpartum?

   a. 2–4 weeks

   b. 6–8 weeks

   c. 12–16 weeks

   d. 16–20 weeks

36–31. Correct statements regarding contraception in breast feeding women in general include which of the following?

   a. Depot medroxyprogesterone lowers the quality of breast milk.

   b. Estrogen-progestin birth control pills do affect the quality of breast milk.

   c. Progestin-only birth control pills do not affect the quantity of breast milk.

   d. Estrogen-progestin birth control pills do not affect the quantity of breast milk.

36–32. Because of deep-vein thrombosis risks, combination hormonal contraception should not be initiated sooner than how many weeks postpartum?

   a. 2 weeks

   b. 4 weeks

   c. 6 weeks

   d. 8 weeks

CHAPTER 36 ANSWER KEY

Question number	Letter answer	Page cited	Header cited
36–1	b	p. 668	Introduction
36–2	c	p. 669	Table 36-1
36–3	a	p. 668	Uterus
36–4	b	p. 668	Uterus
36–5	d	p. 669	Sonographic Findings
36–6	b	p. 670	Afterpains
36–7	b	p. 670	Lochia
36–8	d	p. 670	Subinvolution
36–9	b	p. 670	Late Postpartum Hemorrhage
36–10	b	p. 670	Late Postpartum Hemorrhage
36–11	c	p. 671	Hematological and Coagulation Changes
36–12	b	p. 671	Pregnancy-Induced Hypervolemia
36–13	a	p. 672	Breast Anatomy and Products
36–14	b	p. 672	Breast Anatomy and Products
36–15	a	p. 673	Immunological Consequences of Breast Feeding; Nursing
36–16	a	p. 674	Table 36-3
36–17	c	p. 674	Contraindications to Breast Feeding
36–18	b	p. 674	Drugs Secreted in Milk
36–19	d	p. 674	Drugs Secreted in Milk
36–20	c	p. 675	Breast Engorgement
36–21	b	p. 675	Other Issues with Lactation
36–22	b	p. 675	Other Issues with Lactation
36–23	a	p. 675	Hospital Care
36–24	a	p. 676	Perineal Care
36–25	c	p. 676	Perineal Care
36–26	b	p. 676	Bladder Function
36–27	a	p. 676	Pain, Mood, and Cognition
36–28	c	p. 676	Obstetrical Neuropathies
36–29	b	p. 676	Musculoskeletal Injuries
36–30	b	p. 678	Contraception
36–31	c	p. 678	Contraception
36–32	b	p. 678	Contraception

CHAPTER 37

Puerperal Complications

37–1. Infection causes what percentage of pregnancy-related deaths?

a. 1%

b. 6%

c. 11%

d. 22%

37–2. Which of the following is the most significant risk factor for the development of puerperal uterine infection?

a. Use of epidural

b. Length of labor

c. Route of delivery

d. Number of vaginal examinations

37–3. As a new, young obstetrician-gynecologist, you strive to avoid postcesarean infection in your patients. Which of the following interventions would be most helpful in this pursuit?

a. Changing scalpels after skin incision

b. Changing gloves after delivery of the fetal head

c. Single dose of antibiotics prior to skin incision

d. Copious irrigation of the abdomen before incision closure

37–4. Which of the following is **NOT** a risk factor for puerperal pelvic infection?

a. Obesity

b. General anesthesia

c. Advanced maternal age

d. Meconium-stained amnionic fluid

37–5. Organisms from which group have been implicated in late-onset, indolent metritis?

a. *Chlamydia*

b. *Pseudomonas*

c. *Clostridium*

d. *Staphylococcus*

37–6. You are called to the bedside of a 16-year-old primipara who underwent a cesarean delivery 28 hours ago for nonreassuring fetal status. She is complaining of abdominal cramps and chills. She has a fever of 38.7°C and is not tolerating oral intake. During examination, her lungs are clear, and breasts are soft. She does, however, have uterine and parametrial tenderness. Her hematocrit is stable, white blood cell count is 15,000 cells/μL, and urinalysis is unremarkable. Which of the following is the likely diagnosis?

a. Atelectasis

b. Postpartum metritis

c. Small bowel obstruction

d. Septic pelvic thrombophlebitis

37–7. The management of the patient in Question 37–6 should include all **EXCEPT** which of the following?

a. Antipyretics

b. Blood cultures

c. Intravenous fluids

d. Intravenous broad-spectrum antibiotics

37–8. After 72 hours of intravenous antibiotics, the patient in Question 37–6 has yet to defervesce. She continues to have fevers as high as 38.5°C. Which of the following is the **LEAST** likely explanation for her condition?

a. Drug fever

b. Infected hematoma

c. Parametrial phlegmon

d. Septic pelvic thrombophlebitis

37–9. The patient in Question 37–6 has been receiving intravenous gentamicin and clindamycin. Which of the following statements regarding this regimen is true?

   a. This regimen has a 50% to 60% response rate.

   b. If the gentamicin is administered once daily, serum levels will probably be inadequate.

   c. It may be ineffective in this patient if the offending organism group is *Enterococcus*.

   d. The gentamicin should be changed to metronidazole so *Clostridium difficile* is covered.

37–10. Which of the following statements regarding perioperative prophylaxis at the time of cesarean delivery is **NOT** true?

   a. Prophylactic antimicrobials reduce the pelvic infection rate by 70% to 80%.

   b. There is no benefit to prophylactic antimicrobials in cases of nonelective cesarean delivery.

   c. Single-dose prophylaxis with ampicillin or a first-generation cephalosporin is as effective as a multiple-dose regimen.

   d. Women known to be colonized with methicillin-resistant *Staphylococcus aureus* (MRSA) should be given vancomycin in addition to a cephalosporin.

37–11. Which of the following has been shown to prevent puerperal pelvic infections following cesarean delivery?

   a. Closure of the peritoneum

   b. Changing gloves after delivery of the placenta

   c. Prenatal treatment of asymptomatic vaginal infections

   d. Allowing the placenta to separate and deliver spontaneously

37–12. Which of the following is a risk factor for wound infection?

   a. Anemia

   b. Obesity

   c. Diabetes mellitus

   d. All of the above

37–13. A 29-year-old multipara presents to the emergency room 7 days after a cesarean delivery. She complains of drainage from her incision, fever, and nausea and vomiting. A photograph of her abdomen is provided. The patient's skin is erythematous, and malodorous pus is oozing from the right angle of the incision. Which of the following is the most appropriate management of this patient?

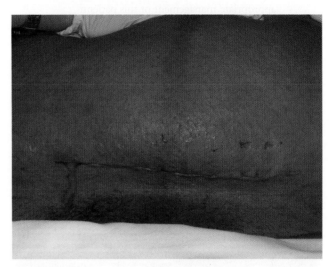

   a. Culture the wound and discharge her home with oral antimicrobial therapy

   b. Culture the wound, start intravenous antimicrobial therapy, open the skin incision fully, and pack with moist gauze

   c. Culture the wound, start intravenous antimicrobial therapy, open the skin incision fully, and place a wound vacuum device

   d. Culture the wound, start intravenous antimicrobial therapy, perform surgical exploration, and provide aggressive supportive care

37–14. For the patient in Question 37–13, you decide to administer intravenous broad-spectrum antimicrobial therapy and perform wound exploration and debridement in the operating room. Purulent material is noted to be issuing from below the fascia. For this reason, the fascia is opened. Pus is also draining from the uterine incision, and a photograph of her uterus is provided here. Which of the following is the most appropriate management of this patient?

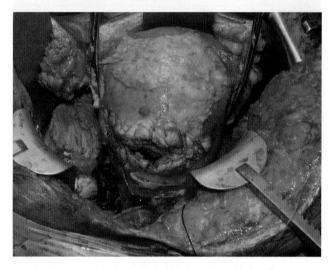

Reproduced with permission from Cunningham FG, Leveno KJ, Bloom SL, et al (eds): Puerperal complications. In Williams Obstetrics, 24th ed. New York, McGraw-Hill, 2014, Fig. 37-4.

a. Abdominal wash out and closure of the patient's fascia, subcutaneous layer, and skin

b. Hysterectomy, abdominal wash out, and closure of the patient's fascia without closure of the skin and subcutaneous layer

c. Debridement of the uterine incision, closure of the uterine incision, abdominal wash out, and closure of both the patient's fascia and superficial layers

d. Reapproximation of the uterine incision with delayed absorbable suture, abdominal wash out, and closure of the patient's fascia without closure of the skin and subcutaneous layer

37–15. Which of the following statements regarding parametrial phlegmon is true?

a. Phlegmons are usually bilateral.

b. Phlegmons typically do not involve the broad ligament.

c. Associated fever typically resolves in 5 to 7 days with antibiotic treatment but may persist longer.

d. A phlegmon should be considered when postpartum fever persists longer than 24 hours despite intravenous antimicrobial therapy.

37–16. An 18-year-old primigravida at 41 weeks' gestation presented to Labor and Delivery for decreased fetal movement. She was found to have oligohydramnios, and an induction of labor was initiated. Twenty-four hours later, the patient was 4 cm dilated with no cervical change for 4 hours, despite adequate contractions. In addition, the patient had been diagnosed with chorioamnionitis, and intravenous antimicrobial therapy was begun. A cesarean delivery was performed for failure to progress. Postpartum, the patient continued to have fever for 5 days despite treatment with intravenous ampicillin, gentamicin, and clindamycin. Which of the following is a reasonable next step in the management of this patient?

a. Surgical exploration to exclude abscess

b. Stop antibiotics and discharge the patient home

c. Continue current management for 5 additional days and then reassess

d. Further evaluate the patient using computed tomography (CT) or magnetic resonance (MR) imaging

37–17. You order a pelvic CT scan for the patient in Question 37–16. An image from that study is provided. What is the most likely diagnosis?

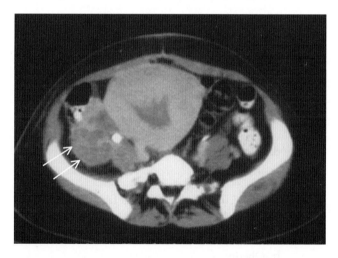

Reproduced with permission from Cunningham FG, Leveno KJ, Bloom SL, et al (eds): Puerperal complications. In Williams Obstetrics, 24th ed. New York, McGraw-Hill, 2014, Fig. 37-7.

a. Pelvic abscess

b. Psoas muscle abscess

c. Ovarian vein thrombosis

d. Retained products of conception

37–18. The patient in Question 37–17 appears quite well despite her continued fevers. Based on her CT findings, which of the following is the most appropriate management of this patient?

a. Continue antibiotics until she is afebrile

b. Stop antibiotics and discharge the patient home

c. Stop antibiotics and start lifelong anticoagulation

d. Continue antibiotics and start a 12-month course of anticoagulation

37–19. Which of the following statements regarding septic pelvic thrombophlebitis is true?

a. Patients complain of severe pain.

b. The overall incidence is 1/10,000 deliveries.

c. Intravenous heparin causes fever to dissipate.

d. The ovarian veins are involved because they drain the upper uterus and therefore, the placental implantation site.

37–20. What percentage of women with septic pelvic thrombophlebitis have clot extending into the vena cava?

a. 1%

b. 5%

c. 10%

d. 25%

37–21. A 22-year-old primipara presents to the emergency room 4 days after a forceps-assisted vaginal delivery complaining of intense perineal pain, fever, and a foul vaginal odor. During examination, infection and dehiscence of a fourth-degree laceration is noted. Which of the following is the most appropriate management of this patient?

a. Oral broad-spectrum antimicrobial therapy and outpatient reevaluation in 3 days

b. Intravenous antimicrobial therapy and hospital admission for observation and sitz baths

c. Intravenous antimicrobial therapy and hospital admission for surgical debridement and local wound care

d. Oral broad-spectrum antimicrobial therapy, placement of a Foley catheter with leg bag, daily sitz baths at home, and outpatient reevaluation in 2 days

37–22. Which of the following is **NOT** a risk factor for episiotomy dehiscence?

a. Smoking

b. Coagulation disorder

c. Human papillomavirus infection

d. Intrapartum antimicrobial therapy

37–23. The patient in Question 37–21 undergoes surgical debridement of her separated and infected fourth-degree laceration. A photograph taken at the end of the surgery is provided. To permit early reapproximation, which of the following is essential postoperatively?

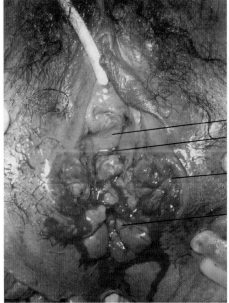

Anterior vaginal wall
Vaginal opening
Disrupted perineum
Rectal mucosa

Reproduced with permission from Cunningham FG, Leveno KJ, Bloom SL, et al (eds): Puerperal infection. In Williams Obstetrics, 23rd ed. New York, McGraw-Hill, 2010, Figure 31-7.

a. Sitz baths completed several times daily

b. Provision of adequate analgesia during each debriding wound scrub

c. A debriding wound scrub completed twice daily with povidone-iodine solution

d. All of the above

37–24. When is an infected episiotomy ready for early repair?

    a. 24 hours after debridement

    b. Once any improvement is seen in the tissue

    c. Once the patient becomes afebrile for 24 hours

    d. When the wound is free of infection and covered by pink granulation tissue

37–25. A 16-year-old primipara is brought to the emergency room three days after having a vaginal delivery. The girl is confused and lethargic. Her mother reports that she has had a fever at home associated with nausea, vomiting, diarrhea, and headache. During examination, you note very mild uterine tenderness and a diffuse macular erythematous rash. The patient is hypotensive, tachycardic, and febrile. Laboratory studies reveal leukocytosis, transaminitis, prolongation of her partial thromboplastin time (PTT), and an elevated creatinine level. Which of the following is the most likely diagnosis?

    a. Cyclospora

    b. Meningitis

    c. Viral hepatitis

    d. Toxic shock syndrome

37–26. When selecting antimicrobial therapy for the patient in Question 37–25, it is important that you select an agent that covers which of the following?

    a. *Staphylococcus aureus*

    b. Group A β-hemolytic *Streptococcus*

    c. Both of the above

    d. Neither of the above

37–27. When is suppurative mastitis most likely to develop?

    a. One week after delivery

    b. Two weeks after delivery

    c. Three weeks after delivery

    d. Eight weeks after delivery

37–28. Which of the following is **NOT** true regarding the symptoms of suppurative mastitis?

    a. Patients report severe pain.

    b. It is almost always bilateral.

    c. Marked engorgement usually precedes inflammation.

    d. Chills or rigor are soon followed by fever and tachycardia.

37–29. What percentage of women with mastitis develop an abscess?

    a. 1%

    b. 5%

    c. 10%

    d. 20%

37–30. A 20-year-old primipara presents to your office 4 weeks after a term spontaneous vaginal delivery. She is breast feeding and reports severe right breast pain. She had a fever at home of 101°F. The patient appears ill. You perform an examination and note a tender right breast fullness, which is warm and erythematous. A photograph is provided below. The patient reports feeding her baby every 3 hours, although the newborn latches poorly on the right breast. She has no complaints regarding her left breast, which appears normal. Which of the following is the most likely diagnosis?

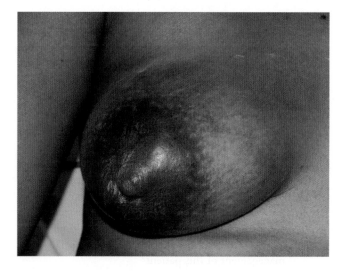

Used with permission from Dr. Emily Adhikari.

    a. Mastitis

    b. Engorgement

    c. Blocked milk duct

    d. Inflammatory breast cancer

37–31. Which of the following is the most appropriate management of the patient in Question 37–30?

a. Milk culture and mammogram

b. Analgesia and frequent breast feeding

c. Milk culture, breast sonography, initiation of antimicrobial therapy, analgesia, and breast feeding/pumping

d. Initiation of antimicrobial therapy, milk culture, and discontinuation of breast feeding or pumping on the right side

37–32. Sonographic examination of the right breast is performed. An image is provided. Which of the following is the most appropriate management of this patient?

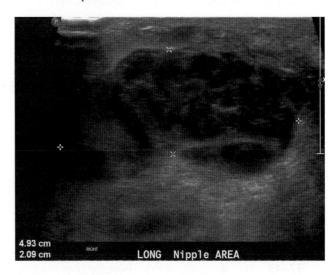

a. Breast biopsy

b. Surgical drainage

c. Increased breast feeding/pumping and discontinuation of antibiotics

d. Continuation of antibiotics for 48 hours with surgical drainage if the patient does not defervesce

CHAPTER 37 ANSWER KEY

Question number	Letter answer	Page cited	Header cited
37–1	c	p. 682	Puerperal Infections
37–2	c	p. 683	Predisposing Factors
37–3	c	p. 683	Cesarean Delivery
37–4	c	p. 683	Other Risk Factors
37–5	a	p. 683	Common Pathogens
37–6	b	p. 684	Pathogenesis and Clinical Course
37–7	b	p. 684	Treatment
37–8	a	p. 684	Treatment
37–9	c	p. 684	Choice of Antimicrobials
37–10	b	p. 685	Perioperative Prophylaxis
37–11	d	p. 685	Other Methods of Prophylaxis
37–12	d	p. 686	Abdominal Incisional Infections
37–13	d	p. 686	Necrotizing Fasciitis
37–14	b	p. 686	Necrotizing Fasciitis
37–15	c	p. 687	Parametrial Phlegmon
37–16	d	p. 688	Imaging Studies
37–17	c	p. 689	Figure 37-7
37–18	a	p. 688	Septic Pelvic Thrombophlebitis
37–19	d	p. 688	Septic Pelvic Thrombophlebitis
37–20	d	p. 688	Septic Pelvic Thrombophlebitis
37–21	c	p. 689	Perineal Infections
37–22	d	p. 689	Perineal Infections
37–23	d	p. 690	Table 37-3
37–24	d	p. 690	Early Repair of Infected Episiotomy
37–25	d	p. 690	Toxic Shock Syndrome
37–26	c	p. 690	Toxic Shock Syndrome
37–27	c	p. 691	Breast Infections
37–28	b	p. 691	Breast Infections
37–29	c	p. 691	Breast Infections
37–30	a	p. 691	Figure 37-8a
37–31	c	p. 691	Breast Infections—Management
37–32	b	p. 692	Breast Abscess

CHAPTER 38

Contraception

38–1. Which of the following is considered long-acting reversible contraception (LARC)?

    a. Copper intrauterine device

    b. Depot medroxyprogesterone acetate

    c. Combination hormonal contraceptive patch

    d. All of the above

38–2. What is the goal of the United States Medical Eligibility Criteria (US MEC) published by the Centers for Disease Control and Prevention?

    a. Guide contraceptive selection for women with comorbidities

    b. Provide legal criteria for contraception provision to minors

    c. Provide financial criteria for Medicaid contraception eligibility

    d. None of the above

38–3. With typical use, which of the following contraceptive methods has the highest failure rate within the first year of use?

    a. Withdrawal

    b. Spermicides

    c. Male condom

    d. Progestin-only pills

38–4. Of U.S. Food and Drug Administration (FDA)-approved intrauterine devices (IUDs), hormone-eluting devices release which of the following?

    a. Norgestimate

    b. Etonogestrel

    c. Norethindrone

    d. Levonorgestrel

38–5. Of U.S. FDA-approved intrauterine devices, which of the following has the longest duration of contraceptive efficacy?

    a. Paragard, copper intrauterine device

    b. Skyla, levonorgestrel-releasing intrauterine device

    c. Mirena, levonorgestrel-releasing intrauterine device

    d. Skyla and Mirena have equivalent durations of efficacy

38–6. The Skyla IUD can be differentiated from the other FDA-approved levonorgestrel-releasing IUD by which of the following characteristics?

    a. White, T-shaped frame

    b. Silver ring atop the stem

    c. Copper bracelets on the lateral T arms

    d. Single braided brown string attached to the T-frame base

38–7. Contraceptive efficacy with this method is believed to result from which of the following?

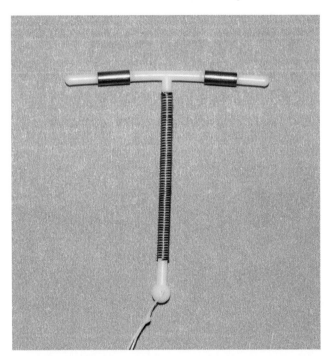

    a. Spermicidal action

    b. Ovulation inhibition

    c. Cervical mucus thickening

    d. All of the above

38–8. During insertion, which of the following increases this IUD-related complication?

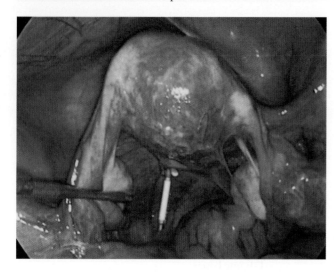

Used with permission from Dr. Kimberly Kho. Reproduced with permission from Werner CL, Moschos E, Griffith WF, et al (eds): Contraception. In Williams Gynecology, 2nd Edition Study Guide. New York, McGraw-Hill, 2012, Q5-9.

   a. Breast feeding

   b. Insertion during menses

   c. Midplane uterine position

   d. None of the above

38–9. Compared with the copper IUD, this intrauterine device offers which of the following long-term advantages?

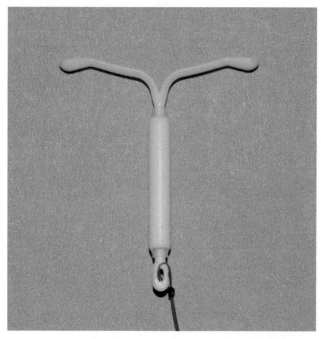

   a. Lower rates of menorrhagia

   b. Longer duration of effective use

   c. Lower rates of ovarian cyst formation

   d. None of the above

38–10. Your patient complains of lower abdominal ache in the months following placement of her IUD. During examination, no IUD strings are seen. Which of the following is the most appropriate next management step?

   a. Obtain KUB radiograph

   b. Reexamine her following her next menses

   c. Perform β-human chorionic gonadotropin (β-hCG) assay

   d. Attempt intrauterine IUD retrieval by means of an IUD hook or forceps

38–11. The patient in Question 38–10 has a negative β-hCG test result. Which of the following is the best next management step?

   a. Diagnostic laparoscopy

   b. Diagnostic hysteroscopy

   c. Transvaginal sonography

   d. Magnetic resonance imaging

38–12. Her sonographic images are shown here, and an arrow indicates a sagittal view of the IUD. Which of the following is the best next clinical step?

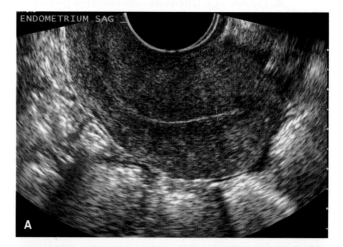

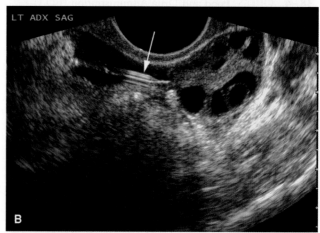

   a. Hysterectomy

   b. Diagnostic laparoscopy

   c. Dilation and curettage

   d. Operative hysteroscopy

38–13. Which of the following statements regarding IUD use and infection are correct?

  a. Prophylaxis with doxycycline 100 mg orally in a single dose is required prior to IUD insertion.

  b. Endocarditis prophylaxis is required for those with mitral valve prolapse prior to IUD insertion.

  c. Negative *Neisseria gonorrhoeae* and *Chlamydia trachomatis* test results are required prior to IUD insertion.

  d. None of the above

38–14. This photograph shows placental membranes following a term delivery. Antenatally, this pregnancy was at increased risk for which of the following?

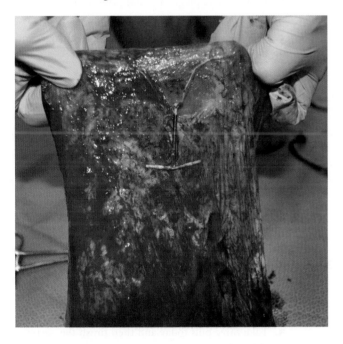

  a. Fetal malformations

  b. Intrauterine infection

  c. Fetal-growth restriction

  d. All of the above

38–15. An asymptomatic woman with 8 weeks of amenorrhea is found to have a positive pregnancy test result, strings of her Mirena IUD visible at the cervical os, and sonographic findings shown here. No adnexal pathology was seen sonographically. She desires to continue the pregnancy if possible. What is the most appropriate management for her?

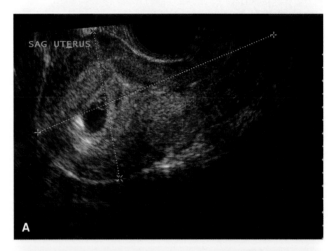

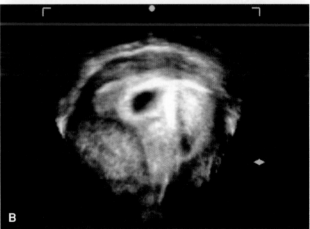

  a. IUD removal

  b. IUD removal and dilatation and curettage

  c. IUD removal and 10-day course of doxycycline

  d. Initiate folate and schedule first prenatal care visit for 2 weeks

38–16. If an intrauterine device is left in situ during pregnancy, what is the risk of this pregnancy complication?

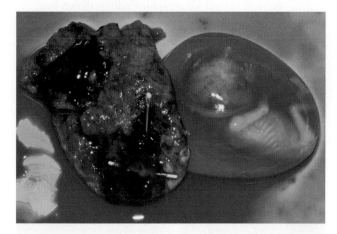

Used with permission from Dr. Clarice Grimes.

    a. 10%

    b. 25%

    c. 50%

    d. 75%

38–17. Which of is true regarding the timing of IUD insertion?

    a. May be inserted immediately following vaginal delivery

    b. May be inserted during the menstrual cycle follicular phase once pregnancy is excluded

    c. May be inserted immediately following dilation and curettage for first-trimester abortion

    d. All of the above

38–18. Which hormone is released from the contraceptive implant currently marketed in the United States?

    a. Norgestimate

    b. Etonogestrel

    c. Norethindrone

    d. Levonorgestrel

38–19. A new patient requests removal of her Implanon implant. You are unable to locate the device by palpation. What is the best next management step?

    a. Sonography

    b. Fluoroscopy

    c. Radiography

    d. Computed-tomography scanning

38–20. Which of the following is a suspected method of efficacy for progestin-containing contraceptive implants?

    a. Endometrial atrophy

    b. Ovulation inhibition

    c. Cervical mucus thickening

    d. All of the above

38–21. According to the US MEC, in addition to pregnancy and current breast cancer, which of the following are absolute contraindications to progestin-releasing implants?

    a. Prior cervical cancer and prior deep-vein thrombosis

    b. Prior ectopic pregnancy and prior deep-vein thrombosis

    c. Prior cervical cancer, prior ectopic pregnancy, and diagnosed depression

    d. None of above

38–22. Rates of which of the following are increased with use of extended cycle hormonal contraception compared with traditional cyclic hormonal contraception use?

    a. Headaches

    b. Escape ovulation

    c. Endometrial cancer

    d. Unpredictable bleeding

38–23. Your patient calls you on Monday stating that she missed taking her birth control pills during the weekend. All **EXCEPT** which of the following are true counseling statements?

    a. Take three pills today and then finish the current pill pack

    b. Take one pill today, finish the pill pack, but add a barrier method until her next menses

    c. Stop pills, use a barrier method until the next menses, then restart a new pack on first day of menses

    d. Discard current pill pack, start new pill pack today, but add an additional barrier method for 7 days

38–24. Drugs whose efficacy may be diminished by combination oral contraceptive pill use include which of the following?

    a. Lisinopril

    b. Macrodantin

    c. Acetaminophen

    d. Metoclopramide

38–25. Which of the following is not a physiologic effect exerted by the estrogen component of combination hormonal contraceptives?

  a. Elevated serum fibrinogen levels

  b. Lowered serum free testosterone levels

  c. Elevated serum follicle-stimulating hormone levels

  d. Lowered serum low-density-lipoprotein (LDL) cholesterol levels

38–26. If prescribing combination oral contraceptive pills to a woman with hypertension, which clinical criteria should be met?

  a. Nonsmoker

  b. Younger than 35 years

  c. Hypertension well controlled

  d. All of the above

38–27. Which of the following is not an absolute contraindication to initiation of combination oral contraceptive pills?

  a. Thrombotic disorders

  b. Two weeks postpartum

  c. Migraines with focal neurologic deficits

  d. Uncomplicated systemic lupus erythematosus with negative antiphospholipid antibody testing

38–28. The relative risk of which of the following cancers has been associated with current combination oral contraceptive pill use?

  a. Ovarian

  b. Melanoma

  c. Cervical

  d. Endometrial

38–29. A proven benefit of combination oral contraceptive pills includes which of the following?

  a. Increased bone density

  b. Improved cognitive memory

  c. Lowered total cholesterol levels

  d. Decreased rates of thromboembolism

38–30. With transdermal contraceptive patch use, the patch should be replaced how frequently?

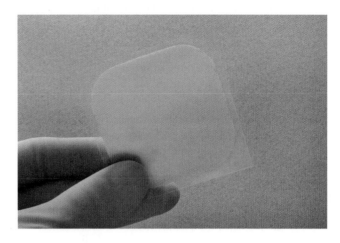

  a. Daily

  b. Weekly

  c. Twice weekly

  d. Every 3 weeks

38–31. With transdermal contraceptive patch use, contraceptive failure may occur in which of the following situations?

  a. Patient weight > 90 kg

  b. Concurrent penicillin antibiotic use

  c. Patch worn while in hot tub or sauna

  d. All of the above

38–32. With this method of contraception, a new ring is used how frequently?

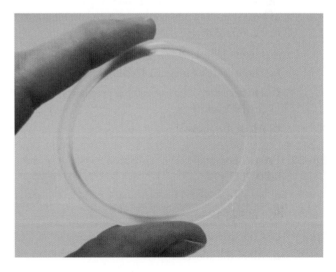

Reproduced with permission from Cunningham FG, Leveno KJ, Bloom SL, et al (eds): Contraception. In Williams Obstetrics, 24th ed. New York, McGraw-Hill, 2014, Figure 38-5.

  a. Daily

  b. Weekly

  c. Monthly

  d. Every 3 months

38–33. Compared with combination oral contraceptive pills, the vaginal contraceptive ring is associated with higher rates of which of the following?

a. Toxic shock syndrome

b. Contraceptive failure

c. Cervical intraepithelial neoplasia

d. None of the above

38–34. Risks and benefits of depot medroxyprogesterone acetate (DMPA) use for longer than 2 years should be evaluated carefully, especially in which of the following patients?

a. Hypertensive women

b. Perimenopausal women

c. Women with a family history of breast cancer

d. Women with a history of simple endometrial hyperplasia

38–35. Potential side effects of DMPA commonly may include which of the following?

a. Amenorrhea

b. Irregular uterine bleeding

c. Delayed return of fertility following DMPA cessation

d. All of the above

38–36. Your patient has diabetes and hypertension but prefers to use "pills" for contraception. She declines an intrauterine device and barrier methods. She is considering a progestin-only contraceptive and favors progestin-only pills. You counsel her regarding the advantages and which of the following disadvantages of progestin-only pills compared with combination oral contraceptives?

a. Higher failure rate

b. Higher rate of irregular bleeding

c. Higher relative rate of ectopic pregnancy with method failure

d. All of the above

38–37. Latex condom efficacy is enhanced by which of the following?

a. Reservoir tip

b. Oil-based spermicide

c. Concurrent female condom use

d. All of the above

38–38. The incidence of which of the following is increased with diaphragm use?

a. Cystocele

b. Cervicitis

c. Urinary tract infection

d. Pelvic inflammatory disease

38–39. Which of the following is **NOT** a variation of periodic abstinence as a family planning method?

a. Withdrawal method

b. Cervical mucus method

c. Calendar rhythm method

d. Temperature rhythm method

38–40. Compared with latex diaphragms, this product offers which advantages?

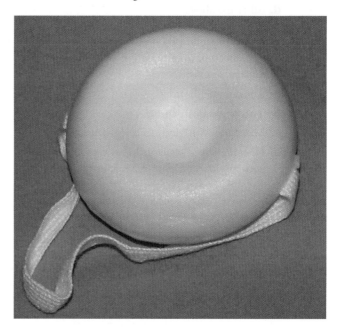

a. Greater efficacy

b. Prescription not required

c. Not associated with subsequent vaginitis

d. Not associated with toxic shock syndrome

38–41. Current methods of emergency contraception include all **EXCEPT** which of the following?

a. Ulipristal acetate

b. Levonorgestrel-releasing IUD

c. Levonorgestrel-containing pills

d. Combination oral contraceptive pills

CHAPTER 38 ANSWER KEY

Question number	Letter answer	Page cited	Header cited
38–1	a	p. 695	Introduction
38–2	a	p. 695	Introduction
38–3	b	p. 696	Table 38-2
38–4	d	p. 696	Long-acting Reversible Contraception: Intrauterine Devices
38–5	a	p. 696	Long-acting Reversible Contraception: Intrauterine Devices
38–6	b	p. 696	Long-acting Reversible Contraception: Intrauterine Devices
38–7	a	p. 697	Contraceptive Action
38–8	a	p. 697	Perforation
38–9	a	p. 699	Menstrual Changes
38–10	c	p. 697	Lost Device
38–11	c	p. 697	Lost Device
38–12	b	p. 697	Lost Device
38–13	d	p. 699	Infection
38–14	b	p. 700	Pregnancy with an IUD
38–15	a	p. 700	Pregnancy with an IUD
38–16	c	p. 700	Pregnancy with an IUD
38–17	d	p. 700	Timing
38–18	b	p. 703	Long-acting Reversible Contraception: Progestin Implants
38–19	a	p. 703	Long-acting Reversible Contraception: Progestin Implants
38–20	d	p. 704	Actions and Side Effects
38–21	d	p. 704	Contraindications to Progestin-Only Contraceptives
38–22	d	p. 705	Administration
38–23	a	p. 705	Administration
38–24	c	p. 708	Table 38-5
38–25	c	p. 708	Metabolic Changes
38–26	d	p. 709	Cardiovascular effects
38–27	d	p. 698	Table 38-3
38–28	c	p. 709	Neoplasia
38–29	a	p. 710	Table 38-6
38–30	b	p. 710	Transdermal Patch
38–31	a	p. 710	Transdermal Patch
38–32	c	p. 710	Transvaginal Ring
38–33	d	p. 710	Transvaginal Ring
38–34	b	p. 711	Actions and Side Effects
38–35	d	p. 711	Actions and Side Effects
38–36	d	p. 711	Progestin-Only Pills
38–37	a	p. 712	Male Condom
38–38	c	p. 712	Diaphragm Plus Spermicide
38–39	a	p. 713	Fertility-Awareness Based Methods
38–40	b	p. 714	Contraceptive Sponge
38–41	b	p. 714	Hormonal Emergency Contraception

CHAPTER 39

Sterilization

39–1. Your patient is a 26-year-old G3P2 who desires permanent sterilization following her upcoming delivery. Her past medical and surgical histories are unremarkable. During your counseling session you quote failures rates for puerperal sterilization; you discuss alternative methods of contraception, including the advantages of vasectomy; and you discuss possible operative and anesthesia complications. Which other preoperative counseling points regarding female tubal sterilization are true?

    a. Ease of sterilization reversal

    b. Higher risk of later menstrual irregularities

    c. Choice of either an abdominal or a hysteroscopic approach for puerperal sterilization

    d. None of the above

39–2. Which of the following aspects of normal postpartum maternal anatomy are not advantageous for puerperal sterilization?

    a. Noninvoluted uterus

    b. Lax anterior abdominal wall

    c. Engorged mesosalpinx vessels

    d. All of the above

39–3. Outcomes associated with performing puerperal tubal sterilization the morning after vaginal delivery include which of the following?

    a. Increases the risk of anesthesia-related complications

    b. Provides longer opportunity to assess neonatal well-being

    c. Increases the risk of postpartum hemorrhage complicating the postoperative course

    d. All of the above

39–4. Although highly effective and shown here, which method is an uncommonly used technique for puerperal sterilization?

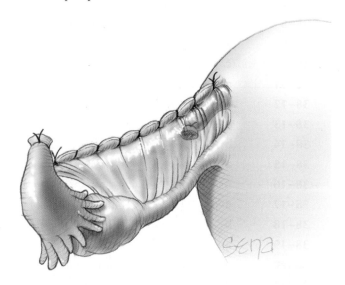

Reproduced with permission from Hoffman BL: Surgeries for benign gynecologic conditions. In Schorge JO, Schaffer JI, Halvorson LM, et al (eds) Williams Gynecology. New York, McGraw-Hill, 2008, Figure 41-24.5.

    a. Uchida

    b. Pomeroy

    c. Parkland

    d. Modified Pomeroy

39–5. Sterilization in the puerperium is typically performed using which of the following anesthetic methods?

    a. Spinal anesthesia

    b. General anesthesia

    c. Incision infiltration

    d. Transversus abdominis plane block

39–6. During puerperal sterilization and following peritoneal cavity entry, the small bowel and omentum continue to drift into your operative field. All **EXCEPT** which of the following techniques can improve visualization?

   a. Enlarge the incision

   b. Use a wider retractor

   c. Place patient in reverse Trendelenburg position

   d. Pack the omentum cephalad with an opened 4 × 4 gauze sponge whose extraabdominal end has been tagged with a hemostat

39–7. Prior to ligation, the fallopian tube is most reliably identified by which of its following attributes?

   a. Fimbria

   b. Pronounced vascularity

   c. Round tubular structure

   d. Location posterior to the uteroovarian ligament

39–8. With the Parkland method of female tubal sterilization, it is recommended that approximately what length of tubal segment be excised to allow adequate separation of tubal stumps?

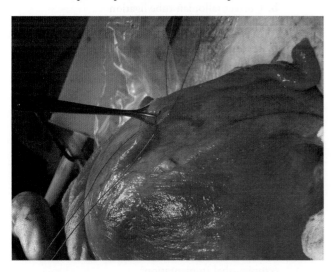

   a. 0.5 cm

   b. 1 cm

   c. 2 cm

   d. 4 cm

39–9. The success of the Pomeroy procedure relies upon the use of what type of suture ligature?

   a. Plain gut

   b. Chromic gut

   c. Synthetic polyglactin braided

   d. Synthetic polydioxanone monofilament

39–10. With this method of interval sterilization, which of the following energy sources is preferred?

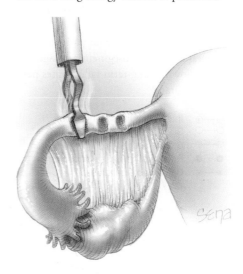

Reproduced with permission from Hoffman BL: Surgeries for benign gynecologic conditions. In Schorge JO, Schaffer JI, Halvorson LM, et al (eds) Williams Gynecology. New York, McGraw-Hill, 2008, Figure 41-29.1.

   a. Harmonic ultrasound

   b. Bipolar electrosurgical coagulation

   c. Unipolar electrosurgical coagulation

   d. Nd:YAG (neodymium-doped yttrium aluminum garnet) laser

39–11. Which of the following is true of nonpuerperal female tubal sterilization performed in the United States?

   a. Commonly performed via minilaparotomy

   b. Commonly performed using general anesthesia

   c. Typically requires overnight hospitalization

   d. None of the above

39–12. Of available methods, which of the following is commonly used for nonpuerperal tubal sterilization in the United States?

   a. Laparoscopic clip application

   b. Laparoscopic supracervical hysterectomy

   c. Distal salpingectomy via posterior colpotomy

   d. Hysteroscopic intratubal quinine instillation

39–13. This image shows the cumulative probability of pregnancy per 1000 procedures by five methods of tubal sterilization using data from the U.S. Collaborative Review of Sterilization (CREST) study. When counseling your patient regarding puerperal bilateral midsegment salpingectomy, which of the following long-term failure rates per procedure is most accurate?

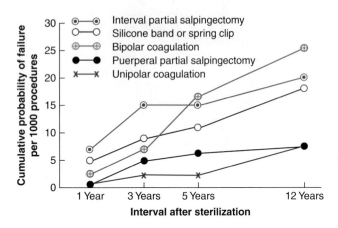

Reproduced with permission from Cunningham FG, Leveno KJ, Bloom SL (eds) Williams Obstetrics, 23rd ed. New York, 2010, Figure 5-15.

a. 1 in 150
b. 1 in 650
c. 1 in 1100
d. 1 in 2000

39–14. Puerperal sterilization failures result most commonly from which of the following?

a. Ligation of incorrect structure
b. Postoperative acute salpingitis
c. Use of absorbable suture for ligation
d. Intercourse too soon following ligation

39–15. This surgical specimen is the result of which intraoperative event during puerperal sterilization?

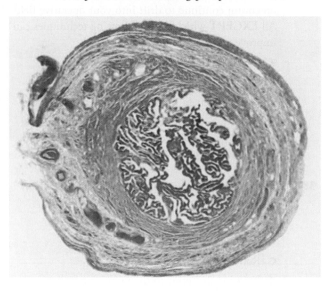

Reproduced with permission from Cunningham FG, Leveno KJ, Bloom SL (eds): Anatomy. In Williams Obstetrics, 23rd ed. New York, 2014, Figure 2-15B.

a. Incidental appendectomy
b. Correct fallopian tube ligation
c. Incorrect round ligament ligation
d. Incorrect uteroovarian ligament ligation

39–16. With Filshie clip application for nonpuerperal female tubal sterilization, which of the following is a possible reason for method failure with this technique?

a. Tubal stump fistula
b. Electrosurgical circuit failure
c. Intercourse too soon after the procedure
d. Surgery scheduled in the follicular phase

39–17. If pregnancy occurs following bilateral bipolar tubal electrosurgical coagulation, what is the rate of ectopic tubal implantation?

a. 10%
b. 30%
c. 50%
d. 75%

39–18. Your patient is a 37-year-old G4P4 who underwent puerperal sterilization 14 months ago and now presents for her annual examination. She has a history of polycystic ovarian syndrome with irregular menses and notes that her last menses was 7 weeks ago. Appropriate management should first be which of the following?

  a. Transvaginal sonographic examination

  b. Serum human chorionic gonadotropin level assessment

  c. Initiation of oral contraceptives for menstrual regulation

  d. Medroxyprogesterone 10 mg daily for 10 days to initiate a withdrawal menses

39–19. Which of the following conditions is increased in women following this procedure compared with those not undergoing this surgery?

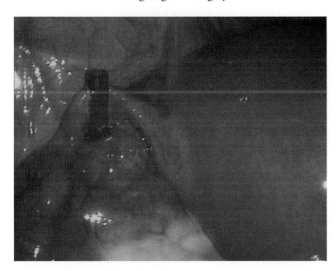

Used with permission from Dr. Michelle Medel.

  a. Risk of ovarian cancer

  b. Incidence of menorrhagia

  c. Risk of pelvic inflammatory disease

  d. None of the above

39–20. Studies support that tubal ligation is a risk for which of the following psychological or sexual side effects?

  a. Regret

  b. Decreased libido

  c. Decreased sexual satisfaction

  d. All of the above

39–21. Your 37-year-old patient underwent bilateral tubal bipolar coagulation for sterilization 7 years ago. Review of her operative report reveals that you coagulated three contiguous spots along a 3-cm length that incorporated most of the tube's isthmic portion. Now in a new relationship, she presents desiring counseling regarding reestablishment of fertility. Which of the following is a correct counseling statement regarding tubal reanastomosis?

  a. Highest pregnancy rates follow ampullary-to-isthmic reanastomosis.

  b. Almost 10 percent of women who conceive following reanastomosis will have an ectopic pregnancy.

  c. Reanastomosis after tubal electrosurgical coagulation has higher pregnancy rates than reanastomosis following Filshie clip application.

  d. All of the above

39–22. This device achieves sterilization by which of the following methods?

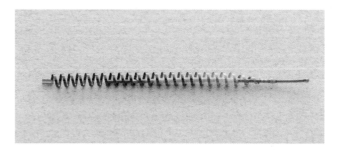

  a. Lies within the cervical canal to secrete spermicide

  b. Wraps around the fallopian tube to occlude the lumen

  c. Is placed within the uterine cavity to agglutinate the endometrium

  d. Is placed within the fallopian tube ostia to promote occlusive tissue ingrowth

39–23. According to Food and Drug Administration recommendations, which of the following imaging procedures is performed after the Essure method of tubal sterilization to document procedure success?

  a. Hysterosalpingography 6 weeks after surgery

  b. Saline infusion sonography 3 months after surgery

  c. Three-dimensional transvaginal sonography 8 weeks after surgery

  d. None of the above

39–24. All **EXCEPT** which of the following are true regarding the Essure method of tubal sterilization?

   a. Requires tissue ingrowth for method success

   b. Requires hysterosalpingography 3 months postprocedure

   c. Requires proximal tubal thermal injury to incite tissue ingrowth

   d. Requires alternative method of contraception until tubal occlusion is documented

39–25. Pregnancy following the Essure method of transcervical tubal sterilization may result from which of the following?

   a. Insert expulsion

   b. Misinterpretation of hysterosalpingogram

   c. Noncompliance with required hysterosalpingogram

   d. All the above

39–26. During vasectomy, which of the following structures is ligated?

   a. Epididymis

   b. Spermatic cord

   c. Ductus deferens

   d. Efferent ductile

39–27. Compared with vasectomy, which of the following is higher with female tubal sterilization?

   a. Cost

   b. Failure rate

   c. Surgical complication rate

   d. All of the above

39–28. To avoid conception following vasectomy, an alternative form of contraception should be used until semen analysis documents aspermia. Complete sperm expulsion from the reproductive tract takes approximately how long?

   a. 1 week

   b. 4 weeks

   c. 8 weeks

   d. 12 weeks

39–29. Most vasectomy failures occur during the first year following the procedure. The cumulative failure rate per 1000 procedures at years 2, 3 and 5 is stable and approximates which of the following?

   a. 10

   b. 50

   c. 80

   d. 125

39–30. Vasectomy failures may result from which of the following?

   a. Recanalization

   b. Incomplete surgical occlusion

   c. Intercourse too soon after the procedure

   d. All of the above

39–31. A long-term complication following vasectomy includes which of the following?

   a. Regret

   b. Atherogenesis

   c. Testicular cancer

   d. All of the above

39–32. Pregnancy rates after vasectomy reversal increase with all **EXCEPT** which of the following?

   a. Microsurgical technique

   b. Younger female partner age

   c. Longer time duration from vasectomy to reversal

   d. Normal sperm quality noted during reversal procedure

CHAPTER 39 ANSWER KEY

Question number	Letter answer	Page cited	Header cited
39–1	d	p. 720	Female Sterilization
39–2	c	p. 720	Puerperal Tubal Sterilization
39–3	b	p. 720	Puerperal Tubal Sterilization
39–4	a	p. 720	Puerperal Tubal Sterilization
39–5	a	p. 720	Surgical Technique
39–6	c	p. 720	Surgical Technique
39–7	a	p. 720	Surgical Technique
39–8	c	p. 721	Figure 39-1
39–9	a	p. 721	Figure 39-2
39–10	b	p. 721	Nonpuerperal (Interval) Surgical Tubal Sterilization
39–11	b	p. 721	Nonpuerperal (Interval) Surgical Tubal Sterilization
39–12	a	p. 721	Nonpuerperal (Interval) Surgical Tubal Sterilization
39–13	a	p. 721	Contraceptive Failure
39–14	a	p. 721	Contraceptive Failure
39–15	b	p. 721	Contraceptive Failure
39–16	a	p. 721	Contraceptive Failure
39–17	c	p. 721	Contraceptive Failure
39–18	b	p. 721	Contraceptive Failure
39–19	d	p. 722	Other Effects
39–20	a	p. 722	Other Effects
39–21	b	p. 722	Reversal of Tubal Sterilization
39–22	d	p. 722	Intratubal Devices
39–23	d	p. 722	Intratubal Devices
39–24	c	p. 722	Intratubal Devices
39–25	d	p. 722	Intratubal Devices
39–26	c	p. 723	Male Sterilization
39–27	d	p. 723	Male Sterilization
39–28	d	p. 723	Male Sterilization
39–29	a	p. 723	Male Sterilization
39–30	d	p. 723	Male Sterilization
39–31	a	p. 724	Long-Term Effects
39–32	c	p. 724	Restoration of Fertility

OBSTETRICAL COMPLICATIONS

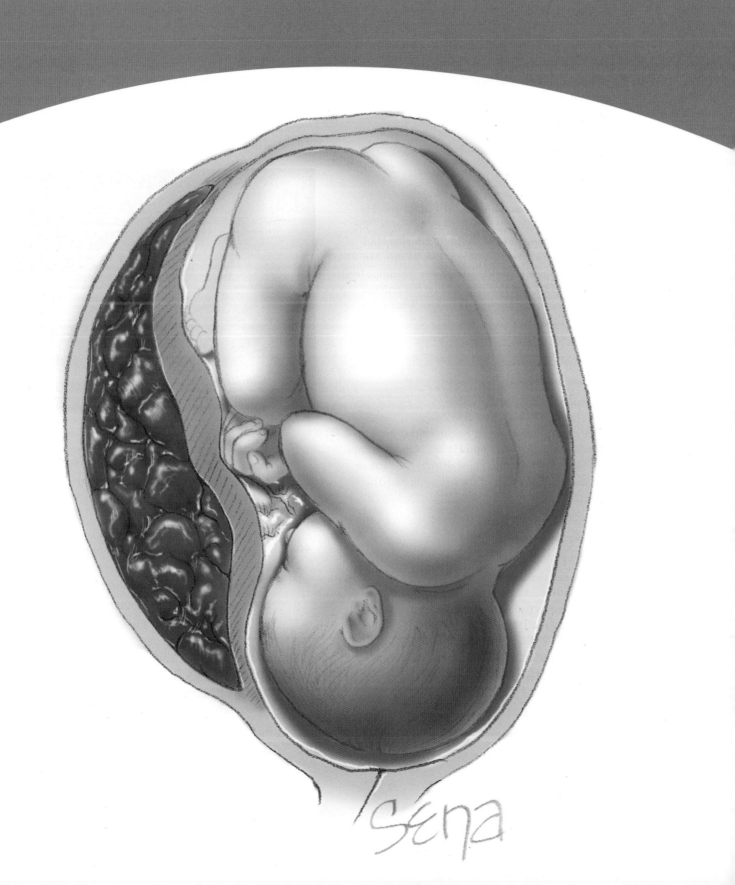

CHAPTER 40

Hypertensive Disorders

40–1. What proportion of maternal deaths can be attributed to hypertensive disorders in pregnancy?

    a. 1 in 2

    b. 1 in 6

    c. 1 in 10

    d. 1 in 20

40–2. A patient has a blood pressure of 110/72 mm Hg on her first prenatal visit at 8 weeks' gestation. She develops hypertension in the third trimester, and at delivery, her blood pressure is 148/94 mm Hg. Urine protein by dipstick is trace, her creatinine level is 0.76 mg/dL, and her hypertension has resolved by the time of her hospital discharge. What is her correct diagnosis?

    a. Preeclampsia

    b. Chronic hypertension

    c. Gestational hypertension

    d. Superimposed preeclampsia

40–3. A patient with antepartum baseline blood pressure measurements of 90/65 mm Hg has blood pressures of 130–140/80–86 mm Hg at delivery. She has an increased risk of which of the following obstetric complications?

    a. Eclampsia

    b. Placental abruption

    c. Nonreassuring fetal heart rate tracing

    d. None of the above

40–4. A multiparous patient who has received no prenatal care presents to Labor and Delivery with a complaint of vaginal bleeding. Her fundal height is 24 cm. Which of the following laboratory tests supports the diagnosis of preeclampsia?

    a. Creatinine 1.14 mg/dL

    b. Platelet count 103,000/μL

    c. Alkaline phosphatase 138 IU/L

    d. Total protein of 258 mg in a 24-hour urine collection

40–5. For the patient in Question 40–4, a sonographic examination is performed to estimate gestational age. One image is shown below. Which of the following may explain the development of preeclampsia in this patient?

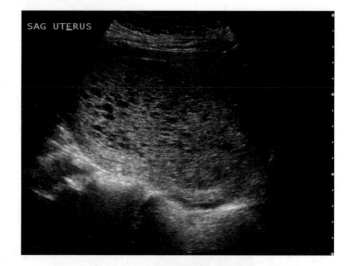

    a. Increased volume of chorionic villi

    b. Extensive remodeling of the spiral arterioles

    c. Increased invasion of extravillous trophoblastic tissue

    d. None of the above

40–6. What is the underlying etiology for proteinuria that is seen with preeclampsia?

    a. Increased capillary permeability

    b. Increased renal artery resistance

    c. Increased glomerular filtration rate

    d. Increased systemic vascular resistance

40–7. All **EXCEPT** which of the following increase a woman's predisposition to develop preeclampsia syndrome?

    a. Obesity

    b. Smoking

    c. Nulliparity

    d. Multiple gestation

40–8. What is a possible explanation for the increased incidence of preeclampsia seen in patients whose pregnancies are complicated by the aneuploidy reflected by the karyotype results shown here?

    a. Increased antiangiogenic factor levels

    b. Increased frequency of placental mosaicism

    c. Higher frequency of spiral arteriole atherosis

    d. Increased levels of oxidative products in the placenta

40–11. Which of the following physiological responses is typically seen in preeclamptic patients?

    a. Increased production of nitric acid

    b. Decreased reactivity to norepinephrine

    c. Increased sensitivity to angiotensin II

    d. All of the above

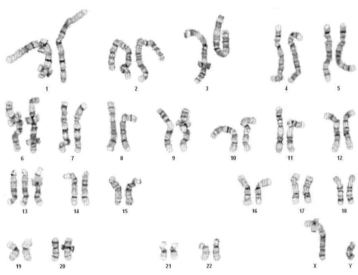

40–9. Shown here, macrophages, which contribute to vessel atherosis, are filled with what substance?

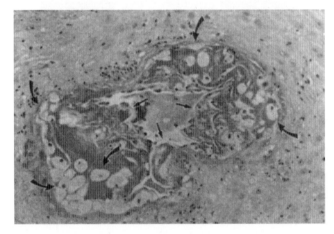

Modified with permission from Cunningham FG, Leveno KJ, Bloom SL, et al (eds): Hypertensive disorders. In Williams Obstetrics, 24th ed. New York, McGraw-Hill, 2014, Figure 40-3A.

    a. Lipids

    b. Interleukins

    c. Nitric oxide

    d. Tumor necrosis factor-α

40–10. Which of the following nutritional supplements has been shown to reduce the incidence of preeclampsia?

    a. Calcium

    b. Vitamin E

    c. Ascorbic acid

    d. None of the above

40–12. The typical blood volume of a gravida at term is 4500 mL. In patients with preeclampsia, which of the following would be the expected blood volume?

    a. 2500 mL

    b. 3200 mL

    c. 4500 mL

    d. 5000 mL

40–13. In patients with preeclampsia, limited blood volume expansion during pregnancy affects maternal cardiac function by which mechanism?

    a. Decreases preload

    b. Increases afterload

    c. Increases stroke volume

    d. Decreases cardiac output

40–14. A neonate is born vaginally after 6 hours of labor and a few minutes of pushing. He has petechiae covering his scalp and chest, and his pediatric nurse notices oozing at the site of a heel stick. His initial platelet count is 32,000/μL. Which of the following maternal hypertensive conditions predisposes to this neonatal condition?

    a. Eclampsia

    b. Preeclampsia

    c. Gestational hypertension

    d. None of the above

40–15. Which of the following is responsible for the clinical sign of preeclampsia seen in the following photograph?

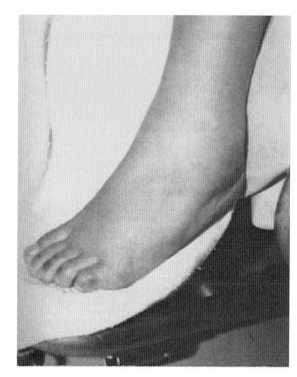

Reproduced with permission from Cunningham FG, Leveno KJ, Bloom SL, et al (eds): Hypertensive disorders. In Williams Obstetrics, 24th ed. New York, McGraw-Hill, 2014, Figure 40-19A.

    a. Endothelial injury

    b. Increased sodium retention

    c. Reduced plasma oncotic pressure

    d. All of the above

40–16. A primigravida delivered 4 hours ago. Her blood pressure was 152/90 mm Hg before delivery, and 1+ proteinuria was found by dipstick. Her delivery was uneventful, and her estimated blood loss was 500 mL. You get a call from her nurse because her urine output for the past 4 hours is only 118 mL. Her BP is 148/88, pulse is 84, she has 12 respirations per minute, and no evidence of ongoing bleeding is noted. Which of the following treatment options is most appropriate for this patient?

    a. Continue observation

    b. Give 10 mg intravenous furosemide

    c. Transfuse 2 units of packed red blood cells

    d. Give 500 mL bolus of intravenous normal saline

40–17. Which of the following leads to increased uric acid levels in patients with preeclampsia?

    a. Increased tubular reabsorption

    b. Increased placental production

    c. Decreased glomerular filtration rate

    d. All of the above

40–18. Your obstetrical patient presents with a blood pressure of 160/104 mm Hg, 3+ proteinuria, and right upper quadrant discomfort at 36 weeks' gestation. Following induction of labor, she delivers vaginally. She has uterine atony, and her estimated blood loss is 1500 mL. Her serum creatinine rises from 0.98 mg/dL predelivery to 1.42 mg/dL. What is the most likely explanation for this finding?

    a. Postpartum hemorrhage

    b. Severe preeclampsia alone

    c. Subcapsular liver hematoma

    d. Dehydration secondary to prolonged induction

40–19. The following computed-tomography image is from a study obtained on a postpartum hypertensive patient with confusion. Cerebral edema was diagnosed. For what associated morbidity is the patient at risk?

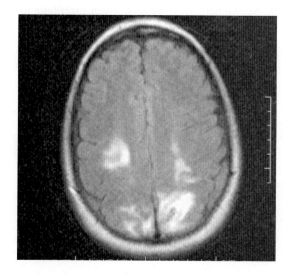

    a. Hemiplegia

    b. Cystic leukomalacia

    c. Retinal artery occlusion

    d. Transtentorial herniation

40–20. All **EXCEPT** which of the following are indicated treatments in the management of the patient discussed in Question 40–19?

a. Mannitol

b. Dexamethasone

c. Intravenous immune globulin

d. Antihypertensive medication

40–21. In a low-risk population, treatment with which of the following medications resulted in a reduced incidence of preeclampsia?

a. Aspirin

b. Pravastatin

c. Hydrochlorothiazide

d. None of the above

40–22. Your obstetrical patient is admitted to the hospital for evaluation of new-onset hypertension at 30 weeks' gestation. All **EXCEPT** which of the following should be part of your evaluation?

a. Maternal weight

b. Cell-free fetal DNA testing

c. Fetal sonographic evaluation

d. Maternal urine protein:creatinine ratio

40–23. The patient in Question 40–22 has blood pressures of 140–150/85–100 mm Hg during the next 5 days. Which of the following should prompt consideration for premature delivery?

a. Headache

b. Worsening pedal edema

c. 3+ proteinuria on dipstick

d. Fetal biophysical profile score of 8

40–24. Three days after admission, the patient in Question 40–23 develops severe preeclampsia and delivery is indicated. Sonographic evaluation reveals a cephalic presentation and estimated fetal weight of 1405 g. If labor induction is attempted, what is the approximate rate of successful vaginal delivery?

a. 10%

b. 30%

c. 50%

d. 80%

40–25. In studies evaluating the antenatal use of labetalol for treatment of early mild preeclampsia, which of the following is reduced?

a. Blood pressure

b. Fetal-growth restriction

c. Length of inpatient hospitalization

d. All of the above

40–26. What is the concern surrounding use of corticosteroids to enhance fetal lung maturation in women with severe hypertension prior to 34 weeks' gestation?

a. It exacerbates maternal hypertension.

b. Time needed for corticosteroid administration may delay delivery.

c. It may trigger eclampsia in women with a genetic predisposition to seizures.

d. It is associated with an increased rate of neonatal intraventricular hemorrhage.

40–27. What salutary effect does dexamethasone possibly have when used in the treatment of HELLP (hemolysis, elevated liver enzymes, low platelet count) syndrome?

a. Decreased maternal mortality rate

b. Decreased rate of acute renal failure

c. Faster aspartate transferase recovery time

d. Increased platelet count in severe thrombocytopenia

40–28. Which of the following explains the findings seen in the chest radiograph below, obtained from a patient with eclampsia?

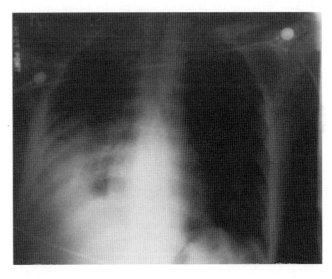

Reproduced with permission from Emerman CL, Anderson E, Cline DM: Community-acquired pneumonia, aspiration pneumonia, and noninfectious pulmonary infiltrates. In Tintinalli JE, Stapczynski JS, Cline DM, et al (eds): Tintinalli's Emergency Medicine: A Comprehensive Study Guide, 7th ed. New York, McGraw-Hill, 2011, Figure 68-4.

a. Pneumothorax

b. Pulmonary edema

c. Pulmonary embolus

d. Aspiration pneumonia

40-29. An eclamptic patient who has received a 4-g loading dose of magnesium sulfate has another seizure. Which of the following medications can be given as adjuvant anticonvulsant therapy?

    a. Midazolam

    b. Thiopental

    c. Additional magnesium sulfate

    d. All of the above

40-30. What is the target magnesium level when used for eclampsia prophylaxis?

    a. 2.0–3.5 mg/dL

    b. 4.8–8.4 mg/dL

    c. 8.4–10.4 mg/dL

    d. None of the above

40-31. What clinical sign or test can be used to detect hypermagnesemia prior to development of respiratory depression?

    a. Heart rate

    b. Patellar reflex

    c. Presence of clonus

    d. Visual field testing

40-32. Which of the following strategies for administering magnesium sulfate for eclampsia prophylaxis should be used in the setting of an elevated serum creatinine?

    a. Give no loading dose and start infusion at 2 g/hr

    b. Give 3-g loading dose followed by 2 g/hr infusion

    c. Give 3-g loading dose, check magnesium level, and then titrate infusion rate

    d. None of the above

40-33. A pregnant patient has a seizure at home and is evaluated by an emergency room physician. He consults with a neurologist who, after excluding other etiologies for the seizure, makes the diagnosis of eclampsia. The neurologist recommends phenytoin for eclampsia prophylaxis to the on-call obstetrician. What is the best response to this recommendation?

    a. Agree and load the patient with phenytoin

    b. Give intravenous loading dose of magnesium sulfate and oral phenytoin

    c. Explain there is a reduction of recurrent seizure activity with magnesium sulfate and start magnesium sulfate

    d. None of the above

40-34. Antenatal use of nitroglycerin to control severe maternal hypertension can lead to which of the following complications?

    a. Fetal acidosis

    b. Fetal oliguria

    c. Fetal cyanide toxicity

    d. Reduced fetal heart rate variability seen during monitoring

40-35. Use of hydroxyethyl starch to expand intravascular volume improves which of the following pregnancy outcomes in women with preeclampsia?

    a. Eclampsia

    b. Fetal death rate

    c. Gestational age at delivery

    d. None of the above

40-36. Preeclampsia is a marker for all **EXCEPT** which of the following morbidities later in life?

    a. Metabolic syndrome

    b. Chronic renal disease

    c. Ischemic heart disease

    d. Nonalcoholic steatohepatitis

CHAPTER 40 ANSWER KEY

Question number	Letter answer	Page cited	Header cited
40–1	b	p. 728	Introduction
40–2	c	p. 728	Terminology and Diagnosis
40–3	d	p. 728	Diagnosis of Hypertensive Disorders
40–4	a	p. 729	Table 40-1
40–5	a	p. 731	Etiopathogenesis; Figure 40-2
40–6	a	p. 731	Preeclampsia Syndrome
40–7	b	p. 731	Preeclampsia Syndrome
40–8	a	p. 733	Immunological Factors
40–9	a	p. 733	Figure 40-3
40–10	d	p. 734	Nutritional Factors
40–11	c	p. 735	Increased Pressor Responses
40–12	b	p. 737	Blood Volume; Figure 40-7
40–13	a	p. 736	Cardiovascular System
40–14	d	p. 738	Neonatal Thrombocytopenia
40–15	d	p. 739	Endocrine Changes; Fluid and Electrolyte Changes
40–16	a	p. 739	Kidney
40–17	d	p. 739	Kidney
40–18	a	p. 740	Acute Kidney Injury
40–19	d	p. 744	Neuroimaging Studies
40–20	c	p. 745	Cerebral Edema
40–21	d	p. 748	Antihypertensive Drugs; Low-Dose Aspirin
40–22	b	p. 749	Evaluation
40–23	a	p. 750	Consideration for Delivery
40–24	b	p. 750	Elective Cesarean Delivery
40–25	a	p. 752	Antihypertensive Therapy for Mild to Moderate Hypertension
40–26	b	p. 754	Glucocorticoids for Lung Maturation
40–27	d	p. 754	Corticosteroids to Ameliorate HELLP Syndrome
40–28	d	p. 756	Immediate Management of Seizure
40–29	d	p. 758	Magnesium Sulfate to Control Convulsions
40–30	b	p. 758	Table 40-11
40–31	b	p. 759	Pharmacology and Toxicology
40–32	d	p. 759	Pharmacology and Toxicology
40–33	c	p. 760	Maternal Safety and Efficacy of Magnesium Sulfate
40–34	c	p. 763	Other Antihypertensive Agents
40–35	d	p. 764	Table 40-13
40–36	d	p. 769	Long-term Consequences

CHAPTER 41

Obstetrical Hemorrhage

41–1. Which of the following is true of obstetrical hemorrhage?

   a. It is the leading cause of maternal death worldwide.

   b. It is no longer a leading cause of maternal death in the United States.

   c. Only 5% of maternal deaths in the United States are due to obstetrical hemorrhage.

   d. All of the above

41–2. Given the diagram shown here, what can be said regarding blood loss at delivery?

   a. It is common to lose more than 500 mL with vaginal delivery.

   b. It is common to lose more than 1000 mL with cesarean delivery.

   c. It is common to lose more than half of maternal blood volume with cesarean hysterectomy.

   d. All of the above

41–3. For a woman measuring 5 ft 0 in. and 120 lb, what is her expected pregravid blood volume?

   a. 3000 mL

   b. 3250 mL

   c. 3500 mL

   d. 3800 mL

41–4. Assuming a 50% increase in blood volume during normal pregnancy, what would the blood volume of the woman from Question 41–2 approximate at 38 weeks' gestation?

   a. 4000 mL

   b. 4500 mL

   c. 5250 mL

   d. 5700 mL

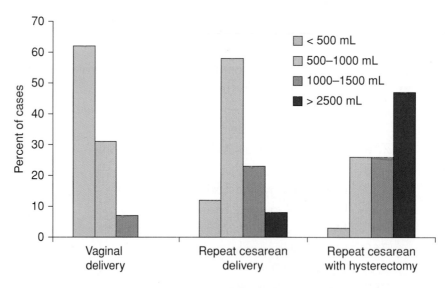

Reproduced with permission from Cunningham FG, Leveno KJ, Bloom SL, et al (eds): Maternal physiology. In Williams Obstetrics, 24th ed. New York, McGraw-Hill, 2014, Figure 41-1.

41-5. Midtrimester bleeding is associated with which of the following?

a. Placenta previa

b. Placental abruption

c. Higher rates of adverse pregnancy outcomes

d. All of the above

41-6. What might delay a practitioner from recognizing dangerous postpartum hemorrhage?

a. Initial catecholamine release after hemorrhage

b. A normal blood pressure in a severely preeclamptic woman

c. Persistent light bleeding during fourth-degree vaginal laceration repair

d. All of the above

41-7. In treating uterine atony after delivery, which of the following is true?

a. Fundal massage should be performed.

b. A 20-unit oxytocin bolus should be administered intravenously.

c. Oxytocin diluted in a crystalloid solution at a concentration of 200 U/min should be administered intravenously.

d. All of the above

41-8. Ms. Jones, a 32-year-old G3P2 gravida with chronic hypertension, had a normal labor that arrested during the second stage at +1 station. She complained of mild dyspnea and fatigue. The fetus had a left occiput anterior presentation and was delivered by forceps. Completion of the third stage followed quickly, and the fundus was noted to be firm. Brisk vaginal bleeding was then noted. What is the most likely cause of bleeding?

a. Uterine atony

b. Uterine rupture

c. Retained placenta

d. Genital tract laceration

41-9. The genital tract of the patient from Question 41-8 was carefully examined, and no lacerations were noted. Prophylactic oxytocin at 200 mU/min was being administered. The examiner then noted that although the fundus felt firm, the lower uterine segment was boggy. Which of the following is suitable treatment in this situation?

a. Hemabate, 250 μg intramuscularly

b. Methergine, 0.2 mg intramuscularly

c. A 20-unit oxytocin intravenous bolus

d. All are suitable

41-10. For Ms. Jones, the patient from Question 41-8, one dose of a uterotonic agent is given and the fundus is massaged. Despite this, she continues to bleed. Which of the following is suitable treatment in this situation?

a. Administer Methergine, 0.2 mg intramuscularly

b. Perform laparotomy to prepare for postpartum hysterectomy

c. Mobilize a team that includes obstetricians, nurses, and anesthesiologists.

d. All of the above

41-11. For Ms. Jones, the patient from Question 41-8, you have provided general anesthesia, evaluated the genital tract again, and administered three doses of Hemabate. Despite this, she continues to bleed, and you have initiated whole blood transfusion. Which of the following is suitable treatment in this situation?

a. Consider laparotomy and uterine compression suture placement

b. Continue to administer Hemabate intramuscularly every 20 minutes

c. Insert a Bakri postpartum balloon or large Foley catheter balloon into the uterine cavity and inflate the balloon

d. All of the above

41-12. For the patient in Question 41-8, despite Bakri balloon placement, heavy uterine bleeding continues. You perform a laparotomy and find an atonic uterus. Which of the following is suitable treatment in this situation?

a. Internal iliac artery ligation

b. Uterine compression suture placement

c. Bilateral uterine artery and uteroovarian pedicle ligation

d. All of the above

41-13. For the patient in Question 41-8, despite these measures, Ms. Jones continues to bleed now from all surgical edges, and the uterus remains atonic. Which of the following is suitable treatment in this situation?

a. Initiate hysterectomy

b. Administer 20-unit oxytocin intravenous bolus

c. Evaluate for dilutional coagulopathy and continue uterine compression

d. All of the above

41–14. For the patient in Question 41–8, after correction of coagulopathy, bleeding stops and the uterus firms. Postoperatively, Ms. Jones is admitted to the intensive care unit, where she is slowly weaned from the ventilator. She is discharged on postoperative day 4. What condition, represented by the histological image of lung shown here, is consistent with the clinical events for Ms. Jones?

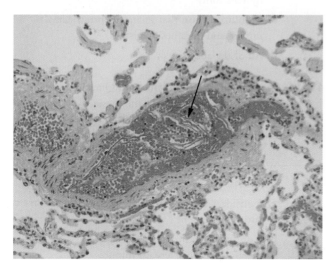

a. Pulmonary embolism
b. Amnionic fluid embolism
c. Primary pulmonary hypertension
d. None of the above

41–15. Which of the following is suitable treatment for this situation?

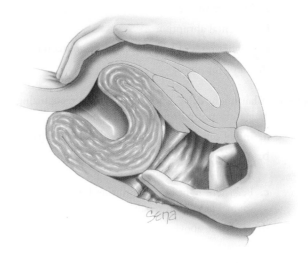

Reproduced with permission from Cunningham FG, Leveno KJ, Bloom SL, et al (eds): Dermatological disorders. In Williams Obstetrics, 23rd ed. New York, McGraw-Hill, 2010, Figure 35-23A.

a. Immediate recognition and calls for assistance improve outcome.
b. If recognized quickly, fundal massage and uterotonic agents are initiated.
c. The patient is evaluated for regional anesthesia, large-bore intravenous access is established, and rapid crystalloid infusion is begun while you wait for blood to arrive.
d. All of the above

41–16. Which of the following statements concerning uterine inversion are true?

a. Placenta accreta is a risk factor.
b. Fundal placental implantation is a risk factor.
c. It has an incidence that approximates 1 in 2000 deliveries.
d. All of the above

41–17. Your patient delivered precipitously and without perineal laceration. During the first hour postpartum, the vulvar mass shown here continues to expand, and the patient complains of significant pain. Evaluation reveals a BP of 90/40 mm Hg, pulse of 120 bpm, and no fever. Which of the following are reasonable management approaches to the condition depicted here?

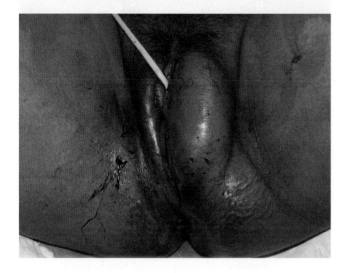

a. Ice packs and observation are planned.

b. This large supralevator hematoma may require angiographic embolization.

c. This likely connects with the ischioanal fossa, and laparotomy is planned to exclude or evacuate a large retroperitoneal hematoma.

d. The point of maximal expansion is incised, clots are evacuated, bleeding points are ligated, and the evacuated space is obliterated by sutures.

41–18. All **EXCEPT** which of the following are associated with primary uterine rupture?

a. Hydramnios

b. Forceps delivery

c. Breech extraction

d. Prior cesarean delivery

41–19. Which of the following has the highest associated relative risk for placental abruption?

a. Thrombophilia

b. Prior abruption

c. Chorioamnionitis

d. Preterm ruptured membranes

41–20. Which of the following regarding placental abruption are true?

a. Classically, it is associated with pain and vaginal bleeding.

b. It is the most frequent cause of clinically significant consumptive coagulopathy.

c. Abruption causing fetal death is usually associated with blood loss that is equivalent to half of maternal blood volume.

d. All the above

41–21. With placental abruption, which condition(s) would preclude vaginal delivery?

a. Intrauterine fetal demise and prior classical cesarean hysterotomy

b. Term fetus at +2 station, brisk vaginal bleeding, and mild coagulopathy

c. Intrauterine fetal demise and a herpes simplex virus ulcer on the maternal perineum

d. All of the above

41–22. Which of the following statements is true concerning placenta previa?

a. A low-lying placenta at 27 weeks' gestation is unlikely to persist until term.

b. Persistent placenta previa is more common in women with prior cesarean deliveries.

c. Approximately 40% of placenta previas that cover the internal cervical os at 20 weeks' gestation will persist until term.

d. All the above

41–23. Placentas that lie within close proximity of the internal cervical os but do not reach it are termed low lying. What is the boundary threshold that defines a low-lying placenta?

a. 1.0 cm

b. 2.0 cm

c. 3.0 cm

d. 4.0 cm

41–24. The incidence of placenta previa increases with which of the following factors?

a. Increasing parity

b. Increasing maternal age

c. Increasing number of cesarean deliveries

d. All of the above

41–25. Histologically, which of the following best describes the villi found at placenta increta sites?

   a. Invade into the myometrium

   b. Attached to the myometrium

   c. Attached to the endometrium

   d. Penetrate through the myometrium

41–26. This picture represents which of the following?

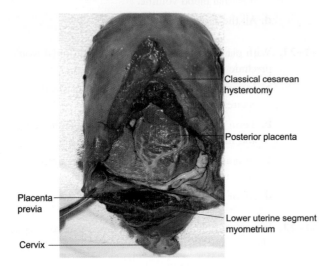

   a. Placenta accreta

   b. Placenta increta

   c. Placenta percreta

   d. Placental abruption

41–27. Using Doppler flow color mapping, as shown here, which two factors are highly predictive of placenta accreta? B = bladder.

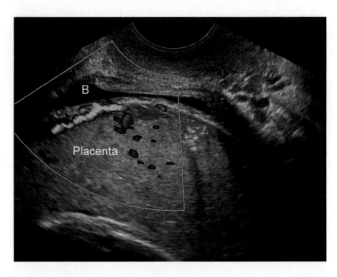

Used with permission from Dr. Christopher Ripperda.

   a. Large intraplacental lakes; fundal placenta

   b. Less than 1 mm between uterine serosa-bladder interface and retroplacental vessels; lateral placenta

   c. Less than 1 mm between uterine serosa-bladder interface and retroplacental vessels; large placental lakes

   d. None of the above

41–28. Management of placenta accreta typically requires which of the following procedures?

   a. Classical cesarean; hysterectomy

   b. Low transverse cesarean; hysterectomy

   c. Classical cesarean; myometrial resection

   d. Low vertical cesarean; myometrial resection

41–29. Which obstetrical conditions can lead to significant consumptive coagulation?

    a. Placental abruption

    b. Amnionic fluid embolism

    c. Gram-negative bacterial sepsis

    d. All of the above

41–30. Above which threshold are serum fibrinogen levels considered adequate to promote coagulation?

    a. 50 mg %

    b. 150 mg %

    c. 250 mg %

    d. 400 mg %

41–31. One of the most important vital signs with obstetrical hemorrhage is which of the following?

    a. Urine output

    b. Blood pressure

    c. Oxygen saturation

    d. Point-of-care hematocrit

41–32. Acute resuscitation of hypovolemia is preferably done with which of the following?

    a. Colloids and ephedrine

    b. Crystalloids and ephedrine

    c. Crystalloids and packed red blood cells

    d. Colloid solutions and packed red blood cells

41–33. With ongoing obstetrical hemorrhage, rapid blood transfusion is typically initiated at which hematocrit threshold?

    a. 20%

    b. 25%

    c. 30%

    d. 35%

41–34. The ideal treatment of hypovolemia from catastrophic hemorrhage is which of the following?

    a. Whole blood

    b. Packed red blood cells

    c. Whole blood and platelets

    d. Packed red blood cells and plasma

41–35. Morbidity from volume replacement with only packed red blood cells and crystalloid infusion would include which of the following?

    a. Thrombocytopenia

    b. Hypofibrinogenemia

    c. Dilutional coagulopathy

    d. All of the above

41–36. Each unit of packed red blood cells raises the hematocrit by what amount?

    a. 2–3%

    b. 3–4%

    c. 4–5%

    d. 5–6%

CHAPTER 41 ANSWER KEY

Question number	Letter answer	Page cited	Header cited
41–1	a	p. 780	Introduction
41–2	d	p. 781	Definition and Incidence
41–3	a	p. 781	Table 41-1
41–4	b	p. 781	Table 41-1
41–5	d	p. 782	Antepartum Hemorrhage
41–6	d	p. 783	Blood Loss Estimation
41–7	a	p. 784	Uterine Atony after Placental Delivery
41–8	d	p. 784	Causes of Obstetrical Hemorrhage
41–9	a	p. 785	Uterotonic Agents
41–10	c	p. 786	Bleeding Unresponsive to Uterotonic Agents
41–11	d	p. 786	Bleeding Unresponsive to Uterotonic Agents
41–12	d	p. 787	Surgical Procedures
41–13	c	p. 787	Surgical Procedures
41–14	b	p. 782	Table 41-2; Amnionic-Fluid Embolism
41–15	a	p. 787	Recognition and Management
41–16	d	p. 787	Uterine Inversion
41–17	d	p. 790	Management
41–18	d	p. 790	Rupture of the Uterus
41–19	b	p. 795	Predisposing Factors
41–20	d	p. 796	Clinical Findings and Diagnosis
41–21	a	p. 798	Vaginal Delivery
41–22	d	p. 799	Placental Migration
41–23	b	p. 800	Classification
41–24	d	p. 801	Incidence and Associated Factors
41–25	a	p. 804	Classification
41–26	b	p. 804	Classification
41–27	c	p. 806	Clinical Presentation and Diagnosis
41–28	a	p. 807	Cesarean Delivery and Hysterectomy
41–29	d	p. 809	Pathological Activation of Coagulation
41–30	b	p. 810	Fibrinogen and Degradation Products
41–31	a	p. 814	Management of Hemorrhage
41–32	c	p. 815	Fluid Resuscitation
41–33	b	p. 815	Blood Replacement
41–34	a	p. 815	Blood Component Products
41–35	d	p. 816	Dilutional Coagulopathy
41–36	b	p. 816	Packed Red Blood Cells

CHAPTER 42

Preterm Labor

42–1. The term *small-for-gestational age* is generally used to designate newborns whose birthweight is less than what percentile?

a. 3%

b. 5%

c. 10%

d. 15%

42–2. The neonatal mortality rate is expected to be lowest for newborns born at which of the following gestational ages?

a. 36 weeks 6 days

b. 37 weeks 4 days

c. 39 weeks 6 days

d. 41 weeks 2 days

42–3. Late-preterm births, defined as those between 34 and 36 weeks' gestation, compose what percentage of all preterm births?

a. 35%

b. 50%

c. 70%

d. 85%

42–4. Which of the following etiologies is largely responsible for the increase in preterm birth rates in the United States during the past 20 years?

a. Triplet pregnancies

b. Spontaneous preterm labor

c. Preterm rupture of fetal membranes

d. Indicated (iatrogenic) preterm birth

42–5. After achieving a birthweight of at least 1000 grams, neonatal survival rates reach 95 percent at approximately what gestational age with regard to newborn sex?

a. 28 weeks for both males and females

b. 30 weeks for both males and females

c. 28 weeks for females and 30 weeks for males

d. 30 weeks for females and 28 weeks for males

42–6. Cesarean delivery for neonates born at the threshold of viability has been demonstrated to protect against which of the following adverse newborn outcomes?

a. Seizures

b. Intraventricular hemorrhage

c. Respiratory distress syndrome

d. None of the above

42–7. Compared with neonates born at term, the risks to those born between 34 and 36 weeks' gestation include which of the following?

a. Increased serious morbidity and mortality rates

b. Equivalent serious morbidity and mortality rates

c. Increased serious morbidity but decreased mortality rates

d. Increased serious morbidity but equivalent mortality rates

42–8. Maternal stress may potentiate preterm labor by which of the following mechanisms involving corticotropin-releasing hormone (CRH)?

a. Increased production of maternal-derived CRH

b. Decreased production of maternal-derived CRH

c. Increased production of placental-derived CRH

d. Decreased production of placental-derived CRH

42–9. A 26-year-old G2P1 presents at 29 weeks' gestation complaining of leaking clear fluid from her vagina. A speculum examination reveals scant pooling of fluid in the posterior vagina, and the microscopic analysis of the fluid reveals the following pattern. You diagnose premature rupture of the fetal membranes (PROM). Of the known risk factors for this condition, which is most commonly identified in such patients?

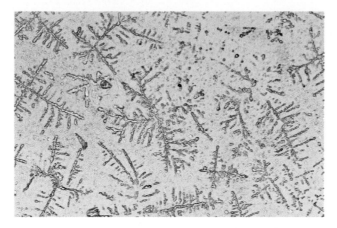

Reproduced with permission from Birnbaumer DM: Microscopic findings. In Knoop KJ, Stack LB, Storrow AB, et al (eds): The Atlas of Emergency Medicine, 3rd ed. New York, McGraw-Hill, 2010, Figure 25.24.

a. Smoking

b. Low socioeconomic status

c. Prior pregnancy complicated by PROM

d. None of the above

42–10. All **EXCEPT** which of the following lifestyle factors has been identified as an antecedent for preterm labor?

a. Frequent coitus

b. Illicit drug use

c. Young maternal age

d. Inadequate maternal weight gain

42–11. A 24-year-old G2P1 at 6 weeks' gestation presents for prenatal care and complains of bleeding, painful gums. Her obstetric history is significant for two prior preterm births. An oral examination reveals the findings noted in the image below. You counsel her that periodontal disease treatment in pregnancy has been proven to have which of the following favorable outcomes?

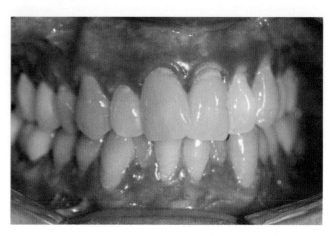

Reproduced with permission from Gonsalves WC, Usatine RP: Gingivitis and Periodontal Disease. In Usatine RP, Smith MA, Chumley H, et al (eds): The Color Atlas of Family Medicine. New York, McGraw-Hill, 2009, Figure 38-1.

a. Improved periodontal health

b. Decreased rates of preterm birth

c. Decreased rates of low birthweight

d. All of the above

42–12. Intervals shorter than how many months between pregnancies have been associated with an increased risk for preterm birth?

a. 18

b. 24

c. 36

d. 48

42–13. A 33-year-old G2P2 is contemplating pregnancy but is hesitant since her two prior deliveries occurred at 28 and 29 weeks' gestation, respectively. You inform her that her risk for a recurrent preterm birth less than 34 weeks' gestation approximates what value?

a. 15%

b. 25%

c. 40%

d. 70%

42–14. A 22-year-old G2P1 at 14 weeks' gestation complains of a malodorous vaginal discharge. A saline preparation of the discharge is prepared, and findings are illustrated in this image. You recommend antimicrobial treatment for this condition for what principal reason?

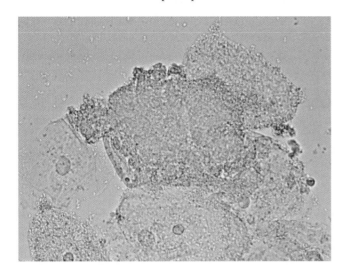

a. Resolution of symptoms

b. Prevention of preterm birth

c. Avoidance of spontaneous abortion

d. Treatment of intraamnionic infection

42–15. Characteristics of Braxton Hicks contractions can include all **EXCEPT** which of the following?

a. Painful

b. Nonrhythmical

c. Irregular pattern

d. Associated with cervical change

42–16. Performance of routine cervical examinations at each prenatal care visit has been demonstrated to effect what outcome?

a. Decreased preterm birth rate

b. Increased interventions for preterm labor

c. Increased rate of premature rupture of fetal membranes

d. None of the above

42–17. Which of the following is true regarding sonographic evaluation of the cervix as a part of the assessment for preterm birth risk?

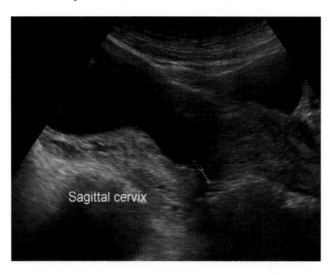

a. Transabdominal approach is preferred to avoid cervical manipulation.

b. In research populations, women with progressively shorter cervices had increased preterm labor rates.

c. Women with prior preterm birth and with cervical lengths equal to 35 mm will benefit from cerclage placement.

d. All of the above

42–18. Potential indications to perform the procedure demonstrated in this image include which of the following?

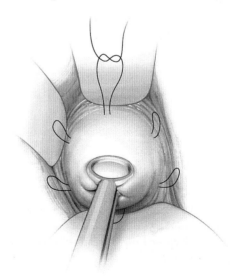

Reproduced with permission from Cunningham FG, Leveno KJ, Bloom SL, et al (eds): Abortion. In Williams Obstetrics, 24th ed. New York, McGraw-Hill, 2014, Figure 18-5C.

a. Recurrent midtrimester losses

b. Short cervix identified sonographically

c. Threatened preterm labor with cervical dilatation

d. All of the above

42–19. 17-Hydroxyprogesterone caproate has been demonstrated in a randomized, controlled trial to decrease the preterm birth rate in women with which of the following characteristics?

  a. Nulliparous

  b. Carrying twins

  c. Prior preterm birth

  d. None of the above

42–20. Based on the known natural history of preterm premature ruptured membranes, approximately what percentage of women will be delivered within 48 hours of membrane rupture when this complication occurs between 24 and 34 weeks' gestation?

  a. 20%

  b. 40%

  c. 70%

  d. 90%

42–21. A 20-year-old primigravida at 18 weeks' gestation presents after she noticed a gush of fluid from her vagina. You confirm the diagnosis of preterm rupture of the fetal membranes. Sonographic evaluation confirms anhydramnios. In the unlikely event that she remains undelivered at a viable gestational age, perinatal survival would be unlikely because of underdevelopment of what organ system?

  a. Brain

  b. Lungs

  c. Heart

  d. Kidneys

42–22. What is the only reliable indicator of clinical chorioamnionitis in women with preterm rupture of the fetal membranes?

  a. Fever

  b. Leukocytosis

  c. Fetal tachycardia

  d. Positive cervical or vaginal cultures

42–23. Several antibiotic regimens have been used to prolong the latency period in women with preterm rupture of the fetal membranes who are attempting expectant management. Which antibiotic should be avoided in this setting because it has been associated with an increased risk of necrotizing enterocolitis in the newborn?

  a. Ampicillin

  b. Amoxicillin

  c. Erythromycin

  d. Amoxicillin-clavulanate

42–24. A 25-year-old primigravida at 34 weeks and 5 days' gestation by certain dating criteria is found to have preterm rupture of the fetal membranes. What is the most appropriate management strategy?

  a. Expedited delivery

  b. Expectant management

  c. Administer a course of corticosteroids followed by delivery

  d. Expectant management unless fetal lung maturity is confirmed

42–25. Corticosteroids administered to women at risk for preterm birth have been demonstrated to decrease rates of respiratory distress if the birth is delayed for at least what amount of time after the initiation of therapy?

  a. 12 hours

  b. 24 hours

  c. 36 hours

  d. 48 hours

42–26. When antimicrobials have been administered to forestall preterm birth in women with preterm labor, rates of which of the following untoward perinatal outcomes have been consistently reduced?

  a. Neonatal death

  b. Cerebral palsy

  c. Chronic lung disease

  d. None of the above

42–27. Although bed rest is commonly prescribed for women deemed to be at increased risk for preterm birth, limited data exist to support a benefit of this recommendation. Which of the following *negative* outcomes have been reported in pregnant women placed on bed rest compared with those without this restriction?

  a. Greater bone loss

  b. Impaired fetal growth

  c. Greater maternal weight gain

  d. Higher rates of preeclampsia

42–28. A 21-year-old primigravida presents at 28 weeks' gestation in active preterm labor, and intravenous terbutaline is administered for tocolysis. Approximately 2 hours after therapy initiation, she begins to cough, and her peripheral oxygen saturation is noted to be 80 percent. The following chest radiograph is obtained. In which of the following clinical settings is the risk for this complication increased?

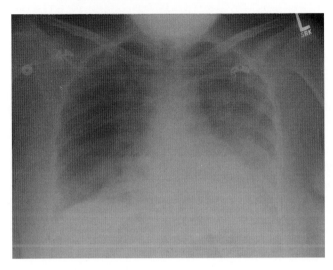

a. Twin pregnancy

b. Maternal sepsis

c. Concurrent administration of corticosteroids

d. All of the above

42–29. What reversible complication can be seen when indomethacin is used for tocolysis longer than 24 to 48 hours?

a. Oligohydramnios

b. Placental abruption

c. Neonatal necrotizing enterocolitis

d. Neonatal intraventricular hemorrhage

42–30. The combination of nifedipine with what other tocolytic agent can potentially cause dangerous neuromuscular blockade?

a. Atosiban

b. Terbutaline

c. Indomethacin

d. Magnesium sulfate

42–31. A 28-year-old primigravida at 27 weeks' gestation presents with regular painful uterine contractions, and her cervix is 8 cm dilated. The fetus has a vertex presentation. The fetal heart rate tracing is reassuring. Which of the following procedures will help decrease the risk for intraventricular hemorrhage in her neonate?

a. Episiotomy

b. Cesarean delivery

c. Forceps-assisted vaginal delivery

d. None of the above

42–32. Although the efficacy is somewhat controversial, intrapartum administration of magnesium sulfate to women who deliver preterm has been demonstrated to reduce rates of which of the following neonatal outcomes?

a. Cerebral palsy

b. Necrotizing enterocolitis

c. Neonatal seizure activity

d. Bronchopulmonary dysplasia

CHAPTER 42 ANSWER KEY

Question number	Letter answer	Page cited	Header cited
42–1	c	p. 829	Introduction
42–2	c	p. 829	Definition of Preterm
42–3	c	p. 829	Definition of Preterm
42–4	d	p. 829	Definition of Preterm
42–5	c	p. 832	Morbidity in Preterm Infants
42–6	d	p. 833	Threshold of Viability
42–7	a	p. 835	Late Preterm Birth
42–8	c	p. 837	Maternal-Fetal Stress
42–9	d	p. 839	Preterm Premature Rupture of Membranes
42–10	a	p. 841	Lifestyle Factors
42–11	a	p. 841	Periodontal Disease
42–12	a	p. 841	Interval between Pregnancies
42–13	c	p. 841	Prior Preterm Birth; Table 42-5
42–14	a	p. 842	Bacterial Vaginosis
42–15	d	p. 842	Symptoms
42–16	d	p. 843	Cervical Change
42–17	b	p. 843	Length
42–18	d	p. 844	Cervical Cerclage
42–19	c	p. 844	Prior Preterm Birth and Progestin Compounds
42–20	d	p. 847	Natural History
42–21	b	p. 848	Risks of Expectant Management
42–22	a	p. 848	Clinical Chorioamnionitis
42–23	d	p. 848	Antimicrobial Therapy
42–24	a	p. 849	Management Recommendations; Table 42-9
42–25	b	p. 850	Corticosteroids for Fetal Lung Maturation
42–26	d	p. 851	Antimicrobials
42–27	a	p. 851	Bed Rest
42–28	d	p. 852	Ritodrine
42–29	a	p. 852	Prostaglandin Inhibitors
42–30	d	p. 853	Calcium Channel Blockers
42–31	d	p. 854	Delivery; Prevention of Neonatal Intracranial Hemorrhage
42–32	a	p. 854	Magnesium for Fetal Neuroprotection

Postterm Pregnancy

43-1. What is the threshold of completed weeks after which a pregnancy is considered prolonged?

    a. 40 weeks

    b. 41 weeks

    c. 42 weeks

    d. 43 weeks

43-2. Which of the following is true regarding calculated gestational age?

    a. Underestimated if based on last menstrual period (LMP) alone

    b. Overestimated if based on first-trimester sonographic examination

    c. Overestimated if based on second-trimester sonographic examination and LMP compared with LMP alone

    d. None of the above

43-3. Rare fetal-placental factors associated with postterm pregnancy include which of the following?

    a. Wilms tumor

    b. Anencephaly

    c. Adrenal hyperplasia

    d. Autosomal-recessive placental sulfatase overproduction

43-4. This graphic suggests which of the following regarding perinatal mortality rates (PMR)?

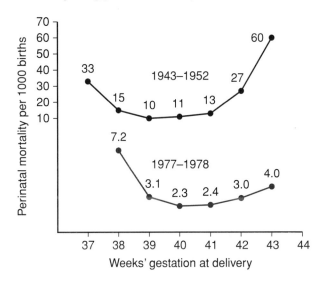

Reproduced with permission from Cunningham FG, Leveno KJ, Bloom SL, et al (eds): Postterm pregnancy. In Williams Obstetrics, 24th ed. New York, McGraw-Hill, 2014, Figure 43-2.

    a. PMR was lowest in 1943–1952.

    b. PMR was higher in 1977–1978.

    c. PMR increases after 41 weeks.

    d. PMR increases after 40 weeks.

43–5. Major causes of death in postterm pregnancy include which of the following?

    a. Placenta accreta

    b. Placental abruption

    c. Unexplained stillbirth in diabetic patients

    d. Cephalopelvic disproportion in prolonged labor

43–6. This graphic illustrates which of the following regarding perinatal mortality rates (PMR)?

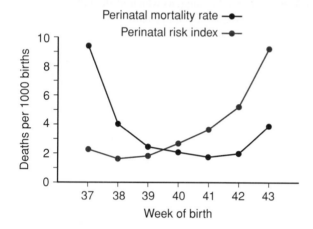

Reproduced with permission from Cunningham FG, Leveno KJ, Bloom SL, et al (eds): Postterm pregnancy. In Williams Obstetrics, 24th ed. New York, McGraw-Hill, 2014, Figure 43-3.

    a. Highest PMR occurs at 43 weeks.

    b. Highest PMR occurs at 38 weeks.

    c. Perinatal risk index, which accounts for risk of all ongoing pregnancies, is highest at 36 weeks

    d. None of the above

43–7. Which of the following is true concerning the syndrome afflicting this infant?

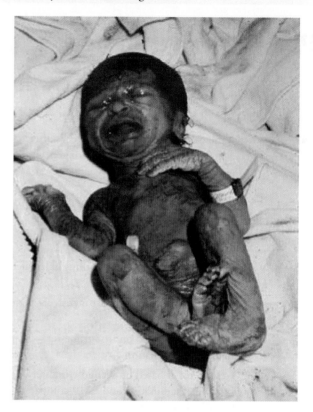

Reproduced with permission from Cunningham FG, Leveno KJ, Bloom SL, et al (eds): Postterm pregnancy. In Williams Obstetrics, 24th ed. New York, McGraw-Hill, 2014, Figure 43-4.

    a. Features include simian crease and low-set ears.

    b. Its incidence in pregnancies between 41 and 43 weeks is 20%.

    c. Neurological deficits are found in 23% of affected newborns.

    d. Associated oligohydramnios substantially increases its likelihood at 42 weeks.

43–8. In postterm gestations, which of the following suggests compromise of fetal oxygenation?

    a. Decreased hematocrit

    b. Proapoptotic gene upregulation

    c. Elevated erythropoietin level

    d. None of the above

43–9. This figure demonstrates which of the following?

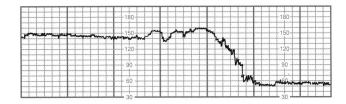

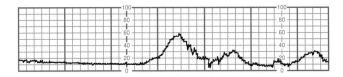

Reproduced with permission from Cunningham FG, Leveno KJ, Bloom SL, et al (eds): Postterm pregnancy. In Williams Obstetrics, 24th ed. New York, McGraw-Hill, 2014, Figure 43-6.

    a. Late deceleration

    b. Variable deceleration

    c. Prolonged deceleration

    d. None of the above

43–10. In postterm pregnancies, which of the following is true of most cases of fetal distress?

    a. Associated with cord occlusion

    b. Associated with prolonged labor

    c. Not correlated with viscous meconium

    d. Caused by uteroplacental insufficiency

43–11. Which of the following increases the risk of meconium aspiration syndrome?

    a. Fetal acidemia

    b. Oligohydramnios

    c. Postterm pregnancy

    d. A and B

43–12. This graphic illustrates which of the following?

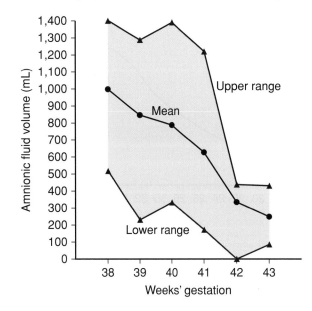

Reproduced with permission from Cunningham FG, Leveno KJ, Bloom SL, et al (eds): Postterm pregnancy. In Williams Obstetrics, 23rd ed. New York, McGraw-Hill, 2010, Figure 37-8.

    a. Amnionic fluid volume decreases from term until 43 weeks.

    b. The largest amount of amnionic fluid is present before term.

    c. The smallest amount of fluid in the upper range is seen at 41 weeks.

    d. The greatest amount of fluid in the lower range is approximately 700 mL at 38 weeks.

43–13. This graphic illustrates which of the following?

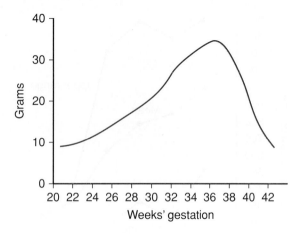

Reproduced with permission from Cunningham FG, Leveno KJ, Bloom SL, et al (eds): Postterm pregnancy. In Williams Obstetrics, 24th ed. New York, McGraw-Hill, 2014, Figure 43-5.

    a. Fetuses lose weight after 40 weeks.

    b. Fetal growth continues until at least 42 weeks.

    c. The peak of fetal growth occurs in the late midtrimester.

    d. Maternal and fetal morbidity associated with macrosomia would be mitigated with timely induction.

43–14. In the presence of macrosomia, which of the following is true?

    a. Early induction decreases maternal and fetal morbidity rates.

    b. Cesarean delivery should be performed for estimated fetal weight > 4000 g.

    c. Cesarean delivery is recommended for estimated fetal weights > 4500 g if there is prolonged second-stage labor.

    d. None of the above

43–15. What percentage of postterm stillbirths are growth-restricted?

    a. 10%

    b. 25%

    c. 33%

    d. 50%

43–16. Concerning an unfavorable cervix, research supports which of the following statements?

    a. A cervical length ≤ 3 cm was predictive of successful induction.

    b. Of women at 42 weeks, 92% have an unfavorable cervix, when defined as a Bishop score < 7.

    c. The risk of cesarean delivery is increased twofold in those with a closed cervix at 42 weeks undergoing labor induction.

    d. All of the above

43–17. Concerning membrane stripping, research supports which of the following statements?

    a. Decreases need for induction

    b. Increases maternal infection rates

    c. Complications include bleeding and pain

    d. All of the above

43–18. This graphic illustrates which of the following?

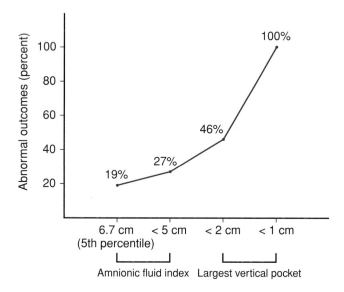

Reproduced with permission from Cunningham FG, Leveno KJ, Bloom SL, et al (eds): Postterm pregnancy. In Williams Obstetrics, 23rd ed. New York, McGraw-Hill, 2010, Figure 37-9.

    a. An AFI < 1 cm had 100% abnormal outcomes.

    b. Abnormal fetal outcomes occur when the AFI is at the 5th centile.

    c. When the AFI is < 2 cm, abnormal outcomes were increased relative to those at 5th centile.

    d. If the largest vertical pocket (LVP) was < 5 cm, the chance of an abnormal outcome was 27%.

43–19. Concerning the station of the vertex in nulliparous pregnancies at the beginning of induction for postterm pregnancy, research supports which of the following statements?

　a. The cesarean delivery rate is directly related to station.

　b. The cesarean delivery rate is 6% if the vertex is at −1 station.

　c. The cesarean delivery rate is 43% if the vertex is at −3 station.

　d. All of the above

43–20. Concerning induction versus fetal testing in prolonged pregnancies, research supports which of the following statements?

　a. Testing is associated with decreased cesarean delivery rates.

　b. Most studies are performed during the 43rd week of gestation.

　c. No differences in perinatal death and cesarean delivery rates are found between the two approaches.

　d. None of the above

43–21. In Alexander's study (2001) comparing induction versus awaiting spontaneous labor at 42 weeks' gestation, investigators found which of the following?

　a. Decreased cesarean delivery rate in the induction group

　b. Increased cesarean delivery rate for fetal distress in the spontaneous labor group

　c. Increased cesarean delivery rate in the induction group related to the use of meperidine analgesia during labor

　d. Increased cesarean delivery rate in the induction group related to nulliparity, epidural anesthesia, and an unfavorable cervix

43–22. Concerning this algorithm that summarizes the American College of Obstetricians and Gynecologists (ACOG) recommendations, which of the following is true?

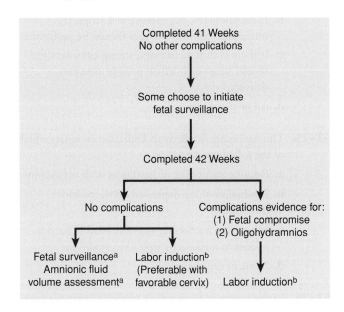

Reproduced with permission from Cunningham FG, Leveno KJ, Bloom SL, et al (eds): Postterm pregnancy. In Williams Obstetrics, 24th ed. New York, McGraw-Hill, 2014, Figure 43-10.

　a. Induction should be performed at 41 completed weeks.

　b. If no complications exist, labor may be induced at 42 completed weeks.

　c. Fetal surveillance should be initiated for a pregnancy with oligohydramnios at 42 completed weeks.

　d. All of the above

43–23. Which of the following is true regarding amnioinfusion?

　a. Requires amniotomy

　b. Reduces late decelerations

　c. Reduces the rate of meconium aspiration syndrome

　d. Does not affect the cesarean delivery rate in postterm fetuses

43–24. Concerning the nulliparous woman with a postterm gestation in early labor, which of the following is true?

   a. If there are repetitive variable decelerations, amnioinfusion is appropriate.

   b. If cephalopelvic disproportion is suspected, immediate cesarean delivery should be performed.

   c. If there is thin meconium, strong consideration should be given to effect prompt cesarean delivery.

   d. All of the above

43–25. The American Academy of Pediatrics supports which of the following practices?

   a. Routine suctioning of newborns with meconium

   b. Intubation of the depressed newborn with meconium

   c. Meconium suctioning after the head is born to minimize meconium aspiration syndrome

   d. None of the above

43–26. In the postterm fetus, which of the following is true regarding amniotomy?

   a. May identify thick meconium

   b. May exacerbate cord compression

   c. Is essential to effect continuous fetal monitoring

   d. A and B

43–27. Your patient is a 32-year-old G3P2 at $40^{6/7}$ weeks' gestation. Her first prenatal visit occurred after 30 weeks' gestation. Examination today reveals a 1-cm dilated cervix, cephalic presentation, no ballotment of the head, and good fetal movement. What is the best next step in the management of this patient?

   a. Nonstress test

   b. Labor induction

   c. Oxytocin challenge test

   d. Sonographic assessment of the amnionic fluid index (AFI)

43–28. One week later, the patient in Question 43–27 returns to your office. Now her examination reveals a 1- to 2-cm dilated cervix, cephalic presentation, and an easily ballottable head. However, she notes decreased fetal movement. Your management plan should include which of the following?

   a. Nonstress test

   b. Labor induction

   c. Oxytocin challenge test

   d. A or B

43–29. With reassuring status by antepartum surveillance verified, what might your next step be for the patient in Question 43-28?

   a. Elective cesarean delivery

   b. Weekly antepartum surveillance

   c. Amniocentesis to verify pulmonary maturity followed by induction

   d. B or C

43–30. Your patient is a 16-year-old G1P0 at 41 weeks' gestation with complaints of decreased fetal movement. Her care started during her first trimester. She has a stated last menstrual period that agrees with 16-week sonographic measurements. Examination reveals a 1- to 2-cm dilated cervix, cephalic presentation, estimated fetal weight of 9 lb, and a ballottable head. What is a reasonable next step?

   a. Nonstress test

   b. Labor induction

   c. Umbilical artery Doppler evaluation

   d. A or B

43–31. After a reassuring nonstress test (NST) result, the patient in Question 43-30 returns to your office 1 week later. Examination now reveals a 2-cm dilated cervix, cephalic presentation, and estimated fetal weight of 9½ lb. Fetal movement is good, and the vertex is ballotable. What is a reasonable next step?

   a. NST

   b. Labor induction

   c. Amnionic fluid surveillance

   d. All of the above

43–32. Your patient is a 22-year-old G1P0 at 42 weeks' gestation by excellent dating criteria. She arrives for induction and cervical examination reveals 1 to 2 cm dilatation, cephalic presentation, and a head that is not ballottable. The estimated fetal weight is 8½ lb. Her fetal heart rate pattern is category II. You perform an amniotomy, place a direct fetal scalp electrode monitor, and encounter viscous meconium. What is an appropriate next step?

   a. Cesarean delivery

   b. Low-dose oxytocin protocol

   c. Place intrauterine pressure catheter

   d. All may be considered.

Reference:

Alexander JM, McIntire DD, Leveno KJ: Prolonged pregnancy: induction of labor and cesarean births. Obstet Gynecol 97:911, 2001

CHAPTER 43 ANSWER KEY

Question number	Letter answer	Page cited	Header cited
43–1	c	p. 862	Introduction
43–2	d	p. 862	Estimated Gestational Age Using Menstrual Dates
43–3	b	p. 863	Incidence
43–4	c	p. 863	Perinatal Mortality
43–5	c	p. 863	Perinatal Mortality
43–6	d	p. 863	Perinatal Mortality
43–7	d	p. 864	Postmaturity Syndrome
43–8	c	p. 864	Placental Dysfunction
43–9	c	p. 865	Fetal Distress and Oligohydramnios
43–10	a	p. 865	Fetal Distress and Oligohydramnios
43–11	d	p. 865	Fetal Distress and Oligohydramnios
43–12	a	p. 865	Fetal Distress and Oligohydramnios
43–13	b	p. 867	Macrosomia
43–14	c	p. 867	Macrosomia
43–15	c	p. 866	Fetal-Growth Restriction
43–16	d	p. 867	Unfavorable Cervix
43–17	c	p. 868	Cervical Ripening
43–18	b	p. 866	Oligohydramnios
43–19	d	p. 868	Station of Vertex
43–20	c	p. 868	Induction versus Fetal Testing
43–21	d	p. 868	Induction versus Fetal Testing
43–22	b	p. 864	Placental Dysfunction
43–23	a	p. 869	Intrapartum Management
43–24	a	p. 869	Intrapartum Management
43–25	b	p. 869	Intrapartum Management
43–26	d	p. 869	Intrapartum Management
43–27	d	p. 866	Oligohydramnios
43–28	a	p. 869	Management Recommendations
43–29	d	p. 869	Management Recommendations
43–30	d	p. 869	Management Recommendations
43–31	d	p. 869	Management Recommendations
43–32	d	p. 869	Intrapartum Management

CHAPTER 44

Fetal-Growth Disorders

44–1. What can be said regarding birthweight in the United States?

   a. All low-birthweight neonates are born preterm.

   b. Of low-birthweight neonates, 3% are born at term.

   c. The percentage of low-birthweight neonates has been decreasing since the mid-1980s.

   d. None of the above

44–2. Given the graphic below, what can be said regarding the velocity of fetal growth at different gestational ages?

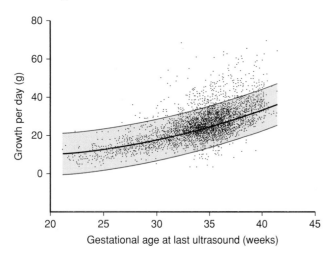

Reproduced with permission from Cunningham FG, Leveno KJ, Bloom SL, et al (eds): Fetal growth disorders. In Williams Obstetrics, 24th ed. New York, McGraw-Hill, 2014, Figure 44-1.

   a. At 24 weeks' gestation, growth averages 5 g/day.

   b. At 34 weeks' gestation, growth averages 25–30 g/day.

   c. There is considerable variation in the velocity of fetal growth.

   d. All of the above

44–3. Elevated C-peptide levels are associated with which of the following?

   a. Hyperinsulinemia

   b. Hypercholesterolemia

   c. Fetal-growth restriction

   d. All of the above

44–4. Amino acids undergo which type of transport from maternal to fetal circulation?

   a. Active transport

   b. Passive diffusion

   c. Facilitated diffusion

   d. None of the above

44–5. This graph depicts the relationship between birthweight percentile and perinatal mortality and morbidity rates. Below which threshold value of birthweight percentile do perinatal mortality rates increase most rapidly?

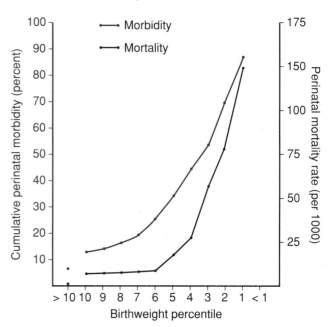

Reproduced with permission from Cunningham FG, Leveno KJ, Bloom SL, et al (eds): Fetal growth disorders. In Williams Obstetrics, 24th ed. New York, McGraw-Hill, 2014, Figure 44-3.

   a. 3

   b. 5

   c. 7

   d. 10

44–6. Symmetrical growth restriction is characterized by a reduction in which of the following?

   a. Head size

   b. Body size

   c. Both body and head size

   d. Both body and femur length

44–7. Which of the following correctly represents current thinking on asymmetrical versus symmetrical growth restriction?

   a. Neonatal morbidity rates are higher with asymmetrical growth restriction.

   b. Uteroplacental insufficiency leads to asymmetrical growth restriction in most cases of preeclampsia.

   c. Assigning specific morbidity to specific fetal-growth restriction patterns is a straightforward process.

   d. None of the above

44–8. Growing evidence suggests that fetal-growth restriction affects organ development, especially which of the following?

   a. Brain

   b. Heart

   c. Kidney

   d. Thyroid

44–9. Compared with appropriately grown fetuses of equivalent gestational age, growth-restricted fetuses have which of the following perinatal advantages?

   a. Lower stillbirth rate

   b. Lower perinatal mortality rate

   c. Lower rate of respiratory distress syndrome

   d. None of the above

44–10. Which of the following is true regarding women with pregravid weights less than 100 lb compared with normal-weight women?

   a. They have a twofold risk of having growth-restricted fetuses.

   b. They have a slightly increased risk of having a fetus with aneuploidy.

   c. The risk of fetal-growth restriction may be modulated by appropriate maternal gestational weight gain.

   d. All of the above

44–11. Which of the following is true regarding maternal nutrition during pregnancy?

   a. Providing micronutrient supplementation to undernourished women consistently lowers rates of small-for-gestational-age newborns.

   b. For all maternal weight categories, excessive maternal weight gain during pregnancy is associated with large-for-gestational-age newborns.

   c. For all maternal weight categories, maternal weight gain in the second and third trimesters that is less than recommended is associated with fetal-growth restriction.

   d. All of the above

44–12. Women screened during pregnancy for psychosocial risk factors compared with pregnant women who do not undergo such screening have which of the following?

   a. Lower preterm birth rates

   b. More appropriate interventions

   c. Lower rates of low-birthweight newborns

   d. All of the above

44–13. Which of the following vascular diseases in women during pregnancy leads to the highest perinatal morbidity rates?

   a. Class F diabetics

   b. Chronic hypertension

   c. Ischemic heart disease

   d. Valvular heart disease

44–14. Which of the following is true concerning diabetes in pregnancy?

   a. Compared with type 1 diabetics, type 2 diabetics have a higher risk of delivering a large-for-gestational-age (LGA) newborn.

   b. Type 1 diabetics have a proportionately higher risk of delivering a small-for-gestational-age (SGA) than an LGA newborn.

   c. Type 1 diabetics without vascular involvement have a proportionately higher risk of delivering an LGA newborn than an SGA one.

   d. None of the above

44–15. Which of the following are true concerning chronic hypoxia?

   a. Women with cyanotic heart disease have a higher rate of growth-restricted fetuses.

   b. Neonates born at lower altitudes have a lower risk of being small for gestational age.

   c. Neonates born at higher altitudes have a lower risk of being large for gestational age.

   d. All of the above

44–16. Regarding maternal anemia, which of the following is true?

    a. It confers a high associated risk of fetal-growth restriction.

    b. Fetal-growth restriction rates are higher in women with sickle-cell trait.

    c. Fetal-growth restriction is related to restricted maternal blood volume expansion.

    d. All of the above

44–17. Which of the following is the primary autoantibody that predicts obstetrical antiphospholipid antibody syndrome?

    a. Lupus anticoagulant

    b. Anticardiolipin antibodies

    c. Anti-beta-glycoprotein-I antibodies

    d. Anti-double-stranded DNA antibodies

44–18. Fetal-growth restriction is associated with all **EXCEPT** which of the following?

    a. Prior infertility

    b. Placental chorangioma

    c. Inherited thrombophilia

    d. Velamentous cord insertion

44–19. The graph below suggests which of the following regarding fetal-growth restriction and multifetal pregnancy?

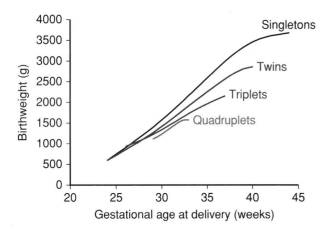

Reproduced with permission from Cunningham FG, Leveno KJ, Bloom SL, et al (eds): Fetal growth disorders. In Williams Obstetrics, 24th ed. New York, McGraw-Hill, 2014, Figure 44-5.

    a. Most growth-restricted neonates result from quadruplet pregnancies.

    b. Fetal-growth restriction can be detected at 20 weeks' gestation in quadruplets.

    c. In multifetal gestations, fetal-growth restriction typically becomes apparent in the early third trimester.

    d. All of the above

44–20. Which of the following drugs are associated with fetal-growth restriction?

    a. Metoclopramide

    b. Diphenhydramine

    c. Cyclophosphamide

    d. Low-dose aspirin

44–21. This growth-restricted newborn was born at 36 weeks' gestation. All **EXCEPT** which of the following are infectious causes of fetal-growth restriction?

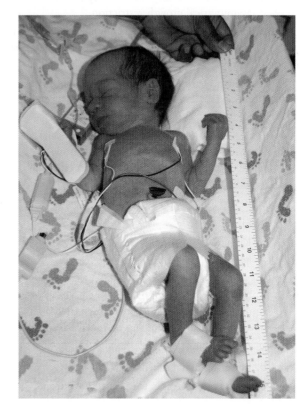

Reproduced with permission from Cunningham FG, Leveno KJ, Bloom SL, et al (eds): Fetal growth disorders. In Williams Obstetrics, 24th ed. New York, McGraw-Hill, 2014, Figure 44-7.

    a. Congenital syphilis

    b. Maternal tuberculosis

    c. First-trimester primary cytomegalovirus infection

    d. Antepartum maternal seroconversion for toxoplasmosis

44–22. In which chromosomal aneuploidy is fetal-growth restriction virtually always present?

    a. 45,X

    b. Trisomy 13

    c. Trisomy 18

    d. Trisomy 21

44–23. Which of the following is true regarding serial fundal height measurements to detect fetal-growth restriction?

    a. Sensitivity < 25%, specificity < 50%

    b. Sensitivity < 35%, specificity > 90%

    c. Sensitivity < 70%, specificity < 50%

    d. Sensitivity < 85%, specificity > 90%

44–24. Which of the following sonographic assessments of fetal-growth restriction is the most predictive of obstetrical outcome?

    a. Biometric growth < 3rd percentile

    b. Biometric growth < 5th percentile

    c. Biometric growth < 3rd percentile and abnormal umbilical artery Doppler velocimetry results

    d. Biometric growth < 5th percentile and absent end-diastolic flow noted during umbilical artery Doppler velocimetry study

44–25. Which of the following is true regarding oligohydramnios?

    a. It is associated with fetal-growth restriction.

    b. It is associated with congenital fetal malformations.

    c. It is associated with a higher cesarean delivery rate.

    d. All of the above

44–26. Which of the following is true concerning the prevention of fetal-growth restriction?

    a. In the United States, malaria prophylaxis assists prevention.

    b. Preconceptional and antepartum smoking cessation assists prevention.

    c. For the gravida with chronic hypertension, antihypertensive therapy assists prevention.

    d. Aspirin therapy assists prevention and is recommended by the American College of Obstetricians and Gynecologists.

44–27. Ms. Smith is a 37-year-old multigravida who presents to your office at 32 weeks' gestation as calculated by her last menstrual period. Her hematocrit is 29 volume percent, and she has sickle-cell trait. During sonographic evaluation, the fetus has biometric values that correlate with a 28-week fetus. What is the most likely explanation?

    a. Aneuploidy

    b. Chronic hypoxia

    c. Poor pregnancy dating

    d. First-trimester cytomegalovirus infection

44–28. For the patient in Question 44–27, when will you reevaluate fetal growth?

    a. 1 week

    b. 2 weeks

    c. 3 weeks

    d. 6 weeks

44–29. Your next obstetrical sonographic evaluation of the patient in Question 44–27 is performed 4 weeks after the first one and now at an estimated gestational age of 36 weeks. The fetus now has measurements similar to a 30-week fetus. Growth restriction seems more likely. What is appropriate at this time?

    a. Delivery

    b. Strict bed rest

    c. Umbilical artery Doppler velocimetry

    d. Sonographic fetal biometry in 1 week

44–30. For the patient in Question 44–27, studies indicate a systolic/diastolic (S/D) ratio of 4, and the patient has an amnionic fluid index (AFI) of 9 cm. What is appropriate at this time?

    a. Delivery

    b. Betamethasone administration

    c. Sonographic fetal biometry in 1 week

    d. Serial umbilical artery Doppler studies and AFI assessment

44–31. For the patient in Question 44–27, during the next week, umbilical artery Doppler velocimetry indicates reversed end-diastolic flow (REDF), and the amnionic fluid index (AFI) is 4 cm. What is appropriate at this time?

    a. Deliver the fetus

    b. Plan delivery at 38 weeks after amniocentesis for pulmonary maturity

    c. Continue serial umbilical artery Doppler studies and AFI assessment

    d. All are reasonable

44–32. According the American College of Obstetricians and Gynecologists, which of the following is the threshold above which macrosomia is defined?

    a. 4000 g

    b. 4250 g

    c. 4500 g

    d. 5000 g

44–33. For the prediction of macrosomia, how does clinical estimation of fetal weight compare with sonographic estimation?

a. Less accurate

b. Similar accuracy

c. Modestly more accurate

d. Significantly more accurate

44–34. In pregnancies with estimated fetal weights > 4000 g after 37 weeks' gestation, prophylactic labor induction has which of the following effects?

a. Increases the cesarean delivery rate

b. Decreases the shoulder dystocia rate

c. Decreases the postpartum hemorrhage rates

d. All of the above

CHAPTER 44 ANSWER KEY

Question number	Letter answer	Page cited	Header cited
44–1	b	p. 872	Introduction
44–2	c	p. 872	Fetal Growth
44–3	a	p. 872	Fetal Growth
44–4	a	p. 872	Fetal Growth
44–5	a	p. 874	Fetal Growth Restriction, Definition
44–6	c	p. 875	Symmetrical versus Asymmetrical Growth Restriction
44–7	a	p. 875	Symmetrical versus Asymmetrical Growth Restriction
44–8	b	p. 876	Fetal Undergrowth
44–9	d	p. 877	Accelerated Lung Maturation
44–10	c	p. 877	Constitutionally Small Mothers
44–11	b	p. 877	Gestational Weight Gain and Nutrition
44–12	d	p. 878	Social Deprivation
44–13	c	p. 878	Vascular Disease
44–14	c	p. 878	Pregestational Diabetes
44–15	d	p. 878	Chronic Hypoxia
44–16	c	p. 878	Anemia
44–17	a	p. 878	Antiphospholipid Antibody Syndrome
44–18	c	p. 879	Inherited Thrombophilias; Infertility; Placental and Cord Abnormalities
44–19	c	p. 879	Multiple Gestations
44–20	c	p. 879	Drugs with Teratogenic and Fetal Effects
44–21	d	p. 879	Maternal and Fetal Infections
44–22	c	p. 880	Chromosomal Aneuploidies
44–23	b	p. 880	Uterine Fundal Height
44–24	c	p. 880	Sonographic Measurements of Fetal Size
44–25	d	p. 881	Amnionic Fluid Volume Measurement
44–26	b	p. 882	Prevention
44–27	c	p. 880	Recognition of Fetal-Growth Restriction
44–28	c	p. 880	Sonographic Measurements of Fetal Size
44–29	c	p. 882	Management
44–30	d	p. 883	Figure 44-9
44–31	a	p. 883	Figure 44-9
44–32	c	p. 885	Empirical Birthweight
44–33	b	p. 885	Diagnosis
44–34	a	p. 886	Prophylactic Labor Induction

CHAPTER 45

Multifetal Pregnancy

45–1. Compared with singleton pregnancies, multifetal gestations have a higher risk of all **EXCEPT** which of the following complications?

    a. Preeclampsia

    b. Hysterectomy

    c. Maternal death

    d. Postterm pregnancy

45–2. Compared with singleton pregnancies, multifetal gestations have an infant mortality rate that is how many times greater?

    a. Twofold

    b. Threefold

    c. Fivefold

    d. Tenfold

45–3. Which of the following mechanisms may prevent monozygotic twins from being truly "identical"?

    a. Postzygotic mutation

    b. Unequal division of the protoplasmic material

    c. Variable expression of the same genetic disease

    d. All of the above

45–4. A patient delivers a twin gestation in which one infant has blood type A and one has type O. The patient and her husband are both type O. A particular phenomenon is proposed as the etiology of the discordant blood types. How would you explain this to the mother?

    a. The proposed phenomenon does not spontaneously occur in humans.

    b. It involves fertilization of one ovum that splits into two during the same menstrual cycle.

    c. It involves fertilization of two ova within the same menstrual cycle, but not at the same coitus.

    d. It involves fertilization of two ova separated in time by an interval as long as or longer than a menstrual cycle.

45–5. When trying to establish chorionicity of the pregnancy shown in the image here, which of the following statements is true?

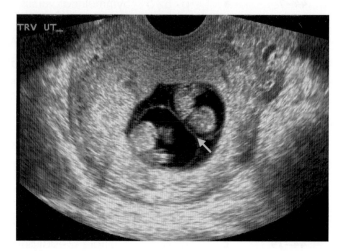

Reproduced with permission from Cunningham FG, Leveno KJ, Bloom SL, et al (eds): Multifetal pregnancy. In Williams Obstetrics, 24th ed. New York, McGraw-Hill, 2014, Figure 45-7B.

    a. There are two placentas.

    b. The twins must be monozygotic.

    c. The twins share the same amnion.

    d. The twins must have arisen from two separate ova.

45–6. Which of the following factors increases the risk for monozygotic twinning?

    a. Increased parity

    b. Increased maternal age

    c. The father is an identical twin.

    d. None of the above

45–7. The first-trimester sonographic image here shows two fetal heads arising from a shared body. How many days after fertilization must the division of this zygote have occurred to lead to the abnormality shown?

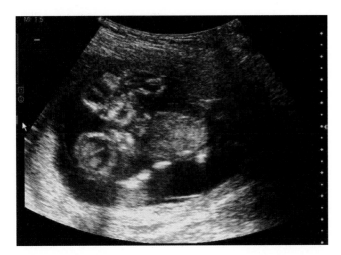

Reproduced with permission from Cunningham FG, Leveno KJ, Bloom SL, et al (eds): Multifetal pregnancy. In Williams Obstetrics, 24th ed. New York, McGraw-Hill, 2014, Figure 45-16.

   a. 0–3 days

   b. 4–7 days

   c. 8–12 days

   d. More than 13 days

45–8. A patient with twins is referred for prenatal care. At the referring clinic, she had several sonographic examinations that establish these to be monochorionic twins. Today, you see only one fetus sonographically. Which of the following statements is false regarding the risk of a vanishing twin?

   a. The risk exceeds 10% in multifetal gestations.

   b. The risk is higher in monochorionic than in dichorionic pregnancies.

   c. This risk is increased if she used assisted reproductive technologies to conceive.

   d. A vanishing twin does not affect first-trimester biomarker testing if it occurs after 10 weeks' gestation.

45–9. What is the approximate risk of triplet or higher-order multifetal gestation if ovarian stimulation and intrauterine insemination is used to achieve pregnancy?

   a. 10%

   b. 20%

   c. 30%

   d. 40%

45–10. What can be confirmed about the placenta being examined in the image here?

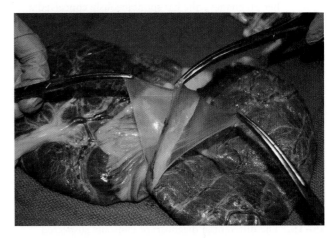

   a. Dizygosity

   b. Monozygosity

   c. One chorion, two amnions

   d. Two chorions, two amnions

45–11. Which of the following is true regarding the rate of monozygotic twinning?

   a. It approximates 1 in 250 worldwide.

   b. It is increased with maternal age and parity.

   c. It is lower for Hispanic women than for white women.

   d. It can be modified by FSH (follicle-stimulating hormone) treatment.

45–12. Which of the following statements is true regarding chorionicity in multifetal pregnancy?

   a. Dichorionic pregnancies are always dizygotic.

   b. Monochorionic membranes should have four layers.

   c. Monochorionic pregnancies are always monozygotic.

   d. Chorionicity is accurately determined by measuring the thickness of the dividing membranes during sonographic examination in the first trimester.

45–13. Among the following choices, which is the strongest risk factor for multifetal pregnancy?

   a. Advanced maternal age

   b. Use of clomiphene citrate

   c. African American ethnicity

   d. Maternal history of being a twin herself

45–14. A patient presents for prenatal care at 12 weeks' gestation and wants to know about specific risks to her pregnancy. She has spontaneously conceived a monochorionic twin gestation. Which statement is false regarding these twins?

    a. They have a higher risk of pregnancy loss than fraternal twins.

    b. Those born at term have a higher risk of cognitive delay than term singletons.

    c. They have twice the risk of malformations compared with singleton pregnancies.

    d. They have a lower risk of pregnancy loss than identical twins conceived with assisted reproductive technologies.

45–15. The differential diagnosis of clinically suspected twins includes all **EXCEPT** which of the following?

    a. Obesity

    b. Hydramnios

    c. Leiomyomas

    d. Blighted ovum

45–16. Regarding maternal adaptations to multifetal pregnancy, which of the following is lower in twin pregnancy compared with that in a singleton pregnancy?

    a. Blood volume expansion

    b. Blood pressure at term

    c. Blood loss at delivery

    d. Systemic vascular resistance

45–17. A fetus that is part of a dichorionic twin pair is estimated to weigh 2000 g at 33 weeks' gestation. What can be said about its growth?

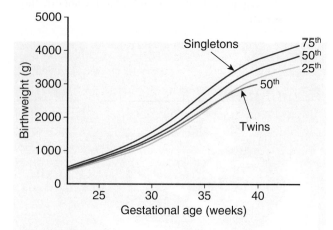

Reproduced with permission from Cunningham FG, Leveno KJ, Bloom SL, et al (eds): Multifetal pregnancy. In Williams Obstetrics, 24th ed. New York, McGraw-Hill, 2014, Figure 45-8.

    a. The fetus already shows growth restriction.

    b. The fetus will be growth restricted at term.

    c. The fetal growth is adequate for gestational age.

    d. Growth differences will not be apparent until delivery.

45–18. Among complications that may be seen in twin pregnancies, which of the following may be seen in dichorionic pregnancies?

    a. Acardiac twin

    b. Fetus-in-fetu

    c. Twin-twin transfusion syndrome

    d. Complete mole with coexisting normal twin

45–19. What is the major cause of increased neonatal morbidity rates in twins?

    a. Preterm birth

    b. Congenital malformations

    c. Abnormal growth patterns

    d. Twin-twin transfusion syndrome

45–20. When diagnosed at 20 weeks' gestation, which of the following statements is true regarding the twin vascular complication seen in the image here?

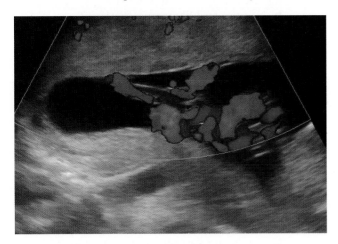

Used with permission from Dr. Jodi Dashe.

a. It precludes vaginal delivery.

b. It implies the twins are conjoined.

c. It has a 50% associated fetal mortality rate.

d. It can be monitored effectively with daily sonography.

45–21. Which are the most common vascular anastomoses seen in monochorionic twin placentas?

a. Deep vein-vein

b. Deep artery-vein

c. Superficial artery-vein

d. Superficial artery-artery

45–22. Which of the following statements is true in twin-reversed-arterial-perfusion (TRAP) sequence?

a. It is caused by a large arteriovenous placental shunt.

b. The donor is at risk of cardiomegaly and high-output heart failure.

c. The most effective treatment is injection of KCl into the recipient twin.

d. Placental arterial perfusion pressure in the recipient exceeds that of the donor.

45–23. A pair of monochorionic twins presents at 20 weeks' gestation with sonographic findings that suggest twin-twin transfusion syndrome. There is significant growth discordance, no bladder is visualized in the smaller twin, neither twin has ascites or hydrops, and umbilical Doppler studies are normal. What would be the assigned Quintero stage?

a. Stage I

b. Stage II

c. Stage III

d. Stage IV

45–24. The recipient cotwin in a monochorionic twin gestation affected by twin-twin transfusion syndrome may experience all **EXCEPT** which of the following neonatal complications?

a. Thrombosis

b. Hypovolemia

c. Kernicterus

d. Heart failure

45–25. What percentage of Quintero stage I cases remain stable without intervention?

a. 25%

b. 50%

c. 75%

d. 90%

45–26. Which of the following therapies for severe twin-twin transfusion syndrome has been shown in a randomized trial to improve survival rates of at least one twin to age 6 months?

a. Septostomy

b. Amnioreduction

c. Selective feticide

d. Laser ablation of vascular anastomoses

45–27. What is the calculated fetal growth discordance of a twin pair where the estimated fetal weight of twin A is 800 g and that of twin B is 600 g?

a. 10%

b. 15%

c. 25%

d. 33%

45–28. A second sonographic evaluation of the twin pair described in Question 45–27 shows 27% discordance. One fetus is male and one is female. Which mechanism is not the likely cause of their discordance?

    a. Unequal placental sharing

    b. Different growth potential

    c. Histological placental abnormality

    d. Suboptimal implantation of one placental site

45–29. With growing discordance, rates of which of the following neonatal complications are increased?

    a. Neonatal sepsis

    b. Necrotizing enterocolitis

    c. Intraventricular hemorrhage

    d. All of the above

45–30. Which of the following is the most important predictor of neurological outcome of the survivor after death of a cotwin?

    a. Chorionicity

    b. Gestational age at time of demise

    c. Malformations present in the deceased twin

    d. Length of time between demise and delivery of survivor

45–31. Which of the following methods of antepartum fetal surveillance has been shown to improve outcomes in twin pregnancies?

    a. Nonstress test

    b. Biophysical profile

    c. Doppler velocimetry of the umbilical artery

    d. None of the above

45–32. Which of the following interventions has been shown to decrease the rate of preterm birth in twins?

    a. Cerclage

    b. Betamimetics

    c. 17-Hydroxyprogesterone caproate

    d. None of the above

45–33. Which of the following findings can predict a lower risk of preterm birth in twins?

    a. Closed cervix on digital examination

    b. Negative fetal fibronectin assessment

    c. Normal cervical length measured by transvaginal sonography

    d. All of the above

45–34. Which is the most common presentation of twins in labor?

    a. Vertex/vertex

    b. Vertex/breech

    c. Breech/vertex

    d. Vertex/transverse

45–35. For twins in labor, risk factors for an unstable fetal lie include all **EXCEPT** which of the following?

    a. Small fetuses

    b. Polyhydramnios

    c. Increased maternal parity

    d. Vertex/vertex presentation

45–36. Which of the following scenarios presents the best opportunity for a vaginal trial of labor?

    a. Nonvertex/vertex presentation

    b. Vertex/nonvertex presentation

    c. Nonvertex second twin whose estimated fetal weight is < 1500 g

    d. Vertex second twin whose estimated fetal weight is > 20% larger than the presenting vertex twin

CHAPTER 45 ANSWER KEY

Question number	Letter answer	Page cited	Header cited
45–1	d	p. 891	Introduction
45–2	c	p. 891	Introduction
45–3	d	p. 892	Dizygotic versus Monozygotic Twinning
45–4	c	p. 892	Superfetation and Superfecundation
45–5	b	p. 896	Sonographic Determination of Chorionicity
45–6	d	p. 892	Frequency of Twinning
45–7	d	p. 893	Figure 45-1
45–8	d	p. 892	The "Vanishing" Twin
45–9	a	p. 895	Infertility Therapy
45–10	d	p. 896	Placental Examination
45–11	a	p. 892	Frequency of Twinning
45–12	d	p. 896	Sonographic Determination of Chorionicity; Genesis of Monozygotic Twins
45–13	b	p. 894	Factors That Influence Twinning
45–14	b	p. 899	Pregnancy Complications; Long-Term Infant Development
45–15	d	p. 896	Clinical Evaluation
45–16	d	p. 898	Maternal Adaptations to Multifetal Pregnancy
45–17	c	p. 899	Low Birthweight; Figure 45-8
45–18	d	p. 902	Aberrant Twinning Mechanisms
45–19	a	p. 900	Preterm Birth
45–20	a	p. 901	Monoamniotic Twins; Figure 45-13
45–21	d	p. 904	Monochorionic Twins and Vascular Anastomoses
45–22	b	p. 908	Acardiac Twin
45–23	b	p. 907	Diagnosis
45–24	b	p. 904	Twin-Twin Transfusion Syndrome
45–25	c	p. 907	Management and Prognosis
45–26	d	p. 907	Management and Prognosis
45–27	c	p. 909	Diagnosis
45–28	a	p. 909	Etiopathogenesis
45–29	d	p. 909	Diagnosis
45–30	a	p. 910	Death of One Fetus
45–31	d	p. 912	Tests of Fetal Well-Being
45–32	d	p. 913	Prevention of Preterm Birth
45–33	d	p. 913	Prediction of Preterm Birth
45–34	a	p. 915	Fetal Presentation
45–35	d	p. 915	Fetal Presentation
45–36	b	p. 916	Cephalic-Noncephalic Presentation

MEDICAL AND SURGICAL COMPLICATIONS

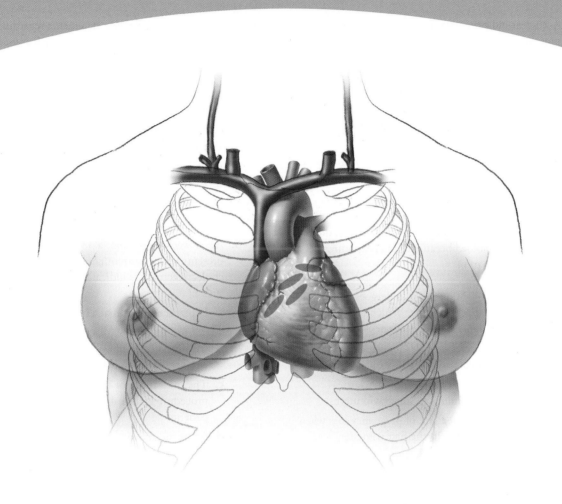

General Considerations and Maternal Evaluation

46–1. A 20-year-old primigravida at 13 weeks' gestation presents with nausea, vomiting, and lower abdominal pain for the past 24 hours. On examination, she has mild guarding in the right lower quadrant of her abdomen. Which of the following statements regarding diagnostic evaluation is most accurate?

a. Magnetic resonance imaging can be used for evaluation of the appendix.

b. Ultrasound is the preferred method of evaluating the appendix during pregnancy.

c. Imaging should not be performed until the patient has been observed for 24 hours.

d. Computed tomography of the maternal abdomen should be avoided because of fetal exposure to ionizing radiation.

46–2. The patient in Question 46–1 undergoes an uncomplicated appendectomy. Which of the following statements is most accurate?

a. She is not at increased risk for excessive adverse pregnancy outcomes.

b. Laparotomy is the preferred approach to minimize risk of injury to the gravid uterus.

c. There is an increased risk of pregnancy loss when surgery is performed in the first trimester.

d. There is an increase in anesthesia-related complications for surgery performed during early pregnancy.

46–3. The increased neonatal death rate seen in gravidas who undergo nonobstetrical surgery is attributable to higher rates of which of the following?

a. Preterm birth

b. Fetal-growth restriction

c. Congenital anomalies in patients with first-trimester procedures

d. Fetal metabolic acidemia associated with emergent cesarean delivery

46–4. Which of the following statements regarding anesthetic agents and teratogenicity is most accurate?

a. There is no evidence that anesthetic agents are harmful.

b. The evidence is contradictory regarding minimal exposure.

c. Halogenated agents carry an increased risk of fetal malformations during the first 8 weeks of pregnancy.

d. Regional anesthesia is the preferred route, as paralytic agents are linked to increased rates of neural-tube defects.

46–5. At 30 weeks' gestation, a 38-year-old multipara presents with recurrent cholelithiasis, and cholecystectomy is indicated. Which of the following is true?

a. Laparoscopic approach is not indicated because of her gestational age.

b. Continuous fetal heart rate monitoring should be employed during the procedure.

c. The indication for the surgical approach of the procedure is the same as for nonpregnant female patients.

d. All of the above

46–6. If insufflation pressures are kept below 20 mm Hg, all **EXCEPT** which of the following are unchanged in women undergoing the procedure depicted below?

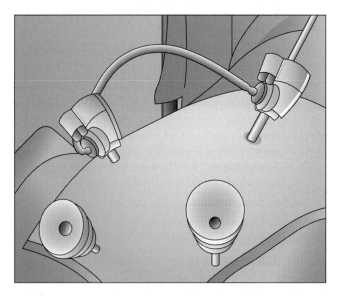

Reproduced with permission from Hoffman BL, Wu D: Introduction to Diagnostic Laparoscopy (update) in Schorge JO, Schaffer JI, Halvorson LM, et al (eds): Williams Gynecology Online. New York, McGraw-Hill, 2009. http://www.accessmedicine.com.

a. Heart rate
b. Cardiac index
c. Mean arterial pressure
d. Systemic vascular resistance

46–7. Which of the following steps in preparation of a patient for laparoscopic surgery differs when the patient is pregnant?

a. Use of general anesthesia
b. Presurgical bowel cleansing
c. Placement of a nasogastric tube
d. Positioning on the surgical table

46–8. Compared with laparoscopy performed in the first trimester, procedures performed later in gestation may use which of the following techniques to reduce surgical complications?

a. Gasless procedure
b. Open entry technique
c. Left upper quadrant port placement
d. All of the above

46–9. Which of the following factors does not affect the dose of ionizing radiation delivered during pregnancy?

a. Type of imaging study
b. Type and age of equipment
c. Distance from radiation source to uterus
d. Gestational age at the time of the procedure

46–10. Which of the following is not a potential effect of radiation exposure during pregnancy?

a. Microcephaly
b. Spontaneous abortion
c. Monozygotic twinning
d. Fetal-growth restriction

46–11. Radiation exposure during which period has the highest risk for lethality?

a. Before implantation
b. During fetal cardiac development
c. During closure of the proximal neural tube
d. None of the above

46–12. The greatest risk for severe mental retardation in humans occurs when high-dose radiation exposure occurs at which of the following gestational ages?

a. Preimplantation
b. 5–8 weeks
c. 8–15 weeks
d. 25–30 weeks

46–13. What is the mean decrease in intelligence quotient (IQ) scores seen with in utero exposure to 100 rads?

a. 5 points
b. 15 points
c. 25 points
d. No change

46–14. Which of the following is an example of a stochastic effect from fetal exposure to ionizing radiation?

a. Childhood cancer
b. Mental retardation
c. Spontaneous abortion
d. Fetal-growth restriction

46–15. What is the preferred method of gastrointestinal tract evaluation during pregnancy?

a. Endoscopy
b. Barium enema
c. Computed tomography
d. Abdominal sonography

46–16. Which of the following is not a reason why it is difficult to calculate fetal exposure during fluoroscopic procedures?

   a. The number of images taken may vary.

   b. The amnionic fluid volume around the fetus is variable.

   c. Total fluoroscopy time for any given procedure is variable.

   d. Amount of time the fetus is within the radiation field is difficult to quantify.

46–17. A 26-year-old woman at 29 weeks' gestation is an unrestrained patient in a motor vehicle accident. She is confused and complaining of a headache. Computed tomographic (CT) scanning of her head is ordered to exclude acute bleeding. What should her family be told about the risk to her fetus from the imaging study?

   a. The risk is negligible.

   b. Computed tomography does not involve ionizing radiation, thus there is no risk.

   c. There is a small risk of ionizing radiation causing childhood cancer with this study, but it is balanced by the necessity of the test.

   d. None of the above

46–18. At 14 weeks' gestation, a patient presents with chest pain and shortness of breath. Using standard protocols for pulmonary embolus evaluation, which of the following statements is the most accurate regarding dosimetry exposure when comparing ventilation-perfusion scans and CT scans?

   a. Exposure is greater with CT scans

   b. Exposure is equivalent for the two types of scans

   c. Exposure is greater with ventilation-perfusion scans

   d. None of the above

46–19. The computed tomography protocol for which of the following conditions is associated with the highest dosimetry exposure to the fetus?

   a. Renal stone

   b. Appendicitis

   c. Pulmonary embolus

   d. Cerebral aneurysm

46–20. Which of the following radionuclide studies delivers the highest dose of radiation to the fetus?

   a. Thyroid scan with ^{131}I at 18 weeks' gestation

   b. Brain scan with ^{99m}Tc DTPA at 15 weeks' gestation

   c. Liver scan using ^{99m}Tc sulfur colloid at 10 weeks' gestation

   d. Abdominal abscess evaluation with ^{67}Ga citrate at 6 weeks' gestation

46–21. A woman given ^{131}I for Graves disease treatment discovers she was pregnant at the time of the administration. Which of the following is a recognized complication in this scenario?

   a. Fetal cretinism

   b. Childhood leukemia

   c. Fetal retinoblastoma

   d. None of the above

46–22. An obstetrician discovers a breast mass in a woman who is having her first prenatal visit at 10 weeks' gestation. The biopsy is positive for cancer, and the breast surgeon would like to perform a sentinel lymphoscintigram during the surgical procedure. Which of the following is an accurate statement?

   a. Pregnancy does not alter the use of ^{99m}Tc-sulfur colloid.

   b. ^{99m}Tc-sulfur should not be used at all during pregnancy.

   c. Surgery and the sentinel lymphoscintigram should be delayed until after 15 weeks' gestation.

   d. Because of fetal concerns, use of the sentinel lymphoscintigram with ^{99m}Tc-sulfur should be based on the individual's risk of tumor spread.

46–23. Which of the following is an advantage of magnetic resonance imaging during pregnancy?

   a. Enhanced soft-tissue contrast

   b. Multiplanar acquisition of images

   c. No ionizing radiation exposure to the fetus

   d. All of the above

46–24. All **EXCEPT** which of the following are true statements regarding contrast agent use with magnetic resonance imaging?

   a. Developmental delay is seen in infants exposed in the third trimester.

   b. There are no documented adverse effects with first-trimester exposure in humans.

   c. Developmental delay is seen in the offspring of animals with prenatal exposure.

   d. Use during pregnancy is not recommended unless there is overwhelming benefit to the patient.

46–25. Which of the following is not a useful application of magnetic resonance imaging during pregnancy?

    a. Renal evaluation for possible urolithiasis

    b. Angiography for suspected pulmonary embolus

    c. Evaluation of a bladder flap mass postoperatively

    d. Evaluation of the uterine wall for placental invasion

46–26. In comparing magnetic resonance (MR) imaging and sonography, which is most accurate for antenatal fetal weight estimation?

    a. MR imaging is more accurate.

    b. Sonography is more accurate.

    c. Sonography and MR imaging are equivalent.

    d. No information is available comparing the two techniques

46–27. Laparoscopic surgery for the condition shown in the image below has been associated with increased rates of which of the following complications?

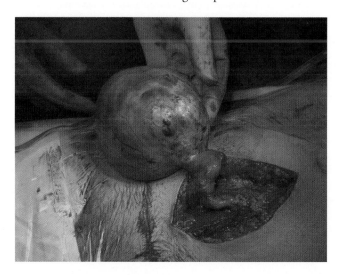

    a. Increased stillbirth rate

    b. Increased preterm delivery

    c. Increased spontaneous abortion

    d. All of the above

46–28. In animal studies, what causes decreased uteroplacental blood flow when intraabdominal insufflation pressures exceeded 15 mm Hg?

    a. Decreased heart rate

    b. Increased cardiac output

    c. Increased perfusion pressure

    d. Increased placental vessel resistance

46–29. A 41-year-old women presents to the emergency room with shoulder pain and nausea. Her electrocardiogram shows ST segment elevation. Cardiac catheterization and angioplasty are performed. Afterward, she is found to be 6 weeks pregnant. Which of the following statements regarding radiation exposure to the embryo is most accurate?

    a. The dose is much less than that for barium enema.

    b. The dose to the embryo is similar to that during cerebral angiography.

    c. The dose during the procedure is similar to that during a barium swallow.

    d. None of the above

46–30. Which of the following has solved problems related to fetal movement during the imaging technique demonstrated below?

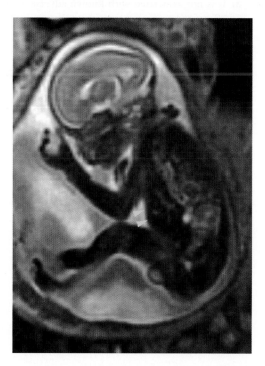

Reproduced with permission from Cunningham FG, Leveno KJ, Bloom SL, et al (eds): Fetal imaging. In Williams Obstetrics, 24th ed. New York, McGraw-Hill, 2014, Fig. 10-44A.

    a. Use of fast-acquisition imaging

    b. Administration of a maternal sedative

    c. Reduction in slice number acquired per study

    d. Timing of study during period of decreased fetal movement

46–31. Which of the following statements is most accurate regarding the imaging modality used below?

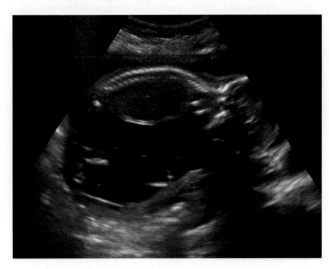

a. It is not associated with known adverse fetal effects.

b. It is associated with very low doses of ionizing radiation.

c. Tracking of total exposure from multiple studies should be performed.

d. Because of known risks to the fetus, its use should be limited during pregnancy.

46–32. Information regarding deterministic effects of ionizing radiation during pregnancy has been obtained from which of the following sources?

a. Animal models

b. Atomic bomb survivors

c. Childhood cancer registries

d. All of the above

CHAPTER 46 ANSWER KEY

Question number	Letter answer	Page cited	Header cited
46–1	a	p. 936	Maternal Indications
46–2	a	p. 927	Surgical Procedures During Pregnancy
46–3	a	p. 927	Perinatal Outcomes
46–4	a	p. 927	Perinatal Outcomes
46–5	c	p. 928	Table 46-2
46–6	b	p. 928	Hemodynamic Effects
46–7	d	p. 928	Technique
46–8	d	p. 928	Technique
46–9	d	p. 930	X-Ray Dosimetry
46–10	c	p. 930	Deterministic Effects of Ionizing Radiation
46–11	a	p. 931	Animal Studies
46–12	c	p. 931	Human Data
46–13	c	p. 931	Human Data
46–14	a	p. 932	Stochastic Effects of Ionizing Radiation
46–15	a	p. 932	Fluoroscopy and Angiography
46–16	b	p. 932	Fluoroscopy and Angiography
46–17	a	p. 933	Computed Tomography
46–18	b	p. 933	Computed Tomography
46–19	b	p. 933	Table 46-7
46–20	a	p. 935	Table 46-8
46–21	a	p. 934	Nuclear Medicine Studies
46–22	a	p. 934	Nuclear Medicine Studies
46–23	d	p. 934	Magnetic Resonance Imaging
46–24	a	p. 935	Contrast Agents
46–25	b	p. 936	Maternal Indications
46–26	a	p. 936	Fetal Indications
46–27	b	p. 928	Perinatal Outcomes
46–28	d	p. 928	Perinatal Outcomes
46–29	a	p. 933	Table 46-6
46–30	a	p. 936	Fetal Indications
46–31	a	p. 937	Table 46-9
46–32	d	p. 930	Deterministic Effects of Ionizing Radiation

CHAPTER 47

Critical Care and Trauma

47–1. Which of the following statements is true of obstetrical patients who require intensive care?

   a. The highest use is before delivery.

   b. The associated mortality rate can reach 10%.

   c. Pulmonary embolus is the most common indication for intensive care.

   d. All of the above

47–2. Which of the following is the most common complication in pregnancy that leads to an intensive care unit admission?

   a. Sepsis

   b. Hemorrhage

   c. Pulmonary embolus

   d. Hypertensive disease

47–3. All **EXCEPT** which of the following monitoring modalities should be routinely used when transporting a critically ill obstetrical patient to another hospital for care?

   a. Electrocardiography

   b. Regular vital signs

   c. Tocodynamic monitoring

   d. Continuous pulse oximetry

47–4. Which of the following physiological changes is typical of pregnancy?

   a. Colloid oncotic pressure increases.

   b. Systemic vascular resistance decreases.

   c. Pulmonary vascular resistance increases.

   d. Left ventricular stroke work index decreases.

47–5. Which of the following statements is true of pulmonary artery catheter monitoring in the acutely ill gravida?

   a. It has been shown to improve survival.

   b. It is essential for the care of patients with severe preeclampsia.

   c. Its use in critically ill obstetrical patients is of limited value.

   d. It aids in the management of patients with low injury-severity scores.

47–6. Which of the following is least likely to contribute to the development of noncardiogenic pulmonary edema in the obstetrical patient?

   a. Sepsis syndrome

   b. Magnesium sulfate administration

   c. Resuscitation during acute hemorrhage

   d. Preeclampsia-related endothelial activation

47–7. A pregnant patient with chronic hypertension develops superimposed preeclampsia. She is diagnosed with pulmonary edema on the first postpartum day. Which of the following statements regarding this complication is true?

   a. Her edema may be cardiogenic.

   b. Her edema may be related to increased capillary permeability.

   c. Brain natriuretic peptide levels are less informative in pregnant patients compared with levels in nonpregnant patients.

   d. All of the above

47–8. Which tocolytic drug has the strongest association with the development of pulmonary edema in obstetrical patients?

   a. Atosiban

   b. Terbutaline

   c. Indomethacin

   d. Magnesium sulfate

47–9. To confirm the diagnosis suggested by the image here, which of the following should not be present?

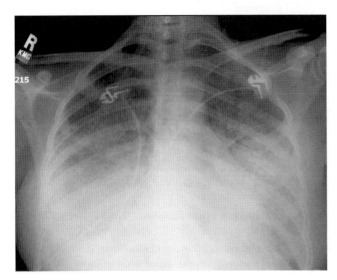

Reproduced with permission from Cunningham FG, Leveno KJ, Bloom SL, et al (eds): Critical care and trauma. In Williams Obstetrics, 24th ed. New York, McGraw-Hill, 2014, Figure 47-1.

    a. Oxygen desaturation

    b. $PaO_2:FiO_2$ ratio < 200

    c. Evidence of heart failure

    d. Severe permeability pulmonary edema

47–10. What is the best way to increase oxygen delivery to peripheral tissues in an obstetrical patient with hemorrhage that is complicated by acute respiratory distress syndrome?

    a. Blood transfusion

    b. Intravenous antibiotics

    c. High-frequency oscillation ventilation

    d. Oxygen therapy to increase arterial Po_2 to 200 mm Hg

47–11. What is the final healing phase of acute respiratory distress syndrome termed?

    a. Fibrotic

    b. Secretory

    c. Exudative

    d. Fibroproliferative

47–12. What would shift the oxyhemoglobin dissociation curve to the right, favoring oxygen delivery to the fetus?

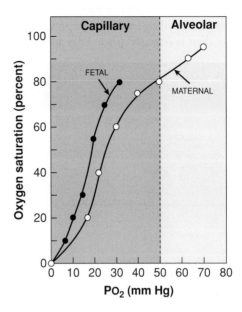

Reproduced with permission from Cunningham FG, Leveno KJ, Bloom SL, et al (eds): Critical care and trauma. In Williams Obstetrics, 24th ed. New York, McGraw-Hill, 2014, Figure 47-2.

    a. Fever

    b. Hypocapnia

    c. Metabolic alkalosis

    d. Decreased 2,3-diphosphoglycerate levels

47–13. What is the approximate mortality risk for an obstetrical patient who requires mechanical ventilation for any amount of time?

    a. 0.5%

    b. 5%

    c. 20%

    d. 40%

47–14. Of infectious causes of acute respiratory distress syndrome, which possible etiology is less likely in an obstetrical patient?

    a. Pneumonia

    b. Pyelonephritis

    c. Chorioamnionitis

    d. Puerperal pelvic infection

47–15. A patient presents to the emergency department 7 days following a cesarean delivery with abdominal tenderness, purulence from her wound, and shortness of breath. Which of the following interventions would most likely lead to the improvement seen in her chest radiographs taken 2 day apart?

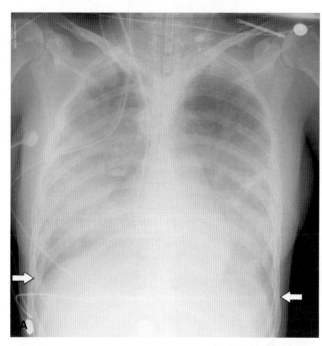

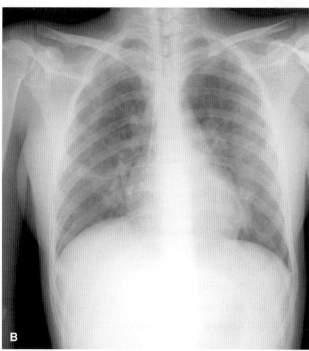

Reproduced with permission from Cunningham FG, Leveno KJ, Bloom SL, et al (eds): Renal and urinary tract disorders. In Williams Obstetrics, 24th ed. New York, McGraw-Hill, 2014, Figure 53-3A&C.

    a. Surfactant therapy

    b. Methylprednisolone therapy

    c. Nitric oxide administration

    d. Positive end-expiratory pressure of 5-15 mm Hg

47–16. Which of the following pathogens is known for its exotoxin that can cause extensive tissue necrosis and gangrene?

    a. *Escherichia coli*

    b. *Proteus mirabilis*

    c. *Staphylococcus aureus*

    d. *Klebsiella pneumoniae*

47–17. Which of the following mediators of sepsis syndrome causes myocardial depression?

    a. Bradykinin

    b. CD4 T cells

    c. Interleukin-6

    d. Tumor necrosis factor-α

47–18. Which of the following clinical signs defines progression from the *warm phase* of septic shock to the *cold phase* of septic shock?

    a. Oliguria

    b. Tachypnea

    c. Leukocytosis

    d. Pulmonary hypertension

47–19. Which intervention is least likely to be beneficial in the treatment of early sepsis?

    a. Correction of anemia

    b. Albumin administration

    c. Broad-spectrum antimicrobials

    d. Aggressive hydration with crystalloid solutions

47–20. A young primigravida presents with fever, tachycardia, hypotension, and uterine tenderness after an attempt at pregnancy termination using abortifacient drugs. Which management decision is most likely to lead to improvement?

    a. Hysterectomy

    b. Diagnostic laparoscopy

    c. Curettage of uterine contents

    d. Uterotonic agent administration

47–21. A 26-year-old G2P1 who is admitted with pyelonephritis has persistent fever after 48 hours of antimicrobial therapy. All **EXCEPT** which of the following are reasonable next steps in the management of this patient?

    a. Blood cultures

    b. Renal sonography

    c. Computed tomography of abdomen

    d. Change of antibiotics based on original urine culture sensitivity

47–22. A G1P1 patient presents 1 week postpartum with fever, abdominal pain, and hypotension. At the time of exploratory laparotomy, the uterus is found to have the soft, bullous outpouchings shown here. Which treatment will most likely lead to survival of this patient?

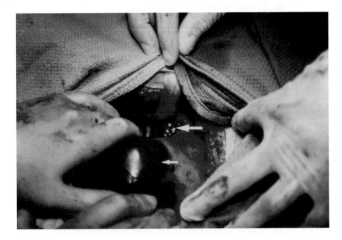

Reproduced with permission from Cunningham FG, Leveno KJ, Bloom SL, et al (eds): Critical care and trauma. In Williams Obstetrics, 24th ed. New York, McGraw-Hill, 2014, Figure 47-7.

a. Hysterectomy

b. Debridement of necrotic tissue

c. Hysterotomy for evacuation of retained placenta

d. Empirical treatment for group A β-hemolytic streptococcus

47–23. What regimen is considered appropriate prophylaxis against *Chlamydia trachomatis* for a sexual assault victim?

a. Cefixime, 400 mg orally as a single dose

b. Azithromycin, 1 g orally as a single dose

c. Erythromycin, 500 mg orally twice daily for 7 days

d. Metronidazole gel 0.75%, 5 g intravaginally daily for 5 days

47–24. What is the most important risk factor for intimate partner homicide?

a. Unwanted pregnancy

b. Use of illicit drugs

c. Prior domestic violence

d. Low socioeconomic status

47–25. A patient presents late in pregnancy for prenatal care and continues to miss appointments. She is typically friendly and pleasant when she comes to her appointments, but today she is quiet during her visit that is attended by her husband. You suspect intimate partner violence. If true, which of the following statements is accurate?

a. She is at increased risk of depression.

b. She is at increased risk for placental abruption.

c. She is at increased risk for a low-birthweight infant.

d. All of the above

47–26. Which of the following is not a risk factor for domestic violence in pregnancy?

a. Poverty

b. Illicit drug use

c. Maternal age > 35

d. Low socioeconomic status

47–27. A patient is involved in a motor vehicle accident and at delivery has the complication seen in the image below. Given this finding, which of the following statements is least likely to be accurate?

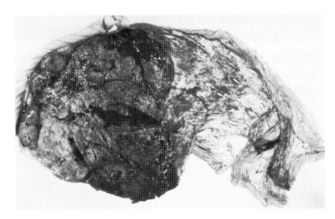

Reproduced with permission from Cunningham FG, Leveno KJ, Bloom SL, et al (eds): Critical care and trauma. In Williams Obstetrics, 24th ed. New York, McGraw-Hill, 2014, Figure 47-11B.

a. The speed of the car was higher than 30 mph.

b. Prior to delivery, the fetal heart rate tracing was nonreassuring.

c. The intrauterine pressure generated by this trauma was more than 500 mm Hg.

d. The patient had contractions every 30 minutes in the first 4 hours after the trauma.

47–28. Which of the following is a critical part of adequate resuscitation of the pregnant patient with cardiac arrest?

  a. Cricoid pressure

  b. Steep Trendelenburg positioning

  c. Left lateral decubitus positioning

  d. All of the above

47–29. What is the likelihood of intact neurological survival for a neonate delivered via perimortem cesarean section 30 minutes after maternal cardiac arrest?

  a. 1%

  b. 8%

  c. 15%

  d. 25%

47–30. A pregnant patient at 34 weeks' gestation presents to the trauma bay in the emergency room after a motor vehicle accident. She was the restrained passenger; the car was traveling approximately 40 mph; and the air bag did not deploy. What complication is least likely to be encountered?

  a. Fetal skull fracture

  b. Maternal bowel injury

  c. Maternal pelvic fracture

  d. Maternal long bone fracture

47–31. What is the most common etiology of all traumatic fetal deaths?

  a. Suicide

  b. Stab wound

  c. Gunshot wound

  d. Motor vehicle collision

47–32. A pregnant patient requires laparotomy after a gunshot wound to the abdomen. Which of the following would make you more likely to deliver the fetus at the time of surgery?

  a. Gestational age of 35 weeks

  b. Reassuring fetal heart rate tracing

  c. Uterine contractions every 20 minutes

  d. Limited evaluation of the injury because of the gravid uterus

47–33. All **EXCEPT** which of the following statements are accurate regarding thermal injuries during pregnancy?

  a. Severe burns usually trigger onset of spontaneous labor.

  b. Pregnancy does not alter maternal outcome after thermal injury.

  c. Fetal mortality rates are typically higher than maternal mortality rates.

  d. A remote history of abdominal burns and contractures conveys a higher risk of preterm birth.

CHAPTER 47 ANSWER KEY

Question number	Letter answer	Page cited	Header cited
47–1	b	p. 940	Obstetrical Intensive Care; Table 47-2
47–2	d	p. 941	Table 47-2
47–3	c	p. 940	Obstetric Critical Care
47–4	b	p. 942	Hemodynamic Changes in Pregnancy
47–5	c	p. 941	Pulmonary Artery Catheter
47–6	b	p. 942	Noncardiogenic Increased Permeability Edema
47–7	d	p. 943	Cardiogenic Hydrostatic Edema
47–8	b	p. 942	Noncardiogenic Increased Permeability Edema
47–9	c	p. 943	Definitions
47–10	a	p. 944	Management
47–11	a	p. 943	Etiopathogenesis
47–12	a	p. 945	Fetal Oxygenation; Figure 47-2
47–13	c	p. 945	Mechanical Ventilation
47–14	a	p. 943	Etiopathogenesis
47–15	d	p. 945	Positive End-Expiratory Pressure
47–16	c	p. 946	Etiopathogenesis
47–17	c	p. 946	Etiopathogenesis
47–18	a	p. 947	Clinical Manifestations
47–19	b	p. 948	Management
47–20	c	p. 948	Surgical Treatment
47–21	a	p. 948	Surgical Treatment
47–22	a	p. 948	Surgical Treatment
47–23	b	p. 952	Table 47-7
47–24	c	p. 951	Physical Abuse—Intimate Partner Violence
47–25	d	p. 951	Physical Abuse—Intimate Partner Violence
47–26	c	p. 951	Physical Abuse—Intimate Partner Violence
47–27	d	p. 953	Placental Injuries—Abruption or Tear; Figure 47-9
47–28	c	p. 956	Cardiopulmonary Resuscitation
47–29	d	p. 956	Cesarean Delivery
47–30	b	p. 951	Automobile Accidents; Other Blunt Trauma
47–31	d	p. 952	Fetal Injury and Death
47–32	d	p. 955	Cesarean Delivery
47–33	d	p. 955	Thermal Injury

CHAPTER 48

Obesity

48–1. Which of the following best describes obesity in the United States?

a. Endemic

b. Epidemic

c. Pandemic

d. Syndemic

48–2. Body mass index (BMI) is defined as which of the following?

a. Height in inches divided by weight in pounds squared.

b. Weight in pounds divided by height in inches squared.

c. Weight in kilograms divided by height in meters squared.

d. Height in meters divided by weight in kilograms squared.

48–3. A 22-year-old G1P0 presents for prenatal care at 8 weeks' gestation. She has a BMI of 26. The National Institutes of Health classifies this patient as which of the following?

a. Normal

b. Overweight

c. Obese–class 1

d. Obese–class 2

48–4. A 19-year-old G1P0 presents for her first prenatal care appointment. She weighs 270 pounds and is 67 inches tall. Using the figure provided, what is the patient's BMI?

a. < 18.5

b. 19–25

c. 25–30

d. > 30.0

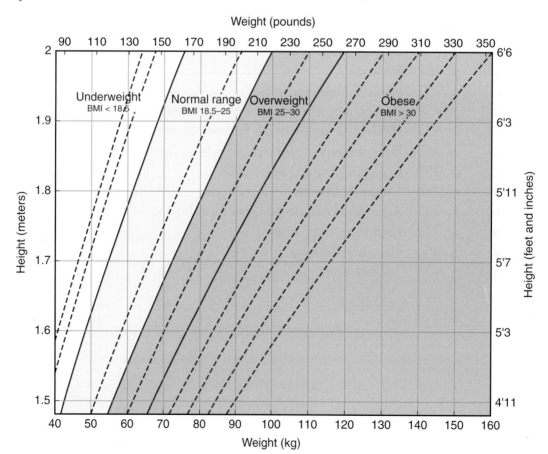

Reproduced with permission from Cunningham FG, Leveno KJ, Bloom SL, et al (eds): Obesity. In Williams Obstetrics, 24th ed. New York, McGraw-Hill, 2014, Fig. 48-1.

48–5. Based on this figure, which of the following statements is true?

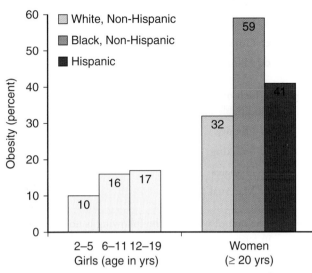

Reproduced with permission from Cunningham FG, Leveno KJ, Bloom SL, et al (eds): Obesity. In Williams Obstetrics, 24th ed. New York, McGraw-Hill, 2014, Fig. 48-2.

  a. The prevalence of obesity increases with age.

  b. Race is not a factor in the prevalence of female obesity.

  c. Obesity is more common in Hispanic women than in black, non-Hispanic women.

  d. Obesity is more common in white, non-Hispanic women than in Hispanic women.

48–6. Which of the following statements regarding adiponectin is not true?

  a. It enhances insulin sensitivity.

  b. It blocks the hepatic release of glucose.

  c. It contributes to the development of hypertension.

  d. It has cardioprotective effects on circulating plasma lipids.

48–7. Which of the following does not contribute to insulin resistance?

  a. Leptin

  b. Resistin

  c. Adiponectin

  d. Tumor necrosis factor-alpha (TNF-α)

48–8. A 35-year-old woman presents to your office for preconceptional counseling. She has chronic hypertension that is controlled with medication. Her blood pressure today is 140/90 mm Hg, and her waist circumference is 36 inches. A fasting glucose level is 115 mg/dL, high-density lipoprotein (HDL) concentration is 60 mg/dL, and triglyceride level is 145 mg/dL. How many criteria does she meet for metabolic syndrome?

  a. 1

  b. 2

  c. 3

  d. 4

48–9. Which of the following is not part of the metabolic syndrome?

  a. Diabetes

  b. Dyslipidemia

  c. Hypertension

  d. Polycystic ovaries

48–10. Nonalcoholic fatty liver disease (NAFLD) contributes what percentage of chronic liver disease cases in Western countries?

  a. 1%

  b. 10%

  c. 25%

  d. 50%

48–11. Rates of which of the following are increased in obese women?

  a. Infertility

  b. Recurrent miscarriage

  c. First-trimester pregnancy loss

  d. All of the above

48–12. A 25-year-old G2P1 at 12 weeks' gestation presents to your office for prenatal care. She has a BMI of 27. Based on the Institute of Medicine's recommendations, how much weight should she gain this pregnancy?

  a. None

  b. 11–20 pounds

  c. 15–25 pounds

  d. 30–40 pounds

48–13. What percentage of women having their first baby gain more weight than recommended?

  a. 1%

  b. 10%

  c. 25%

  d. 75%

48–14. Which of the following adverse pregnancy effects is not of increased prevalence in overweight women compared with women of normal BMI?

    a. Preeclampsia

    b. Urinary infection

    c. Gestational diabetes

    d. Emergency cesarean delivery

48–15. Incidence of which of the following medical problems is not increased with increasing BMI?

    a. Macrosomia

    b. Preeclampsia

    c. Gestational diabetes

    d. All have increased incidence

48–16. You have two similar pregnant women in your practice. Both are 25 years old, primiparous, and free of diabetes and hypertension. One has a BMI of 25, and the other has a BMI of 35. What is the difference in their chances of developing preeclampsia?

    a. Equal risk

    b. A 3% chance versus a 12% chance

    c. A 10% chance versus a 25% chance

    d. A 10% chance versus a 40% chance

48–17. In the study by Weiss and colleagues from 2004, what was the cesarean delivery rate for morbidly obese women?

    a. 10%

    b. 21%

    c. 47%

    d. 62%

48–18. Compared with normal-weight patients, obese women have increased rates of all **EXCEPT** which of the following?

    a. Hypertension

    b. Wound infection

    c. Vaginal delivery

    d. Gestational diabetes

48–19. Which of the following statements regarding obesity and pregnancy is not true?

    a. Obese women are more likely to breast feed.

    b. Postpartum depression rates are increased in obese women.

    c. Obese women have greater weight retention 1 year after delivery.

    d. Second-trimester dilatation and evacuations take longer in obese women.

48–20. Serum levels of which of the following are increased in obese pregnant women?

    a. Insulin

    b. Interleukin-6

    c. C-reactive protein

    d. All of the above

48–21. Which of the following is the highest-ranking modifiable risk factor for stillbirth?

    a. Obesity

    b. Smoking

    c. Diabetes

    d. Maternal age

48–22. The rate of which of the following is not increased in fetuses of obese pregnant women?

    a. Stillbirths

    b. Heart defects

    c. Renal agenesis

    d. Neural-tube defects

48–23. Which of the following has the strongest influence on the prevalence of the condition depicted in this photograph?

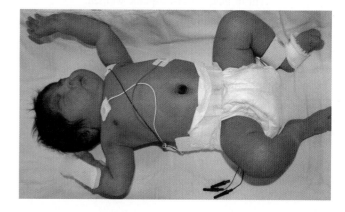

    a. Prepregnancy BMI

    b. Gestational diabetes

    c. Gestational weight gain

    d. Pregestational diabetes

48–24. Which of following contributes to childhood obesity?

    a. Maternal obesity

    b. Maternal gestational diabetes

    c. Maternal-child environment subsequent to birth

    d. All of the above

48–25. During the prenatal care of an obese woman, which of the following commonly collected measures will likely be **LEAST** useful in patient management?

a. Fundal height

b. Urine protein

c. Blood pressure

d. Cervical dilatation

48–26. When performing a cesarean delivery on the obese pregnant woman, which of the following is not an advantage of the incision depicted in this figure?

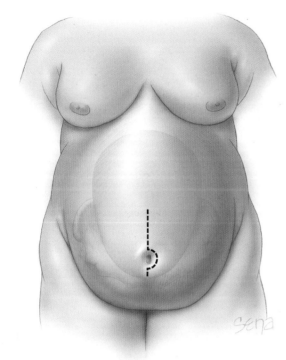

A

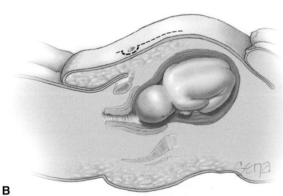

B

Reproduced with permission from Cunningham FG, Leveno KJ, Bloom SL, et al (eds): Obesity. In Williams Obstetrics, 24th ed. New York, McGraw-Hill, 2014, Fig. 48-7A&B.

a. Provides the least intervening tissue

b. Permits access to the lower uterine segment

c. Greatly reduces the chances of wound infection

d. Prevents moisture from collecting on the incision

48–27. Regarding cesarean delivery in obese women, which of the following should be done to reduce the chances of wound disruption?

a. Vertical skin incision

b. Weight loss during the pregnancy

c. Closure of the subcutaneous layer

d. All of the above

48–28. Which of the following is not recommended by the American College of Obstetricians and Gynecologists to lower thromboembolic complications in the obese parturient?

a. Hydration

b. Early mobilization

c. Compression stockings

d. Full anticoagulation with heparin

48–29. Which of the following complications is more likely in a pregnant woman who has undergone bariatric surgery?

a. Diabetes

b. Preeclampsia

c. Large-for-gestational age neonate

d. Small-for-gestational age neonate

48–30. Which of the following complications is more common after Roux-en-Y gastric bypass than after gastric banding?

a. Hypertension

b. Cesarean delivery

c. Gestational diabetes

d. Small-for-gestational age newborn

48–31. A 30-year-old G3P2 at 14 weeks' gestation presents for prenatal care. She reports that she had bariatric surgery 2 years ago, losing 100 pounds. You correctly counsel her which of the following?

a. She is at increased risk for diabetes.

b. She is at increased risk for hypertension.

c. She does not need to see her bariatric doctor during the pregnancy.

d. She needs to be assessed for vitamin deficiencies, and she may need vitamin B_{12}, vitamin D, or calcium supplementation.

48–32. When caring for a pregnant woman who has undergone bariatric surgery, vigilance for which of the following is essential?

a. Appendicitis

b. Bowel obstruction

c. Acute cholecystitis

d. Gastroesophageal reflux disease

CHAPTER 48 ANSWER KEY

Question number	Letter answer	Page cited	Header cited
48–1	a	p. 961	Obesity
48–2	c	p. 961	Definitions
48–3	b	p. 961	Definitions
48–4	d	p. 962	Figure 48-1
48–5	a	p. 962	Figure 48-2
48–6	c	p. 961	Adipose Tissue as an Organ System
48–7	c	p. 962	Adipocytokines in Pregnancy
48–8	c	p. 963	Table 48-1
48–9	d	p. 962	Metabolic Syndrome
48–10	c	p. 963	Nonalcoholic Fatty Liver Disease
48–11	d	p. 964	Pregnancy and Obesity
48–12	c	p. 965	Maternal Weight Gain and Energy Requirement
48–13	d	p. 965	Maternal Weight Gain and Energy Requirement
48–14	d	p. 965	Table 48-3
48–15	d	p. 966	Figure 48-5
48–16	b	p. 966	Figure 48-6
48–17	c	p. 965	Maternal Morbidity
48–18	c	p. 965	Maternal Morbidity
48–19	a	p. 965	Maternal Morbidity
48–20	d	p. 966	Preeclampsia
48–21	a	p. 967	Perinatal Mortality
48–22	c	p. 967	Perinatal Morbidity
48–23	a	p. 967	Perinatal Morbidity
48–24	d	p. 967	Fetal Programming and Childhood Morbidity
48–25	a	p. 968	Prenatal Care
48–26	c	p. 968	Figure 48-7
48–27	c	p. 968	Surgical and Anesthetic Concerns
48–28	d	p. 968	Surgical and Anesthetic Concerns
48–29	d	p. 969	Bariatric Surgery
48–30	d	p. 969	Table 48-4
48–31	d	p. 969	Recommendations
48–32	b	p. 969	Recommendations

Cardiovascular Disorders

49–1. What percent of pregnancies are complicated by heart disease?

   a. 0.1%

   b. 1%

   c. 4%

   d. 8%

49–2. Which of the following parameters increases by 40 percent in pregnancy?

   a. Heart rate

   b. Cardiac output

   c. Mean arterial pressure

   d. Left ventricular stroke work index

49–3. Which aspect of cardiac physiology does not change in pregnancy?

   a. Mean arterial pressure

   b. Pulmonary vascular resistance

   c. Left ventricular contractility

   d. Left ventricular stroke work index

49–4. Which of the following is never a normal finding in pregnancy?

   a. Dyspnea

   b. Systolic murmur

   c. Diastolic murmur

   d. Exercise intolerance

49–5. When encountered in an obstetrical patient, which of the following are considered expected variations from the nonpregnant state?

   a. Larger cardiac silhouette seen on chest radiograph

   b. Tricuspid regurgitation seen during echocardiography

   c. Increased left atrial end-diastolic dimensions seen during echocardiography

   d. All of the above

49–6. All **EXCEPT** which of the following are electrocardiogram changes seen in normal pregnancy?

   a. Increased voltage

   b. 15-degree left axis deviation

   c. Premature atrial contractions

   d. ST segment changes in inferior leads

49–7. A pregnant woman with preexisting cardiac disease is comfortable at rest but cannot stand up to brush her teeth without experiencing chest pain. What is her New York Heart Association classification?

   a. I

   b. II

   c. III

   d. IV

49–8. Excluding those associated with Marfan syndrome, which congenital heart lesions carry the greatest risk of heritability?

   a. Aortic stenosis

   b. Pulmonary stenosis

   c. Tetralogy of Fallot

   d. Coarctation of the aorta

49–9. A pregnant patient at 13 weeks' gestation has known heart disease. All **EXCEPT** which of the following are predictive of poor outcomes in pregnancy?

   a. Prior stroke

   b. Cardiac symptoms at rest

   c. Ejection fraction of 30%

   d. Mitral valve area of 2.5 cm^2

49–10. Which of the following statements is true regarding antepartum and intrapartum care of patients with cardiovascular disease?

   a. Vaginal delivery is preferred.

   b. Spinal blockade is the recommended anesthetic.

   c. These patients should avoid pneumococcal vaccination.

   d. Invasive monitoring with pulmonary artery catheter is required.

49–11. A patient with prior valve replacement heart surgery presents for prenatal care. Her chest radiograph lateral view is shown here and arrows point to her St. Jude valve. With mechanical valves, what is the maternal mortality rate in pregnancy?

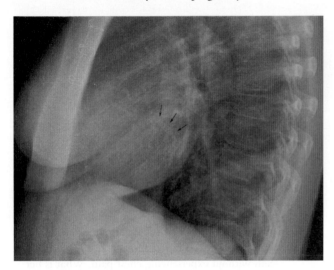

a. 0.1–0.4%

b. 3–4%

c. 7–9%

d. 12–15%

49–12. In a pregnant woman with a mechanical heart valve, which of the following anticoagulation regimens would be considered inadequate for prevention of thromboembolism involving the prosthesis?

a. Warfarin

b. Low-dose unfractionated heparin

c. Adjusted-dose unfractionated heparin

d. Adjusted-dose low-molecular-weight heparin

49–13. Which of the following anticoagulants is not compatible with breast feeding?

a. Warfarin

b. Unfractionated heparin

c. Low-molecular-weight heparin

d. All are compatible

49–14. If a patient requires cardiac bypass for valve replacement during pregnancy, which of the following can she expect?

a. Fetal death rate of 5%

b. Minimal miscarriage risk

c. Maternal mortality rate of 20%

d. Maternal mortality rate similar to nonpregnant women

49–15. A pregnant patient with mitral stenosis requires percutaneous transcatheter balloon dilatation of the mitral valve. What can you tell the patient as part of your presurgical counseling?

a. It is preferred to open surgical repair.

b. Left atrial pressures will improve as the mitral valve area increases.

c. Balloon dilatation is successful in more than 90 percent of procedures.

d. All of the above

49–16. A patient who had a heart transplant as a child is now considering pregnancy. What complications can she expect during pregnancy?

a. A tissue rejection risk less than 5%

b. A high likelihood of vaginal delivery

c. A risk of hypertension that approximates 50%

d. A heart that will not undergo the normal physiologic changes of pregnancy

49–17. A patient in labor gives a history of mitral stenosis. She is asymptomatic and currently taking a beta blocker, but she is not sure why her doctor recommended it. What complication is the prophylactic beta blocker trying to prevent in these patients?

a. Irregular heart rhythm

b. Mural thrombus formation

c. Tachycardia leading to pulmonary edema

d. Left ventricular hypertrophy and dilatation

49–18. The patient whose heart is seen in this image has systemic lupus erythematosus and has had a prior stroke. The left atrium (LA) and left ventricle (LV) are identified, and the arrows point to noninfectious inflammatory vegetations on the mitral leaflets. Which of the following is the likely condition associated with her mitral insufficiency?

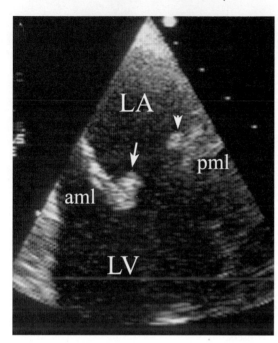

Modified with permission from Roldan CA: Connective tissue disease and the heart. In Crawford MH (ed): Current Diagnosis & Treatment: Cardiology, 3rd ed. New York, McGraw-Hill, 2009, Figure 33-2.

    a. Antiphospholipid antibodies

    b. Infarction of the papillary muscle

    c. Calcification of the mitral annulus

    d. None of the above

49–19. A patient with critical aortic stenosis presents to the labor and delivery unit, and her cervix is 6-cm dilated. All **EXCEPT** which of the following are suitable management steps?

    a. Limit activity

    b. Provide narcotic epidural anesthesia

    c. Perform pulmonary artery catheterization

    d. Decrease cardiac preload by limiting intravenous fluids

49–20. For patients with congenital heart disease, what is the most common adverse cardiovascular event encountered in pregnancy?

    a. Arrhythmia

    b. Heart failure

    c. Thromboembolic event

    d. Cerebrovascular hemorrhage

49–21. Which congenital defect is associated most often with "paradoxical embolism"?

    a. Eisenmenger syndrome

    b. Atrial septal defect

    c. Patent ductus arteriosus

    d. Ventricular septal defect

49–22. A patient with the congenital lesion shown in this figure is now pregnant. She has not had surgery to correct her lesion, and her hematocrit is 68 volumes percent. Her expected risk for pregnancy loss approximates which of the following?

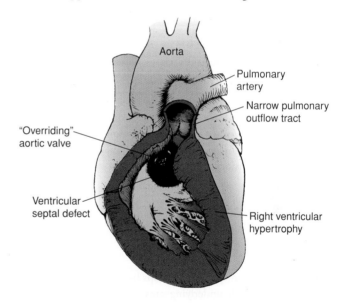

Reproduced with permission from Harris IS, Foster E: Congenital heart disease in adults. In Crawford MH (ed): Current Diagnosis & Treatment: Cardiology, 3rd ed. New York, McGraw-Hill, 2009, Figure 28-23.

    a. 40%

    b. 60%

    c. 80%

    d. 100%

49–23. This echocardiography image shows a short-axis view of the heart of a female with Eisenmenger syndrome. A markedly dilated pulmonary artery (PA) is seen. All **EXCEPT** which of the following are common underlying defects that lead to this condition?

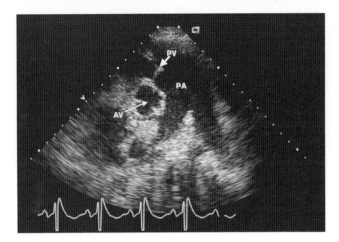

Reproduced with permission from Harris IS, Foster E: Congenital heart disease in adults. In Crawford MH (ed): Current Diagnosis & Treatment: Cardiology, 3rd ed. New York, McGraw-Hill, 2009, Figure 28-26B.

    a. Atrial septal defect

    b. Valvular heart disease

    c. Patent ductus arteriosus

    d. Ventricular septal defect

49–24. Which World Health Organization classification best categorizes patients with idiopathic pulmonary hypertension?

    a. I

    b. II

    c. III

    d. IV

49–25. A pregnant patient develops heart failure without an identifiable underlying cause. If she does not recover baseline cardiac function by 6 months postpartum, which of the following best approximates her 5-year mortality rate?

    a. 5%

    b. 20%

    c. 40%

    d. 80%

49–26. What is the most common cause of heart failure during pregnancy and the puerperium?

    a. Obesity

    b. Viral myocarditis

    c. Valvular heart disease

    d. Chronic hypertension with severe preeclampsia

49–27. An obese primigravida develops acute dyspnea while in labor. Her chest radiograph is shown here. What intervention will most likely resolve her symptoms?

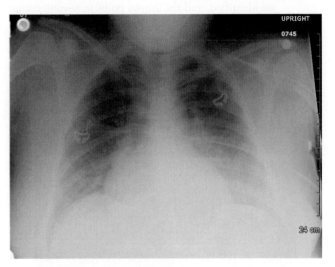

    a. Intravenous furosemide

    b. Intravenous hydralazine

    c. 3 L oxygen by face mask

    d. Therapeutic heparinization

49–28. With infective endocarditis, what is the most common causative organism in intravenous drug users?

    a. *Enterococcus* species

    b. *Staphylococcus aureus*

    c. *Streptococcus viridans*

    d. *Staphylococcus epidermidis*

49–29. Which of the following is an adequate intravenous regimen for prophylaxis of bacterial endocarditis for the at-risk patient in labor who is penicillin allergic?

    a. Cefazolin, 1 g

    b. Ceftriaxone, 1 g

    c. Clindamycin, 600 mg

    d. All are adequate

49–30. Patients with QT prolongation are at risk of developing which of the following arrhythmias?

    a. Atrial fibrillation

    b. Torsades de pointes

    c. Wolff-Parkinson-White

    d. Paroxysmal supraventricular tachycardia

49–31. Which of the following is a threshold for aortic root size above which a patient with Marfan syndrome is at higher risk of dissection during pregnancy?

    a. 20 mm

    b. 30 mm

    c. 40 mm

    d. 50 mm

49–32. A 42-year-old gravida at 32 weeks' gestation with diabetes presents with chest pain and has an abnormal electrocardiogram. All **EXCEPT** which of the following statements are correct regarding the evaluation and management of suspected myocardial infarction in pregnancy?

    a. The patient should be delivered immediately.

    b. The patient should be started on a beta blocker.

    c. The patient should receive daily low-dose aspirin.

    d. Troponin levels can be used to aid diagnosis in pregnancy.

CHAPTER 49 ANSWER KEY

Question number	Letter answer	Page cited	Header cited
49–1	b	p. 973	Introduction
49–2	b	p. 973	Cardiovascular Physiology; Table 49-1
49–3	c	p. 973	Cardiovascular Physiology
49–4	c	p. 974	Diagnosis of Heart Disease; Table 49-2
49–5	d	p. 975	Diagnostic Studies
49–6	a	p. 976	Electrocardiography
49–7	c	p. 976	Classification of Functional Heart Disease
49–8	a	p. 976	Congenital Heart Disease in Offspring; Table 49-4
49–9	d	p. 976	Classification of Functional Heart Disease
49–10	a	p. 977	Peripartum Management Considerations
49–11	b	p. 979	Valve Replacement before Pregnancy
49–12	b	p. 979	Anticoagulation
49–13	d	p. 979	Recommendations for Anticoagulation
49–14	d	p. 980	Cardiac Surgery During Pregnancy
49–15	d	p. 980	Mitral Valvotomy During Pregnancy
49–16	c	p. 981	Pregnancy after Heart Transplantation
49–17	c	p. 981	Mitral Stenosis
49–18	a	p. 982	Mitral Insufficiency
49–19	d	p. 983	Aortic Stenosis
49–20	a	p. 984	Congenital Heart Disease
49–21	b	p. 984	Atrial Septal Defects
49–22	d	p. 985	Cyanotic Heart Disease
49–23	b	p. 985	Eisenmenger Syndrome
49–24	a	p. 987	Table 49-8
49–25	d	p. 988	Cardiomyopathies; Prognosis
49–26	d	p. 990	Heart Failure
49–27	a	p. 990	Heart Failure: Management
49–28	b	p. 990	Infective Endocarditis
49–29	d	p. 991	Table 49-10
49–30	b	p. 992	Prolonged QT Interval
49–31	c	p. 993	Effect of Pregnancy on Marfan Syndrome
49–32	a	p. 994	Myocardial Infarction During Pregnancy

CHAPTER 50

Chronic Hypertension

50–1. A 36-year-old primigravida has a 2-year history of chronic hypertension that is well controlled with medication. She monitors her blood pressure at home, and at her 16-week appointment, she is thrilled to report a drop in her blood pressure. What is the best response to this information?

    a. She should discontinue her medication at this time.

    b. Chronic hypertension typically improves early in pregnancy.

    c. This finding predicts a favorable prognosis for her pregnancy.

    d. None of the above

50–2. Which of the following factors may influence blood pressure?

    a. Race

    b. Weight

    c. Gender

    d. All of the above

50–3. Which of the following blood pressure measurements meets the criteria for "prehypertension" as defined by the Joint National Committee 7?

    a. Diastolic blood pressure 70–80 mm Hg

    b. Diastolic blood pressure 90–95 mm Hg

    c. Systolic blood pressure 120–130 mm Hg

    d. Systolic blood pressure 140–150 mm Hg

50–4. An African-American patient presents for her annual gynecologic examination and has a blood pressure reading of 142/92 mm Hg. After checking it at home several more times, she calls to report persistent readings of 140–150/90–100 mm Hg. What medication is appropriate as initial therapy for most nonpregnant patients?

    a. Enalapril

    b. Labetalol

    c. Losartan

    d. Hydrochlorothiazide

50–5. What is the target blood pressure you are attempting to achieve with this therapy?

    a. < 120/90 mm Hg

    b. < 130/80 mm Hg

    c. < 140/90 mm Hg

    d. < 150/100 mm Hg

50–6. Which of the following factors is an indication for evaluation of renal function in a patient with chronic hypertension who is considering pregnancy?

    a. Age of 45 years

    b. Preexisting diabetes mellitus

    c. Hypertension duration of 3 years

    d. All of the above

50–7. How should a patient whose blood pressure is 120/80 mm Hg at her annual examination be counseled?

    a. Initiate 30 minutes of daily exercise

    b. Limit alcohol consumption to two drinks per day

    c. Start pravastatin to reduce her cardiovascular risk

    d. Plan no recommendation as her blood pressure is normal

50–8. A new patient with chronic hypertension presents to discuss future pregnancy. She brings additional records with her, including a copy of this image, which depicts her cerebrovascular accident from 3 years ago. What is the most appropriate response to her question regarding pregnancy outcomes?

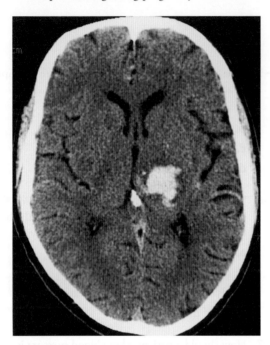

Reproduced with permission from Ropper AH, Samuels MA: Cerebrovascular diseases. In Adams & Victor's Principles of Neurology, 9th ed. New York, McGraw-Hill, 2009, Figure 34-21.

a. Her risk for recurrence approaches 80%.

b. Pregnancy is relatively contraindicated.

c. Outcomes are good if blood pressure is controlled prior to conception.

d. If her serum creatinine level is < 2.5 mg/dL, the pregnancy should be uneventful.

50–9. The diagnosis of chronic hypertension is supported when hypertension is present prior to what threshold gestational age?

a. 8 weeks

b. 14 weeks

c. 20 weeks

d. 24 weeks

50–10. Which of the following comorbidities is most frequently seen in pregnant women with chronic hypertension?

a. Hypothyroidism

b. Pregestational diabetes

c. Systemic lupus erythematosus

d. Antiphospholipid antibody syndrome

50–11. The chest radiograph below was obtained from a patient with chronic hypertension 1 day after delivery at 38 weeks' gestation. Which of the following statements is true regarding this condition?

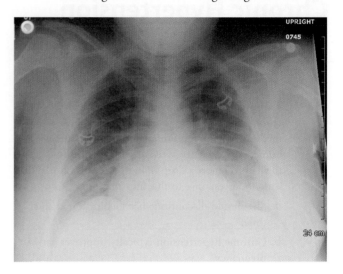

a. It occurs in approximately 1% of gravidas with chronic hypertension.

b. It is most often seen in gravidas with a history of cardiomyopathy.

c. It is the most frequent delivery complication seen in women with chronic hypertension.

d. None of the above

50–12. Administration of which of the following antihypertensive medications may contribute to development of the condition seen in Question 50–11?

a. Losartan

b. Nifedipine

c. Lisinopril

d. Hydralazine

50–13. Which of the following postpartum events predisposes to development of the condition in Question 50–11?

a. Increased peripheral resistance

b. Increased left-ventricular workload

c. Increased intravascular fluid volume

d. All of the above

50–14. What treatment is indicated when this develops postpartum?

a. Digoxin

b. Furosemide

c. Hydralazine

d. Fluid restriction

50–15. The risk of maternal death is increased by what degree in women with chronic hypertension?

    a. Twofold

    b. Fivefold

    c. Tenfold

    d. Fiftyfold

50–16. What is the risk of the following pregnancy complication in women with chronic hypertension?

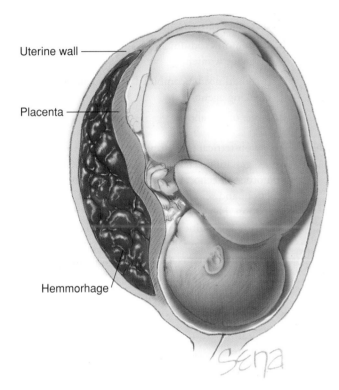

Reproduced with permission from Cunningham FG, Leveno KJ, Bloom SL, et al (eds): Obstetrical hemorrhage. In Williams Obstetrics, 23rd ed. New York, McGraw-Hill, 2010, Figure 35-4.

    a. 0.1%

    b. 0.3–0.5%

    c. 1–2%

    d. 10%

50–17. For women with chronic hypertension, what additional factor further increases the risk of the event shown in Question 50–16?

    a. Oligohydramnios

    b. Maternal smoking

    c. Multifetal gestation

    d. Pregestational diabetes

50–18. What dietary supplement may reduce the incidence the event shown in Question 50–16?

    a. Vitamin C

    b. Vitamin E

    c. Folic acid

    d. Omega-3 fatty acids

50–19. Serum assays for which of the following can accurately predict the development of superimposed preeclampsia in a patient with chronic hypertension?

    a. Inhibin

    b. Pregnancy-associated plasma protein A

    c. Vascular endothelial growth factor receptor 1

    d. None of the above

50–20. Results from randomized controlled trials suggest what benefit is gained from low-dose aspirin use during pregnancy in women with chronic hypertension?

    a. No benefit

    b. Reduced preterm birth rates

    c. Reduced maternal mortality rates

    d. Reduced fetal-growth restriction rates

50–21. A patient with no prenatal care presents to Labor and Delivery in the third trimester with a complaint of decreased fetal movement for 1 day. She takes an unknown medication for chronic hypertension. What is the risk of stillbirth in a gravida with chronic hypertension?

    a. 1 per 20 births

    b. 1–2 per 100 births

    c. 1–2 per 1000 births

    d. 1 per 5000 births

50–22. The fetal heart rate tracing for the patient in Question 50-21 is shown below. Sonographic evaluation is performed, and her amnionic fluid index is 2.3 cm, which is markedly abnormal. What class of antihypertensive medications may be responsible for this finding?

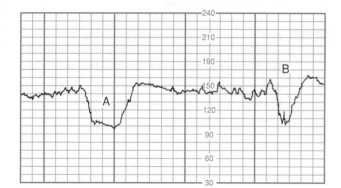

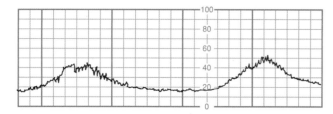

Reproduced with permission from Cunningham FG, Leveno KJ, Bloom SL, et al (eds): Intrapartum assessment. In Williams Obstetrics, 24th ed. New York, McGraw-Hill, 2014, Figure 24-21.

    a. Loop diuretics

    b. β-Adrenergic receptor blockers

    c. Calcium-channel blocking agents

    d. Angiotensin-converting enzyme inhibitors

50–23. A 30-year-old G3P2 presents for prenatal care. Her prior pregnancies have both been complicated by mild gestational hypertension near term. She is currently 12 weeks pregnant, and her blood pressure is 146/88 mm Hg. Which of the following is the most appropriate next step in her management?

    a. Continued observation

    b. Begin treatment with methyldopa

    c. Begin treatment with hydrochlorothiazide

    d. None of the above

50–24. Which of the following pregnancy complications is reduced when antihypertensive therapy is started during pregnancy?

    a. Preterm delivery

    b. Maternal morbidity

    c. Development of severe hypertension

    d. Neonatal intensive care admissions

50–25. Thiazide medications have which of the following side effects that limit their use in pregnancy?

    a. Postural hypotension

    b. Reduced volume expansion

    c. Oligohydramnios in the third trimester

    d. Teratogenicity when taken in the first trimester

50–26. Which of the following is a true statement regarding the use of oral hydralazine as an antihypertensive agent?

    a. It is an effective monotherapy in pregnancy.

    b. It promotes sodium and water diuresis in pregnant women.

    c. It should not be combined with calcium-channel blocking agents.

    d. None of the above

50–27. A new obstetrical patient presents for care at 8 weeks' gestation. Her blood pressure is 146/92. You order an echocardiogram, assess baseline renal function, and send her to an ophthalmologist for evaluation. Her eye examination is normal, and her serum creatinine level is 0.71 mg/dL. Her echocardiogram reveals moderate left ventricular hypertrophy. What is the most appropriate next step in her management?

    a. Start antihypertensive therapy

    b. Proceed with routine prenatal care

    c. Repeat the entire evaluation in the second trimester

    d. Plan expectant management with biweekly blood pressure checks

50–28. Regarding the patient in Question 50-27, what is her risk of developing superimposed preeclampsia?

    a. 5%

    b. 10%

    c. 20–30%

    d. 50%

50–29. If the patient from Question 50-27 actually develops superimposed preeclampsia, what is the likelihood she will deliver before 37 weeks' gestation?

    a. 2%

    b. 10%

    c. 20%

    d. 50%

50–30. All **EXCEPT** which of the following support the diagnosis of superimposed preeclampsia?

    a. Decreased platelet count

    b. Increased serum creatinine level

    c. Elevated serum alkaline phosphatase level

    d. Elevated serum aspartate aminotransferase level

50–31. According to the American College of Obstetricians and Gynecologists, what antenatal assessment has been conclusively shown to be of benefit in the management of pregnancies complicated by chronic hypertension?

    a. Nonstress testing

    b. Biophysical profile

    c. Umbilical artery Doppler studies

    d. Serial sonographic evaluations of fetal growth

50–32. Which of the following medications is preferred for intrapartum prevention of eclampsia?

    a. Phenytoin

    b. Midazolam

    c. Phenobarbital

    d. Magnesium sulfate

CHAPTER 50 ANSWER KEY

Question number	Letter answer	Page cited	Header cited
50–1	b	p. 1000	Introduction
50–2	d	p. 1000	General Considerations
50–3	c	p. 1001	Table 50-1
50–4	d	p. 1001	Table 50-1
50–5	c	p. 1001	Treatment and Benefits for Nonpregnant Adults
50–6	b	p. 1001	Preconceptional Counseling
50–7	a	p. 1001	Treatment and Benefits for Nonpregnant Adults; Table 50-2
50–8	b	p. 1001	Preconceptional Counseling
50–9	c	p. 1002	Diagnosis and Evaluation in Pregnancy
50–10	b	p. 1002	Associated Risk Factors
50–11	d	p. 1003	Maternal Morbidity and Mortality
50–12	b	p. 1006	Calcium-Channel Blocking Agents
50–13	d	p. 1008	Postpartum Hypertension
50–14	b	p. 1008	Postpartum Hypertension
50–15	b	p. 1003	Maternal Morbidity and Mortality
50–16	c	p. 1004	Placental Abruption
50–17	b	p. 1004	Placental Abruption
50–18	c	p. 1004	Placental Abruption
50–19	d	p. 1004	Prevention of Superimposed Preeclampsia
50–20	a	p. 1004	Prevention of Superimposed Preeclampsia
50–21	b	p. 1004	Perinatal Morbidity and Mortality
50–22	d	p. 1006	Angiotensin-Converting Enzyme Inhibitors
50–23	a	p. 1005	Blood Pressure Control
50–24	c	p. 1005	Blood Pressure Control
50–25	b	p. 1005	Diuretics
50–26	d	p. 1005	Vasodilators
50–27	a	p. 1007	Recommendations for Therapy in Pregnancy
50–28	c	p. 1007	Pregnancy-Aggravated Hypertension or Superimposed Preeclampsia
50–29	d	p. 1007	Pregnancy-Aggravated Hypertension or Superimposed Preeclampsia
50–30	c	p. 1007	Pregnancy-Aggravated Hypertension or Superimposed Preeclampsia
50–31	d	p. 1007	Fetal Assessment
50–32	d	p. 1007	Intrapartum Consideration

CHAPTER 51

Pulmonary Disorders

51–1. What percentage of pregnant women have chronic asthma?

a. 1%

b. 4%

c. 14%

d. 20%

51–2. What happens to vital capacity in pregnancy?

a. Increases by 20%

b. Decreases by 25%

c. Increases by 40%

d. Decreases by 45%

51–3. What effect does progesterone have on tidal volume?

a. Increases by 20%

b. Decreases by 25%

c. Increases by 40%

d. Decreases by 45%

51–4. What happens to carbon dioxide production in pregnancy?

a. Increases by 20%

b. Decreases by 25%

c. Increases by 30%

d. Decreases by 40%

51–5. What happens to residual volume in pregnancy?

a. Increases by 20%

b. Decreases by 20%

c. Increases by 40%

d. Decreases by 40%

51–6. Which of the following statements regarding physiologic pulmonary changes in pregnancy is true?

a. Basal oxygen consumption decreases.

b. Ventilation is increased by more frequent breathing.

c. Ventilation is increased because of deeper breathing.

d. Ventilation is increased because of increased chest wall compliance.

51–7. A pregnant patient reports asthma symptoms 3 days per week, and she is awakened by these approximately twice per month. Between exacerbations, her FEV_1 (forced expiratory volume in 1 second) is ≥ 80 percent of predicted. Her asthma is best classified by which of the following descriptors?

a. Intermittent

b. Mild persistent

c. Moderate persistent

d. Very severe persistent

51–8. A pregnant patient reports asthma symptoms that prompt daily use of her inhaler, and she is awakened by these symptoms approximately twice weekly. Between exacerbations, her FEV_1/FVC (forced expiratory volume in 1 second/forced vital capacity) is reduced by 5 percent. Her asthma is best classified by which of the following descriptors?

a. Intermittent

b. Mild persistent

c. Moderate persistent

d. Very severe persistent

51–9. Which of the following best characterizes persistent asthma?

a. Symptoms once daily

b. $FEV_1 < 60\%$ of predicted

c. Some limitation of normal activities

d. Single, daily use of short-acting β-agonists for symptoms

51–10. A 25-year-old G1P0 at 20 weeks' gestation presents with an asthma exacerbation. Her FEV_1 is 50 percent. Her Pco_2 is normal, and her Po_2 is decreased. These values are very concerning and likely reflect which of the following?

a. She is in respiratory failure.

b. She has a significant metabolic acidosis.

c. A normal Pco_2 indicates fatigue and early CO_2 retention.

d. A fetus cannot survive when the mother's FEV_1 drops to 50%.

51–11. Up to what percentage of women with mild or moderate asthma will have an intrapartum exacerbation?

a. 2%

b. 20%

c. 40%

d. 60%

51–12. The fetal response to maternal hypoxemia is which of the following?

a. Decreased cardiac output

b. Increased umbilical blood flow

c. Decreased systemic vascular resistance

d. Decreased pulmonary vascular resistance

51–13. Which of the following is a sign of a potentially fatal asthma attack?

a. Tachycardia

b. Central cyanosis

c. Labored breathing

d. Prolonged expiration

51–14. Which of the following statements regarding pulmonary function testing is true?

a. An FEV_1 of 50% correlates with severe disease.

b. The peak expiratory flow rate increases in normal pregnancy.

c. A woman's baseline pulmonary function tests should be determined when symptomatic.

d. Pulmonary function testing should be routine in the management of chronic and acute asthma.

51–15. The recommended treatment for mild persistent asthma symptoms includes a short-acting β-agonist and which other agent(s)?

a. No other agent

b. Low-dose inhaled corticosteroids (ICs)

c. Low-dose ICs, and a long-acting β-agonist

d. High-dose ICs, and a long-acting β-agonist

51–16. The recommended treatment for severe persistent asthma symptoms includes a short-acting β-agonist and which other agent(s)?

a. Low-dose inhaled corticosteroids (ICs)

b. Low-dose ICs, and a long-acting β-agonist

c. High-dose ICs, and a long-acting β-agonist

d. High-dose ICs, a long-acting β-agonist, and oral corticosteroids

51–17. Which of the following does not describe theophylline?

a. Methylxanthine

b. Bronchodilator

c. Corticosteroid

d. Antiinflammatory agent

51–18. Which of the following is effective for acute asthma?

a. Zileuton

b. Cromolyn

c. Montelukast

d. Epinephrine

51–19. A 19-year-old G2P1 at 23 weeks' gestation presents with an asthma exacerbation. Her FEV_1 is 35%, and she is afebrile and otherwise well. You treat her with an inhaled β-agonist treatment and inhaled corticosteroids. After three doses of the inhaled β-agonist, the patient has an oxygen saturation of 94% and an FEV_1 of 45%. Which of the following is the best next management step?

a. Transfer to the intensive care unit for status asthmaticus

b. Discharge her home with a short-acting β-agonist inhaler and schedule a 2-week follow-up office appointment

c. Admit for additional treatment with inhaled β-agonists and intravenous corticosteroids and observe for respiratory distress

d. Discharge her home with β-agonist and corticosteroid nebulizer treatments and with broad-spectrum antibiotics for presumed pneumonia

51–20. A pregnant woman is treated for an asthma exacerbation at 37 weeks' gestation with a regimen that included systemic corticosteroid therapy. She presents again at 39 weeks with labor. Which of the following would not be part of your management plan?

a. Epidural anesthesia, when and if desired by the patient

b. Determination of FEV_1 upon admission to Labor and Delivery

c. Treatment of postpartum hemorrhage with carboprost tromethamine

d. Hydrocortisone 100 mg intravenously every 8 hours during labor and for 24 hours after delivery

51–21. On average, how long does the cough of acute bronchitis persist?

    a. 1–2 days

    b. 3–4 days

    c. 5–7 days

    d. 10–20 days

51–22. Which of the following is not a risk factor for pneumonia?

    a. Asthma

    b. Pregnancy

    c. Binge drinking

    d. Chronic bronchitis

51–23. Which of the following most commonly causes pneumonia?

    a. Influenza A

    b. *Mycoplasma pneumoniae*

    c. *Legionella pneumophila*

    d. *Chlamydophila pneumoniae*

51–24. Which of the following statements regarding pneumonia is true?

    a. Chest radiography is essential for diagnosis.

    b. Chest radiography accurately predicts the etiology.

    c. The responsible pathogen can be identified in most cases.

    d. Sputum cultures are recommended in all suspected cases of pneumonia.

51–25. A 19-year-old G1P0 at 22 weeks' gestation with no significant past medical history presents with cough, fever, and chest pain on inspiration for 3 days. She has a fever of 38.5°C, has 22 respirations per minute, and is oxygenating well. The patient's chest radiograph is provided here. The best treatment for this patient is which of the following?

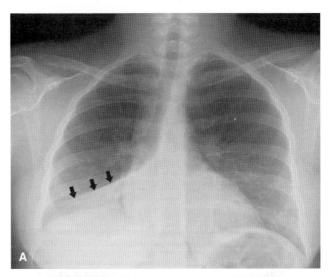

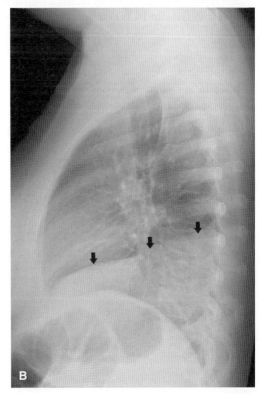

Reproduced with permission from Cunningham FG, Leveno KJ, Bloom SL, et al (eds): Pulmonary disorders. In Williams Obstetrics, 24th ed. New York, McGraw-Hill, 2014, Figure 51-3.

    a. Vancomycin

    b. Moxifloxacin

    c. Azithromycin

    d. Levofloxacin and vancomycin

51–26. What percentage of women with pneumonia develop pleural effusion?

   a. 2%

   b. 20%

   c. 40%

   d. 60%

51–27. A 25-year-old G3P2 at 19 weeks' gestation presents with fever, cough, myalgias, and nausea for 2 days. Her two children at home have also been sick. By rapid test, the patient is diagnosed with influenza A. The best treatment regimen for this patient is which of the following?

   a. Amantadine for 5 days

   b. Amantadine for 10 days

   c. Oseltamivir for 5 days

   d. Oseltamivir and amantadine for 10 days

51–28. A 33-year-old G3P0 at 18 weeks' gestation presents for prenatal care. She is brought to the clinic by a deputy as she is currently incarcerated on drug charges. The patient came to this country 1 year ago. She reports having previously received the bacille Calmette-Guérin (BCG) vaccine. By her history, she has multiple risks for tuberculosis. Which of the following is the best initial test for this patient?

   a. Chest radiography

   b. Sputum collection

   c. Tuberculin skin test

   d. Interferon-gamma release assay (IGRA)

51–29. A 30-year-old G2P1 at 15 weeks' gestation presents with cough, fever, and weight loss. She has recently immigrated to the United States from Mexico. You send a QuantiFERON-TB Gold, which yields a positive result. The patient's chest radiography is provided below. Sputum is positive for acid-fast bacilli. Which of the following is the correct diagnosis for this patient?

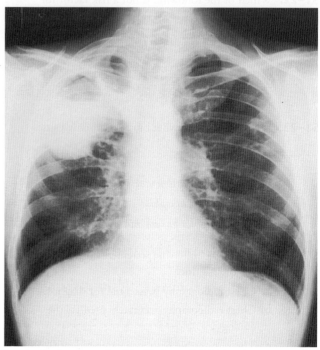

Reproduced with permission from Phan VD, Poponick JM: Tuberculosis. In Tintinalli JE, Stapczynski JS, Cline DM, et al (eds): Tintinalli's Emergency Medicine: A Comprehensive Study Guide, 7th ed. New York, McGraw-Hill, 2011, Figure 70-2.

   a. Sarcoidosis

   b. Active tuberculosis

   c. Latent tuberculosis

   d. Extrapulmonary tuberculosis

51–30. Which of the following is the best management plan for the patient in Question 51–29?

   a. Initiate isoniazid

   b. Initiate isoniazid and rifampin

   c. Initiate isoniazid, rifampin, ethambutol, pyrazinamide, and pyridoxine

   d. Delay treatment until after delivery, then initiate isoniazid, rifampin, and pyridoxine

51–31. A 38-year-old G1P0 at 22 weeks' gestation presents for prenatal care. The patient has active sarcoidosis, and a photograph of her hands is provided here. Regarding sarcoidosis in pregnancy, you correctly counsel her which of the following?

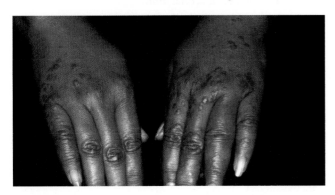

Reproduced with permission from Wolff K, Johnson RA (eds): The skin in immune, auto-immune, and rheumatic disorders. In Fitzpatrick's Color Atlas and Synopsis of Clinical Dermatology, 6th ed. New York, McGraw-Hill, 2009, Figure 14-51.

    a. Perinatal outcomes are poor.

    b. Disease progression in pregnancy is common.

    c. Severe disease warrants serial determination of pulmonary function.

    d. All common treatment modalities are absolutely contraindicated in pregnancy.

51–32. This image shows five classes of genetic mutations affecting a peptide that ultimately functions in epithelial-cell membrane transport of electrolytes. These mutations cause which of the following diseases?

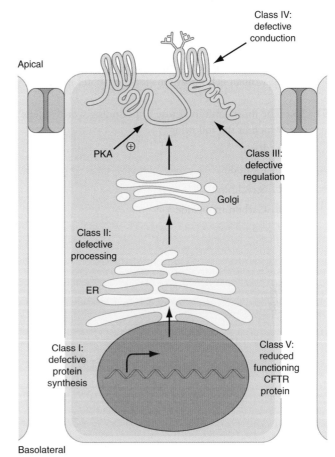

Reproduced with permission from Boucher RC: Cystic fibrosis. In Longo DL, Fauci AS, Kasper DL, et al (eds): Harrison's Principles of Internal Medicine, 18th ed. New York, McGraw-Hill, 2012, Figure 259-1.

    a. Sarcoidosis

    b. Cystic fibrosis

    c. Maple syrup urine disease

    d. Primary ciliary dyskinesia

51–33. The organism most strongly associated with cystic fibrosis is which of the following?

    a. *Burkholderia cepacia*

    b. *Staphylococcus aureus*

    c. *Pseudomonas aeruginosa*

    d. *Haemophilus influenzae*

51–34. Which of the following statements regarding cystic fibrosis is true?

    a. Disease severity is quantified by pulmonary function studies.

    b. When the FEV_1 is at least 40%, women tolerate pregnancy well.

    c. The best predictor of pregnancy outcome in women with cystic fibrosis is nutritional status.

    d. Diabetes in pregnancy is less likely if the affected woman is homozygous for the $\Delta F508$ mutation.

51–35. The most common cause of poisoning worldwide is which of the following?

    a. Ricin

    b. Cyanide

    c. Strychnine

    d. Carbon monoxide

51–36. Fetal heart tracing findings in cases of maternal carbon monoxide poisoning include all **EXCEPT** which of the following?

    a. Elevated baseline

    b. Absence of accelerations

    c. Marked beat-to-beat variability

    d. Decreased beat-to-beat variability

CHAPTER 51 ANSWER KEY

Question number	Letter answer	Page cited	Header cited
51–1	b	p. 1011	Pulmonary Disorders
51–2	a	p. 1011	Pulmonary Disorders
51–3	c	p. 1011	Pulmonary Disorders
51–4	c	p. 1011	Pulmonary Disorders
51–5	b	p. 1011	Pulmonary Disorders
51–6	c	p. 1011	Pulmonary Disorders
51–7	b	p. 1012	Clinical Course
51–8	c	p. 1012	Clinical Course
51–9	b	p. 1012	Clinical Course
51–10	c	p. 1012	Clinical Course
51–11	b	p. 1013	Effects of Pregnancy on Asthma
51–12	a	p. 1014	Fetal Effects
51–13	b	p. 1014	Clinical Evaluation
51–14	d	p. 1014	Clinical Evaluation
51–15	b	p. 1014	Management of Chronic Asthma
51–16	c	p. 1014	Management of Chronic Asthma
51–17	c	p. 1014	Management of Chronic Asthma
51–18	d	p. 1014	Management of Chronic Asthma
51–19	c	p. 1015	Management of Acute Asthma
51–20	c	p. 1015	Labor and Delivery
51–21	d	p. 1015	Acute Bronchitis
51–22	b	p. 1016	Bacterial Pneumonia
51–23	a	p. 1016	Incidence and Causes
51–24	a	p. 1016	Diagnosis
51–25	c	p. 1016	Management
51–26	b	p. 1016	Management
51–27	c	p. 1018	Management
51–28	d	p. 1020	Diagnosis
51–29	b	p. 1020	Diagnosis
51–30	c	p. 1021	Active Infection
51–31	c	p. 1022	Sarcoidosis and Pregnancy
51–32	b	p. 1022	Cystic Fibrosis
51–33	c	p. 1022	Pathophysiology
51–34	a	p. 1022	Pregnancy with Cystic Fibrosis
51–35	d	p. 1023	Carbon Monoxide Poisoning
51–36	c	p. 1024	Treatment

CHAPTER 52

Thromboembolic Disorders

52–1. What is the approximate incidence of thromboembolic events per pregnancy?

a. 1/10

b. 1/100

c. 1/1000

d. 1/10,000

52–2. Which of the following statements is correct regarding the timing of pregnancy-related deep-vein thrombosis (DVT) and pulmonary embolism (PE)?

a. DVT and PE are more common antepartum.

b. DVT and PE are more common postpartum.

c. DVT is more common antepartum, and PE is more common postpartum.

d. PE is more common antepartum, and DVT is more common postpartum.

52–3. All **EXCEPT** which of the following physiologic alterations predispose to venous thrombosis in pregnancy?

a. Lower extremity venous stasis

b. Decreased plasminogen activity

c. Endothelial cell injury at delivery

d. Increased synthesis of clotting factors

52–4. Which of the following risk factors for developing thromboembolism in pregnancy is most important?

a. Cesarean delivery

b. Multifetal gestation

c. Postpartum hemorrhage

d. Personal history of thrombosis

52–5. Approximately what percentage of thromboembolic events that occur during pregnancy can be attributed to an inherited or acquired thrombophilia?

a. 1%

b. 15%

c. 50%

d. 75%

52–6. The mutations that cause antithrombin deficiency are almost always inherited in what fashion?

a. X-linked dominant

b. X-linked recessive

c. Autosomal dominant

d. Autosomal recessive

52–7. Understanding pregnancy physiology is essential to diagnose protein S deficiency. Concentrations of which of the following decline substantially during normal pregnancy?

a. Free protein S

b. Total protein S

c. Functional protein S

d. All of the above

52–8. During his first day of life, a seemingly healthy neonate who was delivered at term suddenly develops fever and diffuse skin lesions as shown in the figure. This is most likely a manifestation of what thrombophilic condition?

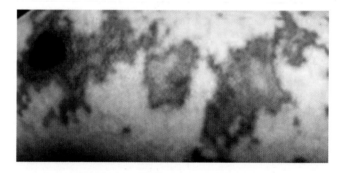

Reproduced with permission from Wolff K, Goldsmith LA, Katz SI, et al: Fitzpatrick's Dermatology in General Medicine, 7th ed. New York, McGraw-Hill, 2008, Figure 180-1C.

a. Homozygous prothrombin mutation

b. Homozygous protein S deficiency

c. Heterozygous protein C deficiency

d. Heterozygous factor V Leiden mutation

52–9. Which of the following inherited thrombophilia syndromes is most prevalent?

a. Protein S deficiency

b. Antithrombin deficiency

c. Factor V Leiden mutation

d. Prothrombin G20210A mutation

52–10. Which of the following pregnancy-related complications are increased in women who are heterozygous carriers of the factor V Leiden mutation?

a. Preeclampsia

b. Placental abruption

c. Fetal-growth restriction

d. None of the above

52–11. All **EXCEPT** which of the following can be causes of elevated homocysteine levels?

a. Folate deficiency

b. Vitamin D deficiency

c. Vitamin B_6 deficiency

d. Methylene-tetrahydrofolate reductase mutation

52–12. The American College of Obstetricians and Gynecologists currently recommends assessment of women for hyperhomocysteinemia and the methylene tetrahydrofolate reductase mutation in what clinical situations?

a. Folic acid deficiency

b. First venous thromboembolism

c. Recurrent venous thromboembolism

d. None of the above

52–13. All **EXCEPT** which of the following women illustrate clinical criteria that would prompt antiphospholipid syndrome laboratory screening?

a. A 33-year-old G2P1 with a 12-week fetal demise.

b. A 41-year-old G2P1 with a history of eclampsia at 36 weeks in her prior pregnancy.

c. A 26-year-old G5P1 at 6 weeks' gestation with spontaneous abortions in her last three pregnancies.

d. A 29-year-old G1P0 at 29 weeks' gestation undergoing induction for severe fetal-growth restriction.

52–14. Which of the following thrombophilic conditions have been most consistently associated with adverse pregnancy outcomes?

a. Factor V Leiden mutation

b. Antiphospholipid syndrome

c. Antithrombin mutation

d. Prothrombin G20210A mutation

52–15. A 32-year-old G2P1 at 29 weeks' gestation presents for a routine prenatal care visit with no complaints. During a routine examination, you note that her legs have the following appearance. Which of the following statements is true regarding this condition in pregnancy?

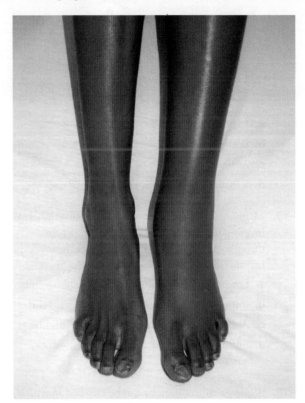

a. Most cases are on the right side.

b. A positive Homans sign is virtually diagnostic.

c. Most cases are located in the iliofemoral veins.

d. Symptoms typically correlate with the degree of vessel involvement.

52–16. The patient described in Question 52–15 undergoes compression ultrasonography of the lower extremity with the following findings. The calipers delineate a vessel lumen. What next step is most appropriate in her management?

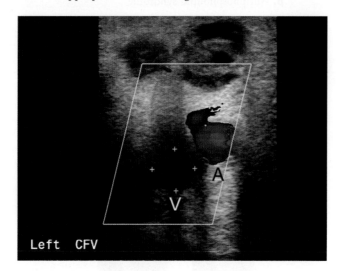

a. Venography

b. Embolectomy

c. Anticoagulation

d. Ventilation-perfusion scan

52–17. Magnetic resonance imaging is a useful adjunctive imaging technique for diagnosing deep-vein thrombosis for all **EXCEPT** which of the following reasons?

a. Lower cost than compression ultrasonography

b. Improved evaluation of the iliofemoral veins

c. Ability to diagnosis nonthrombotic conditions

d. Ability to reconstruct pelvic venous system anatomy

52–18. D-Dimer concentrations can be elevated in which of the following pregnancy-related complications?

a. Preeclampsia

b. Placenta previa

c. Gestational diabetes

d. Prurigo of pregnancy

52–19. This image obtained during venography shows a filling defect (*arrows*) in the popliteal vein. Although this modality remains the gold standard for diagnosing deep-vein thrombosis, it is used infrequently for all **EXCEPT** of the following reasons?

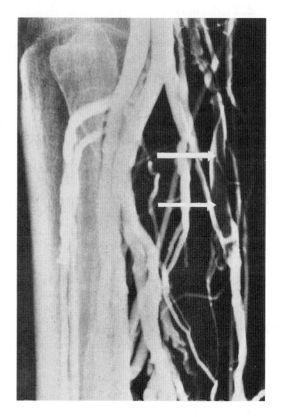

Reproduced with permission from Liem TK, Moneta GL: Venous and lymphatic disease. In Brunicardi FC, Andersen DK, Billiar TR, et al (eds): Schwartz's Principles of Surgery, 9th ed. New York, McGraw-Hill, 2010, Figure 24-8.

a. It is invasive.

b. Intravenous contrast is required.

c. It has a low negative-predictive value.

d. It increases the risk for procedure-associated thrombosis.

52–20. Anticoagulation in pregnancy should preferentially be accomplished with which medication?

a. Warfarin

b. Dabigatran

c. Unfractionated heparin

d. Low-molecular-weight heparin

52–21. Pulmonary embolism occurs in approximately what percentage of patients with untreated deep-vein thrombosis?

    a. 10%

    b. 35%

    c. 60%

    d. 85%

52–22. If unfractionated heparin is selected as the treatment for thromboembolism, the initial intravenous dose is continued for at least how many days before converting to subcutaneous dosing?

    a. 2

    b. 5

    c. 10

    d. 14

52–23. In women who are fully anticoagulated with low-molecular-weight heparin, periodic monitoring of anti-factor Xa levels is particularly important when which of the following comorbidities is present?

    a. Pneumonia

    b. Renal insufficiency

    c. Chronic hypertension

    d. Gestational diabetes

52–24. Women receiving therapeutic doses of low-molecular-weight heparin should not receive neuraxial blockade (e.g., epidural anesthesia) for how long after the last dose was administered?

    a. 12 hours

    b. 24 hours

    c. 36 hours

    d. 48 hours

52–25. The risk for heparin-induced osteoporosis is increased by all **EXCEPT** which of the following?

    a. Cigarette smoking

    b. African American race

    c. Anticoagulation longer than 6 months

    d. Unfractionated heparin as the anticoagulant

52–26. What is the most common presenting symptom in patients with a pulmonary embolus?

    a. Cough

    b. Dyspnea

    c. Syncope

    d. Chest pain

52–27. Results from which of the following tests, when normal, effectively exclude a diagnosis of pulmonary embolism?

    a. Chest radiograph

    b. Electrocardiogram

    c. Oxygen saturation

    d. None of the above

52–28. Circulatory collapse requires obstruction of at least what percentage of the pulmonary vascular tree?

    a. 25%

    b. 50%

    c. 75%

    d. 90%

52–29. Which of the following clinical findings in the setting of pulmonary embolism increases the mortality rate?

    a. Hypoxia

    b. Hemoptysis

    c. Marked elevation of D-dimers

    d. Right ventricular dysfunction

52–30. What is the procedure-related mortality rate with pulmonary angiography?

    a. 0.005%

    b. 0.05%

    c. 0.5%

    d. 5%

52–31. A 35-year-old G4P3 with three prior cesarean deliveries presents at 39 weeks' gestation complaining of ruptured fetal membranes and shortness of breath. During preoperative evaluation, she is noted to have tachycardia and hypoxia, and computed tomographic (CT) angiography is emergently performed. One image from this study is shown here, and the arrow points to a filling defect. Which of the following is the most appropriate next step?

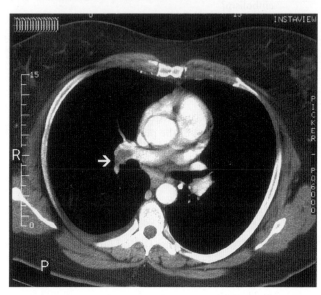

Reproduced with permission from Cunningham FG, Leveno KJ, Bloom SL, et al (eds): Thromboembolic disorders. In Williams Obstetrics, 24th ed. New York, McGraw-Hill, 2014, Figure 38-5.

    a. Pulmonary angiography

    b. Thrombolytic administration

    c. Placement of a vena cava filter

    d. Unfractionated heparin infusion

52–32. Which of the following statements is accurate regarding the use of thrombolytics in pregnancy?

    a. They should be avoided entirely.

    b. They should be avoided in the last trimester.

    c. They should be avoided in the first trimester.

    d. They should be administered when clinically indicated irrespective of pregnancy timing.

CHAPTER 52 ANSWER KEY

Question number	Letter answer	Page cited	Header cited
52–1	c	p. 1028	Introduction
52–2	c	p. 1028	Introduction
52–3	b	p. 1028	Pathophysiology
52–4	d	p. 1028	Pathophysiology
52–5	c	p. 1028	Pathophysiology
52–6	c	p. 1030	Antithrombin Deficiency
52–7	d	p. 1031	Protein S Deficiency
52–8	b	p. 1031	Protein S Deficiency
52–9	c	p. 1031	Activated Protein C Resistance—Factor V Leiden Mutation
52–10	d	p. 1031	Activated Protein C Resistance—Factor V Leiden Mutation
52–11	b	p. 1032	Hyperhomocysteinemia
52–12	d	p. 1032	Hyperhomocysteinemia
52–13	b	p. 1033	Antiphospholipid Antibodies
52–14	b	p. 1033	Thrombophilias and Pregnancy Complications
52–15	c	p. 1035	Deep-Vein Thrombosis—Clinical Presentation
52–16	c	p. 1036	Deep-Vein Thrombosis—Compression Ultrasonography/Management
52–17	a	p. 1036	Deep-Vein Thrombosis—Magnetic Resonance Imaging
52–18	a	p. 1036	Deep-Vein Thrombosis—D-Dimer Screening Tests
52–19	c	p. 1036	Deep-Vein Thrombosis—Venography
52–20	d	p. 1036	Deep-Vein Thrombosis—Management
52–21	c	p. 1036	Deep-Vein Thrombosis—Management
52–22	b	p. 1037	Unfractionated Heparin
52–23	b	p. 1038	Low-Molecular-Weight Heparin
52–24	b	p. 1039	Labor and Delivery
52–25	b	p. 1040	Heparin-Induced Osteoporosis
52–26	b	p. 1040	Pulmonary Embolism—Clinical Presentation
52–27	d	p. 1040	Pulmonary Embolism—Clinical Presentation
52–28	c	p. 1041	Massive Pulmonary Embolism
52–29	d	p. 1041	Massive Pulmonary Embolism
52–30	c	p. 1043	Intravascular Pulmonary Angiography
52–31	c	p. 1044	Vena Cava Filter
52–32	d	p. 1044	Thrombolysis

CHAPTER 53

Renal and Urinary Tract Disorders

53–1. Which of the following statements regarding the physiologic changes of pregnancy is true?

   a. Glomerular filtration decreases.

   b. Effective renal plasma flow increases.

   c. Serum creatinine concentration increases.

   d. Glomeruli become larger because of an increased number of cells (hyperplasia).

53–2. Which of the following is a threshold for proteinuria in pregnancy, above which levels are considered abnormal?

   a. 50 mg/day

   b. 100 mg/day

   c. 200 mg/day

   d. 300 mg/day

53–3. A serum creatinine level in pregnancy that persistently exceeds what threshold value should prompt a suspicion for intrinsic renal disease?

   a. 0.3 mg/dL

   b. 0.5 mg/dL

   c. 0.7 mg/dL

   d. 0.9 mg/dL

53–4. A 27-year-old G1P0 at 14 weeks' gestation presents for prenatal care. She reports having donated a kidney to a family member 2 years ago. She has no other significant medical history. In regard to her having only one kidney, which of the following is true?

   a. She has a significantly increased risk for developing preeclampsia.

   b. She is likely to manifest severe edema in the third trimester.

   c. She will require close monitoring for frequent electrolyte abnormalities.

   d. If her renal function is normal, she can expect to have a normal pregnancy.

53–5. An asymptomatic 17-year-old G1P0 at 16 weeks' gestation presents for her first prenatal visit, and a urine culture is sent as part of routine care. The results show > 100,000 gram-negative rods. The diagnosis is which of the following?

   a. Cystitis

   b. Pyelonephritis

   c. Diverticulitis

   d. Asymptomatic bacteriuria

53–6. If the patient in Question 53–5 is not treated, what is the chance that she will develop a symptomatic infection during pregnancy?

   a. 5%

   b. 10%

   c. 25%

   d. 50%

53–7. The patient in Question 53–5 refuses any treatment that she must take over multiple days. Which of the following regimens would be an acceptable single-dose oral treatment?

   a. Ampicillin, 2 g

   b. Ciprofloxacin, 250 mg

   c. Nitrofurantoin, 100 mg

   d. Trimethoprim-sulfamethoxazole, 160/800 mg

53–8. After treatment of the patient in Question 53–5, what is her risk of recurrence?

   a. 10%

   b. 30%

   c. 50%

   d. 70%

53–9. Lower urinary tract symptoms with pyuria but a sterile urine culture are likely due to which pathogen?

   a. *Escherichia coli*

   b. *Proteus mirabilis*

   c. *Chlamydia trachomatis*

   d. *Klebsiella pneumoniae*

53–10. What is the leading cause of septic shock in pregnancy?

   a. Pneumonia

   b. Pyelonephritis

   c. Breast abscess

   d. Chorioamnionitis

53–11. A 16-year-old G1P0 at 22 weeks' gestation presents to the emergency room complaining of fever, nausea with vomiting, chills, dysuria, and flank pain. Her temperature is 102°F, and right costovertebral angle tenderness is noted. A urinalysis reveals many leukocytes, many bacteria, small blood, and large ketones. The patient's urine culture will most likely reveal what organism? An image of the organism is provided here.

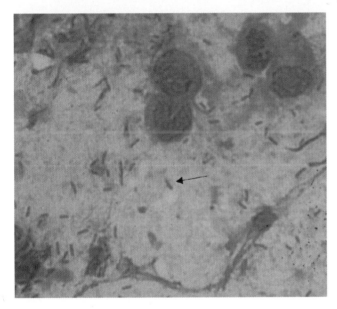

Reproduced with permission from Levinson W: Gram-negative rods related to the enteric tract. In Review of Medical Microbiology and Immunology, 12th ed. New York, McGraw-Hill, 2012, Figure 18-1.

   a. *Escherichia coli*

   b. *Proteus mirabilis*

   c. *Chlamydia trachomatis*

   d. *Klebsiella pneumoniae*

53–12. For the patient in Question 53–11, which of the following best describes appropriate management?

   a. Discharge her home with oral antibiotics, antiemetics, and close surveillance

   b. 23-hour inpatient observation with intravenous antimicrobials and fluid restriction to prevent pulmonary edema

   c. One dose of intravenous antimicrobials in the emergency room, discharge home, oral antibiotics, and close surveillance

   d. Hospitalization, intravenous antimicrobial therapy and hydration, close monitoring of vital signs, and evaluation of electrolytes

53–13. You admit the patient in Question 53–11. Intravenous antimicrobial therapy and hydration with crystalloid solutions are begun. The next day, she is tachypneic and her oxygen saturation is low. She is hypotensive, continues to spike high temperatures, and appears ill. You initiate oxygen via face mask. What is the next step in your management?

   a. Chest radiograph

   b. Renal sonography

   c. Modification of antimicrobial therapy

   d. Computed tomographic chest angiography

53–14. A chest radiograph for the patient in Question 53–11 is provided here. The most likely diagnosis is which of the following?

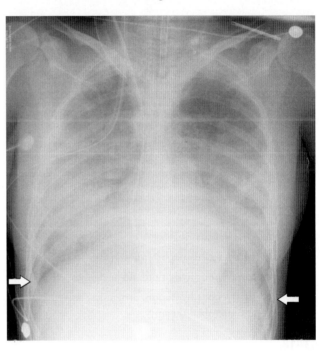

Reproduced with permission from Cunningham FG, Leveno KJ, Bloom SL, et al (eds): Maternal physiology. In Williams Obstetrics, 24th ed. New York, McGraw-Hill, 2014, Figure 53-3A.

   a. Pulmonary embolism

   b. Mild pulmonary edema

   c. Community-acquired pneumonia

   d. Acute respiratory distress syndrome

53–15. After discharge from the hospital for acute pyelonephritis, patients should receive oral antimicrobial treatment for how long?

   a. 3–5 days

   b. 7–14 days

   c. 21–28 days

   d. Oral antimicrobial therapy is not necessary.

53–16. Which of the following promotes nephrolithiasis?

    a. Hydration

    b. Low-sodium diet

    c. Low-calcium diet

    d. Thiazide diuretics

53–17. A 24-year-old G2P1 at 15 weeks' gestation presents to the emergency room with severe pain that radiates from her back to lower abdomen. The patient is afebrile, and urinalysis only reveals red blood cells. One of the patient's renal sonograms is provided here. What is the best management plan for this patient?

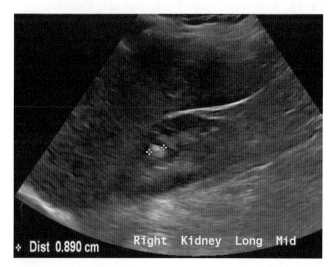

    a. Ureteral stenting

    b. Percutaneous nephrolithotomy

    c. Intravenous hydration and analgesics

    d. Intravenous hydration, analgesics, and antimicrobial therapy

53–18. The rate of which of the following obstetrical complications is not increased in renal transplant recipients treated with cyclosporine and tacrolimus?

    a. Preeclampsia

    b. Preterm birth

    c. Fetal malformation

    d. Fetal-growth restriction

53–19. A 26-year-old woman who underwent renal transplant 1 year ago presents for preconceptional counseling. You recommend she delay pregnancy until which of the following benchmarks is achieved?

    a. Her creatinine ranges from 2 to 3 mg/dL.

    b. She has been in good general health for 1 to 2 years.

    c. She documents no evidence of graft rejection for 3 months.

    d. All of the above

53–20. Obstetrical management of a pregnant renal transplant recipient should include which of the following?

    a. Glucose tolerance testing

    b. Renal function monitoring

    c. Fetal-growth restriction surveillance

    d. All of the above

53–21. Which of the following statements is not true regarding polycystic kidney disease, the autosomal dominant disease demonstrated in the image here?

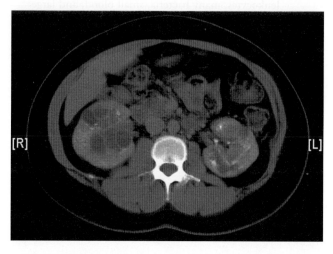

Reproduced with permission from Smith MA: Polycystic kidney disease. In Usatine RP, Smith MA, Chumley H, et al (eds): The Color Atlas of Family Medicine. New York, McGraw-Hill, 2009, Figure 67-1.

    a. Most cases are caused by a mutation on chromosome 8.

    b. Ten percent of patients die from berry aneurysm rupture.

    c. It causes 5–10% of end-stage renal disease in the United States.

    d. One third of patients have coexistent asymptomatic hepatic cysts.

53–22. Which of the following does not cause acute nephritic syndrome?

    a. IgA nephropathy

    b. Infective endocarditis

    c. Systemic lupus erythematosus

    d. Focal segmental glomerulosclerosis

53–23. Of the following, which is the most common cause of nephrotic syndrome?

    a. Amyloidosis

    b. Minimal change disease

    c. Membranous glomerulonephritis

    d. Focal segmental glomerulosclerosis

53–24. Select the correct statement regarding nephrotic syndrome.

   a. Heavy proteinuria is the hallmark.

   b. There is increased risk of thromboembolism.

   c. In pregnancy, prognosis is dependent on the degree of hypertension and renal insufficiency.

   d. All of the above

53–25. Which of the following is not a known complication of nephrotic syndrome in pregnancy?

   a. Preeclampsia

   b. Polycythemia

   c. Preterm birth

   d. Peripheral edema

53–26. Which of the following contributes the most to end-stage renal disease requiring dialysis and transplant?

   a. Diabetes

   b. Hypertension

   c. Glomerulonephritis

   d. Polycystic kidney disease

53–27. A 22-year-old G1P0 at 14 weeks' gestation with a history of type 1 diabetes presents for prenatal care. Her diabetes is poorly controlled, and her serum creatinine is 3.5 mg/dL. While counseling her regarding the prognosis of this pregnancy, how would you categorize her renal impairment?

   a. Mild renal insufficiency

   b. Moderate renal insufficiency

   c. Severe renal insufficiency

   d. None of the above

53–28. For the patient in Question 53–27, her pregnancy-induced hypervolemia will surely be reduced by the renal insufficiency. This patient will likely expand her blood volume by what amount?

   a. 0%

   b. 10%

   c. 25%

   d. 55%

53–29. Which of the following would not be part of your pregnancy management plan for the patient in Question 53–27?

   a. Low-protein diet

   b. Excellent glucose control

   c. Frequent blood pressure monitoring

   d. Serial sonographic examinations to follow fetal growth

53–30. When managing a pregnant woman on dialysis, which of the following is an important modification?

   a. Reduce doses of daily oral multivitamins

   b. Stop erythropoietin because of harmful fetal effects

   c. Add additional bicarbonate and less calcium to dialysate

   d. Extend dialysis to 5–6 times weekly to avoid hypotension

53–31. A 24-year-old G1P0 at 37 weeks' gestation presents to Labor and Delivery complaining of headache, lower abdominal pain, and decreased fetal movement. Her initial blood pressure is 140/90, and no fetal heart tones are seen sonographically. She has 4+ urine protein. The patient is diagnosed with severe preeclampsia and with fetal demise due to a suspected placental abruption. You send a panel of laboratory tests, start magnesium sulfate infusion, transfuse 2 units of packed red blood cells, and induce labor. The patient has a prompt vaginal delivery with an estimated 1 L blood loss. Postpartum, her urine output is 20 mL/hr, heart rate is 120 beats per minute, and blood pressure is 90/60. Which of the following is your plan of management?

   a. Initiate dopamine drip

   b. Administer a loop diuretic

   c. Provide a one-time intravenous bolus of crystalloid solution

   d. Replace intravascular volume with crystalloid solution and blood

53–32. The condition depicted in this renal sonogram can cause all **EXCEPT** which of the following complications?

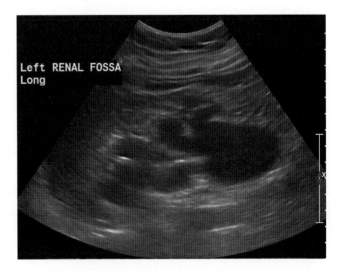

   a. Oliguria

   b. Hypotension

   c. Renal failure

   d. Elevated serum creatinine

53–33. Regarding the condition depicted in this photograph, all **EXCEPT** which of the following statements are true during pregnancy?

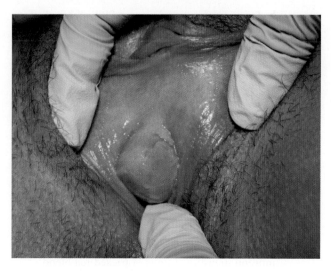

Photograph contributed by Gracy Jilson, WHNP.

a. It is usually managed surgically.

b. Recurrent urinary tract infections may develop.

c. Urine can collect within the sac and dribble out.

d. It originates from an enlarging paraurethral gland abscess that ruptures into the urethral lumen and leaves a persistent diverticular sac and ostium into the urethra.

CHAPTER 53 ANSWER KEY

Question number	Letter answer	Page cited	Header cited
53–1	b	p. 1051	Pregnancy-Induced Urinary Tract Changes
53–2	d	p. 1051	Assessment of Renal Function During Pregnancy
53–3	d	p. 1051	Assessment of Renal Function During Pregnancy
53–4	d	p. 1052	Pregnancy after Unilateral Nephrectomy
53–5	d	p. 1053	Asymptomatic Bacteriuria
53–6	c	p. 1053	Significance
53–7	a	p. 1053	Table 53-1
53–8	b	p. 1053	Treatment
53–9	c	p. 1054	Cystitis and Urethritis
53–10	b	p. 1054	Acute Pyelonephritis
53–11	a	p. 1054	Clinical Findings
53–12	d	p. 1055	Table 53-2
53–13	a	p. 1055	Table 53-2
53–14	d	p. 1055	Figure 53-3
53–15	b	p. 1054	Management
53–16	c	p. 1056	Nephrolithiasis
53–17	c	p. 1057	Management
53–18	c	p. 1057	Pregnancy Outcomes
53–19	b	p. 1057	Pregnancy Outcomes
53–20	d	p. 1058	Management
53–21	a	p. 1058	Polycystic Kidney Disease
53–22	d	p. 1059	Table 53-3
53–23	d	p. 1060	Table 53-4
53–24	d	p. 1059	Nephrotic Syndromes
53–25	b	p. 1059	Pregnancy
53–26	a	p. 1060	Chronic Renal Disease
53–27	c	p. 1060	Chronic Renal Disease
53–28	c	p. 1061	Pregnancy and Chronic Renal Disease
53–29	a	p. 1062	Management
53–30	d	p. 1062	Dialysis During Pregnancy
53–31	d	p. 1064	Prevention
53–32	b	p. 1064	Obstructive Renal Failure
53–33	a	p. 1064	Urethral Diverticulum

CHAPTER 54

Gastrointestinal Disorders

54–1. Which of the following diagnostic studies are considered safe to use in pregnancy?

    a. Cystoscopy

    b. Flexible sigmoidoscopy

    c. Endoscopic retrograde cholangiopancreatography

    d. All of the above

54–2. All **EXCEPT** which of the following are common indications for surgery during pregnancy?

    a. Appendicitis

    b. Adnexal mass

    c. Cholecystitis

    d. Nephrolithiasis

54–3. Which of the following is preferred treatment to maintain adequate nutrition in a pregnant patient with nausea and vomiting?

    a. Hyperalimentation

    b. Parenteral feeding

    c. Enteral alimentation

    d. Dextrose-containing solutions

54–4. Which of the following is the most common serious complication of parenteral feeding?

    a. Hemothorax

    b. Pneumothorax

    c. Catheter sepsis

    d. Brachial plexus injury

54–5. What is the approximate incidence of laparotomy and laparoscopy for nonobstetrical indications in pregnancy?

    a. 1:50

    b. 1:100

    c. 1:500

    d. 1:1000

54–6. Which of the following statements is true regarding nonobstetrical surgery in pregnancy?

    a. There is increased risk of stillbirth.

    b. There is increased risk of cerebral palsy.

    c. There is increased risk of preterm delivery.

    d. There is no increase in long-term risks to the fetus or the mother.

54–7. In cases of severe hyperemesis gravidarum, all **EXCEPT** which of the following initial complications are common?

    a. Acidosis

    b. Dehydration

    c. Hypokalemia

    d. Mild transaminitis

54–8. What organism has a proposed association with hyperemesis gravidarum?

    a. *Helicobacter pylori*

    b. *Bacteroides fragilis*

    c. *Clostridium difficile*

    d. *Streptococcus viridans*

54–9. A serious complication seen in hyperemesis gravidarum is shown here. What is the likely cause of this finding?

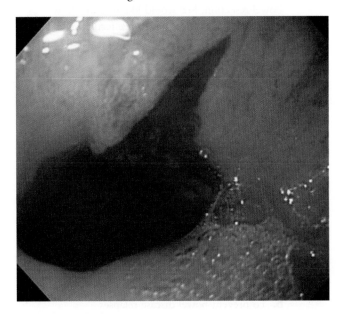

Reproduced with permission from Song LM, Topazian M: Gastrointestinal endoscopy. In Longo DL, Fauci AS, Kasper DL, et al (eds): Harrison's Principles of Internal Medicine, 18th ed. New York, McGraw-Hill, 2012, Figure 291-20.

    a. Dehydration

    b. *Helicobacter pylori* infection

    c. Persistent vomiting

    d. Vitamin K deficiency

54–10. Which vitamin deficiency in hyperemesis gravidarum could lead to fetal intracranial hemorrhage?

    a. Thiamine

    b. Vitamin A

    c. Vitamin D

    d. Vitamin K

54–11. Which vitamin deficiency in hyperemesis gravidarum is associated with confusion, ocular findings, and ataxia?

    a. Thiamine

    b. Vitamin A

    c. Vitamin D

    d. Vitamin K

54–12. Which of the following interventions is the preferred initial treatment of hyperemesis gravidarum?

    a. Glucocorticoids

    b. Enteral nutrition

    c. Hyperalimentation

    d. Antiemetics and intravenous hydration

54–13. All **EXCEPT** which of the following medications are safe to use in pregnancy for the treatment of reflux esophagitis?

    a. Cimetidine

    b. Omeprazole

    c. Misoprostol

    d. Calcium carbonate

54–14. What is the rate of hospital readmission in patients with hyperemesis gravidarum?

    a. 5%

    b. 15%

    c. 30%

    d. 45%

54–15. What is the main mechanism underlying reflux esophagitis in pregnancy?

    a. Increased gastric emptying

    b. Excessive gastric acid production

    c. Relaxation of the upper esophageal sphincter

    d. Relaxation of the lower esophageal sphincter

54–16. A pregnant patient with history of swallowing problems presents with dysphagia, chest pain, and vomiting. A barium swallow done just prior to pregnancy revealed these images. What is the patient's diagnosis?

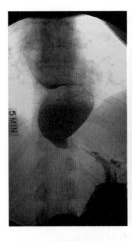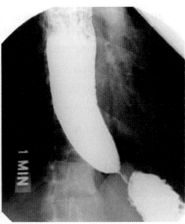

Reproduced with permission from Kahrilas PJ, Hirano I: Diseases of the esophagus. In Longo DL, Fauci AS, Kasper DL, et al (eds): Harrison's Principles of Internal Medicine, 18th ed. New York, McGraw-Hill, 2012, Figure 292-5.

    a. Achalasia

    b. Hiatal hernia

    c. Peptic ulcer disease

    d. Diaphragmatic hernia

54–17. A pregnant patient presents with peptic ulcer disease. She is symptomatic, and a urea breath test is positive. Which of the following treatment options should be avoided in this patient?

a. Amoxicillin, 1000 mg twice daily

b. Metronidazole, 500 mg twice daily

c. Clarithromycin, 500 mg twice daily

d. Tetracycline, 500 mg four times daily

54–18. A pregnant patient presents with diarrhea for 3 days. She is not febrile, has not had bloody stools, and is able to drink liquids without vomiting. Which of the following drugs is indicated?

a. Ciprofloxacin

b. Metronidazole

c. Bismuth subsalicylate

d. Trimethoprim-sulfamethoxazole

54–19. A pregnant patient is referred to you because of concurrent Crohn disease. Which of the following is true regarding her disease?

a. It conveys a 3–5% risk of cancer.

b. A proctocolectomy would be curative.

c. It involves the deep layers of small and large bowel.

d. It is typically associated with antineutrophil cytoplasmic antibody.

54–20. Options for the treatment of inflammatory bowel disease in pregnancy include all **EXCEPT** which of the following medications?

a. Infliximab

b. Mesalamine

c. Methotrexate

d. Glucocorticoids

54–21. If one partner of a couple has inflammatory bowel disease, which of the following is a known potential cause of subfertility in this couple?

a. Development of rectovaginal fistulas

b. Use of immune modulators as treatment

c. Sperm abnormalities caused by sulfasalazine

d. None of the above

54–22. Which of the following statements is true regarding inflammatory bowel disease in pregnancy?

a. Relapses are usually mild.

b. Pregnancy increases the likelihood of a flare.

c. Most treatments are discontinued during pregnancy.

d. Active disease in early pregnancy increases the likelihood of poor pregnancy outcome.

54–23. A patient with Crohn disease presents for preconceptional counseling. The patient is currently in remission, but her surgeon has recommended bowel resection. She would like to know how this surgery will affect her future fertility and pregnancies. Which of the following statements should be part of her counseling?

a. She can expect her fertility to decrease if she has surgery.

b. She will need to be delivered by cesarean section if she conceives.

c. Laparoscopic anastomosis compared with anastomosis via laparotomy has a higher subsequent fertility rate.

d. None of the above

54–24. Why is high-dose folic acid supplementation indicated in pregnant patients with inflammatory bowel disease?

a. To prevent fetal cardiac defects

b. To prevent bowel disease relapses

c. To counteract the antifolate actions of sulfasalazine

d. To act synergistically with calcium in the prevention of osteoporosis

54–25. A pregnant patient presents in the early first trimester while taking the immune modulator infliximab to treat her Crohn disease. Which of the following statements is true regarding this drug?

a. It is considered safe in pregnancy.

b. It is associated with fetal-growth restriction.

c. It is associated with higher rates of congenital skeletal defects.

d. All of the above

54–26. What is the most common cause of intestinal obstruction in pregnancy and the puerperium?

a. Volvulus

b. Adhesions

c. Carcinoma

d. Intussusception

54–27. Cases of bowel obstruction in pregnancy are least likely to occur during which of the following time frames?

a. Early first trimester

b. Midpregnancy

c. Third trimester

d. Immediately postpartum

54–28. A patient in the midtrimester presents with colicky abdominal pain, nausea, and vomiting. At laparotomy, surgical findings are similar to those shown here. What is her likely diagnosis?

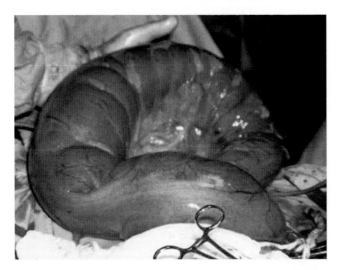

Reproduced with permission from Cunningham FG, Leveno KJ, Bloom SL, et al (eds): Gastrointestinal disorders. In Williams Obstetrics, 24th ed. New York, McGraw-Hill, 2014, Figure 54-4.

    a. Perforation

    b. Crohn disease

    c. Colonic volvulus

    d. Ulcerative colitis

54–29. What is the incidence of appendicitis in pregnancy?

    a. 1:500

    b. 1:1500

    c. 1:5000

    d. 1:10,000

54–30. During what part of pregnancy is a patient most likely to be diagnosed with a *ruptured* appendix?

    a. First trimester

    b. Second trimester

    c. Third trimester

    d. Postpartum

54–31. What are the most reproducible findings in a pregnant woman with appendicitis?

    a. Fever

    b. Anorexia

    c. Nausea and vomiting

    d. Persistent abdominal pain and tenderness

54–32. Which method(s) may be appropriately used in pregnancy for appendicitis diagnosis?

    a. Transvaginal sonography

    b. Computed tomography (CT)

    c. Magnetic resonance (MR) imaging

    d. All of the above

54–33. A second-trimester pregnant patient presents with appendicitis. One of her MR images is shown here that displays the appendix with surrounding edema (*arrow*), the adjacent right ovary (*arrowhead*), and fetus (*carets*). Which of the following statements is accurate regarding this condition?

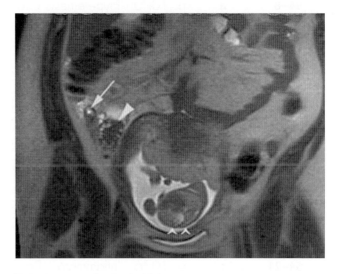

Used with permission from Dr. April Bailey.

    a. The risk of spontaneous abortion is increased.

    b. Accuracy of diagnosis improves with increasing gestational age.

    c. Surgical evaluation is best postponed until the second trimester.

    d. Tocolytics decrease the risk of preterm labor associated with this complication.

CHAPTER 54 ANSWER KEY

Question number	Letter answer	Page cited	Header cited
54–1	d	p. 1069	Diagnostic Techniques
54–2	d	p. 1070	Laparotomy and Laparoscopy
54–3	c	p. 1070	Nutritional Support
54–4	c	p. 1070	Nutritional Support
54–5	c	p. 1070	Laparotomy and Laparoscopy
54–6	d	p. 1070	Laparotomy and Laparoscopy
54–7	a	p. 1070	Hyperemesis Gravidarum
54–8	a	p. 1070	Hyperemesis Gravidarum
54–9	c	p. 1071	Complications
54–10	d	p. 1071	Complications
54–11	a	p. 1071	Complications
54–12	d	p. 1072	Management
54–13	c	p. 1072	Gastroesophageal Reflux Disease
54–14	c	p. 1072	Management
54–15	d	p. 1072	Gastroesophageal Reflux Disease
54–16	a	p. 1073	Achalasia
54–17	d	p. 1073	Peptic Ulcer
54–18	c	p. 1074	Acute Diarrhea
54–19	c	p. 1075	Inflammatory Bowel Disease, Table 54-4
54–20	c	p. 1076	Ulcerative Colitis and Pregnancy
54–21	c	p. 1076	Inflammatory Bowel Disease and Fertility
54–22	d	p. 1076	Inflammatory Bowel Disease and Pregnancy
54–23	c	p. 1076	Inflammatory Bowel Disease and Fertility
54–24	c	p. 1076	Ulcerative Colitis and Pregnancy
54–25	a	p. 1077	Crohn Disease and Pregnancy
54–26	b	p. 1078	Intestinal Obstruction
54–27	a	p. 1078	Intestinal Obstruction
54–28	c	p. 1078	Intestinal Obstruction, Figure 54-4
54–29	b	p. 1078	Appendicitis
54–30	c	p. 1078	Appendicitis
54–31	d	p. 1079	Diagnosis
54–32	d	p. 1079	Diagnosis
54–33	a	p. 1079	Pregnancy Outcomes

CHAPTER 55

Hepatic, Biliary, and Pancreatic Disorders

55–1. All **EXCEPT** which of the following liver-related changes are physiologic in pregnancy?

a. Asterixis

b. Palmar erythema

c. Spider angiomas

d. Elevated serum alkaline phosphatase levels

55–2. What is the underlying pathophysiology of intrahepatic cholestasis of pregnancy?

a. Acute hepatocellular destruction

b. Incomplete clearance of bile acids

c. Microvascular thrombus accumulation

d. Eosinophil infiltration of the liver

55–3. Which of the following clinical features are characteristic of intrahepatic cholestasis of pregnancy?

a. Maculopapular rash

b. Nausea and vomiting

c. Generalized pruritis

d. Serum transaminase levels > 500 U/L

55–4. Which of the following viral infections has been associated with a marked increase in the risk for intrahepatic cholestasis of pregnancy?

a. Hepatitis C

b. Hepatitis B

c. Cytomegalovirus

d. Human immunodeficiency virus

55–5. A 42-year-old primigravida presents at 35 weeks' gestation with several new complaints. Most bothersome is yellowing of her sclera. After performing a thorough history, physical, and laboratory evaluation, you make a diagnosis of intrahepatic cholestasis of pregnancy. Approximately what percentage of women with this condition will develop jaundice?

a. < 1%

b. 10%

c. 50%

d. > 90%

55–6. Referring to the patient described in Question 55–5, which of the following medications is most appropriate to initiate?

a. Hydroxyzine

b. Cholestyramine

c. Diphenhydramine

d. Ursodeoxycholic acid

55–7. The patient from Question 55–5 reports that she has been reading about intrahepatic cholestasis of pregnancy and understands that the condition may be associated with stillbirth. You explain that the association is somewhat ambiguous but that one plausible reason may involve which of the following fetal complications?

a. Cardiac arrest

b. Hepatocellular injury

c. Hypoxic encephalopathy

d. Disseminated intravascular coagulation

55–8. All **EXCEPT** which of the following statements regarding acute fatty liver of pregnancy are true?

a. It occurs in about 1 in 10,000 pregnancies.

b. Recurrence in subsequent pregnancies is common.

c. It is the most common cause of liver failure in pregnancy.

d. All statements are true.

55–9. Which mutation patterns of the enzymes of fatty acid oxidation have classically been associated with maternal acute fatty liver of pregnancy?

a. Homozygous mutation in the fetus and mother

b. Heterozygous mutation in the fetus and mother

c. Homozygous mutation in the fetus; heterozygous mutation in the mother

d. Heterozygous mutation in the fetus; homozygous mutation in the mother

55–10. From an etiopathogenesis perspective, acute fatty liver of pregnancy is analogous to what childhood illness?

　a. Reye syndrome

　b. Biliary atresia

　c. Autoimmune hepatitis

　d. Epstein-Barr virus infection

55–11. All **EXCEPT** which of the following are clinical characteristics that increase the risk for acute fatty liver of pregnancy?

　a. Nulliparity

　b. Female fetus

　c. Twin gestation

　d. Third trimester

55–12. A 33-year-old G2P1 presents at 35 weeks' gestation with complaints of nausea and vomiting. Laboratory evaluation reveals markedly elevated transaminase levels, renal dysfunction, and coagulopathy. A peripheral smear is performed and is shown here. What is the underlying etiology of the blood smear findings in this patient?

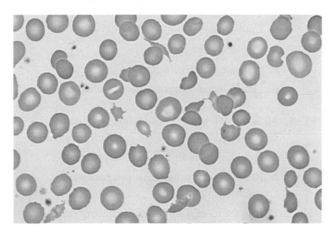

Reproduced with permission from Lichtman MA, Beutler E, Kipps TJ: Color atlas III: Red cell morphology. In Williams Hematology, 7th ed. New York, McGraw-Hill, 2006, Plate III-3.

　a. Autoimmune antibody binding

　b. Lowered capillary oxygen tension

　c. Decreased cholesterol production

　d. Increased destruction in the spleen

55–13. As a part of the evaluation for the patient described in Question 55–12, you want to confirm the suspected diagnosis with imaging. Which of the following modalities is most appropriate?

　a. Sonography

　b. Computed tomography

　c. Magnetic resonance imaging

　d. None of the above

55–14. You stabilize the patient described in Question 55–12 and correct her coagulopathy. After this, you induce labor, and she has a vaginal delivery. On postpartum day 2, she appears to be doing well, but you notice that her urine output has increased to approximately 800 mL per hour. What is the most likely cause of this condition?

　a. Pituitary tumor

　b. Acute tubular necrosis

　c. Hypothalamic dysfunction

　d. Elevated serum vasopressinase concentrations

55–15. Although it can be dangerous if coagulopathy is not adequately addressed, what is the approximate cesarean delivery rate in women who have acute fatty liver of pregnancy?

　a. 10%

　b. 30%

　c. 60%

　d. 90%

55–16. This image shows a hepatocellular carcinoma filling the left side of this cirrhotic liver. What is the most common cause of liver cancer?

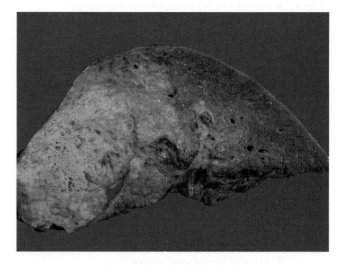

Reproduced with permission from Kemp WL, Burns DK, Brown TG: Pathology of the liver, gallbladder, and pancreas. In Pathology: The Big Picture. New York, McGraw-Hill, 2008, Figure 15-14A.

　a. Alcohol abuse

　b. Hemochromatosis

　c. Chronic viral hepatitis

　d. Primary biliary cirrhosis

55–17. All **EXCEPT** which of the following clinical findings would indicate a severe course of acute hepatitis that should prompt hospitalization?

   a. Hyperglycemia

   b. Hypoalbuminemia

   c. Central nervous symptoms

   d. Prolonged prothrombin time

55–18. Which of the following statements regarding acute viral hepatitis is correct?

   a. Jaundice is usually the presenting symptom.

   b. Serum transaminase levels correspond with disease severity.

   c. Low-grade fever is more common with hepatitis A infection.

   d. Bilirubin levels typically fall as transaminase levels rise.

55–19. Complete clinical recovery is **LEAST** likely to occur following acute infection with which of the following?

   a. Hepatitis A

   b. Hepatitis B

   c. Hepatitis C

   d. Hepatitis E

55–20. Which type of hepatitis virus is represented here?

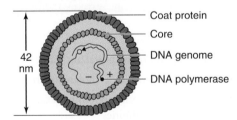

Virus particle

Modified with permission from Ryan K et al. Sherris Medical Microbiology, 3rd ed. Originally published by Appleton & Lange. Copyright 1994 McGraw-Hill.

   a. Hepatitis A

   b. Hepatitis B

   c. Hepatitis C

   d. Hepatitis E

55–21. After infection with hepatitis B, what is the first detectable serological marker?

   a. HBs antigen

   b. HBe antigen

   c. Anti-HBs antibody

   d. IgM anti-HB core antibody

55–22. Chronic hepatitis B infection is most likely to develop in which of the following patients?

   a. A newborn

   b. An 8-year-old child

   c. A 32-year-old healthy woman

   d. All are equally likely to develop chronic infection

55–23. Approximately what percentage of patients infected with hepatitis C will have no identifiable risk factors?

   a. 10%

   b. 33%

   c. 66%

   d. 90%

55–24. What is the primary adverse perinatal outcome in women infected with hepatitis C?

   a. Stillbirth

   b. Low birthweight

   c. Admission to intensive care unit

   d. Vertical transmission of hepatitis C virus

55–25. Which of the following statements regarding breast feeding in women infected with hepatitis B (HBV) and C (HCV) is correct?

   a. It is contraindicated in both.

   b. It is contraindicated only in HBV infection.

   c. It is contraindicated only in HCV infection.

   d. Neither is a contraindication.

55–26. Which of the following statements regarding hepatitis E is correct?

   a. It is a DNA virus.

   b. No effective vaccine is available.

   c. It is transmitted by sexual contact.

   d. Affected pregnant women are at increased risk for mortality compared with affected nonpregnant women.

55–27. Rates of which of the following complications appear to be increased in pregnant women with autoimmune hepatitis?

   a. Preeclampsia

   b. Hepatitis flares

   c. Maternal mortality

   d. All of the above

55–28. Steatohepatitis is most common in women of which ethnic group?

   a. Asian

   b. Hispanic

   c. White

   d. African American

55–29. The following image depicts the typical nodular, fibrotic appearance of a cirrhotic liver. What is the most common cause of this condition in the general population?

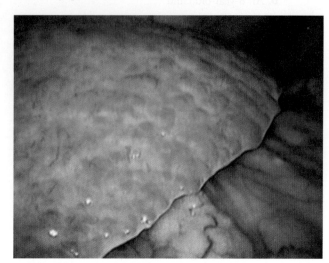

Reproduced with permission from Geller DA, Goss JA, Tsung A: Liver. In Brunicardi FC, Andersen DK, Billiar TR, et al (eds): Schwartz's Principles of Surgery, 9th ed. New York, McGraw-Hill, 2010, Figure 31-16A.

a. Viral hepatitis

b. Alcohol exposure

c. Autoimmune hepatitis

d. Nonalcoholic fatty liver disease

55–30. Women with cirrhosis who become pregnant are at increased risk for all **EXCEPT** of the following untoward outcomes?

a. Preterm birth

b. Gestational diabetes

c. Fetal-growth restriction

d. Rupture of splenic artery aneurysms

55–31. Which of the following management strategies is recommended for sonographically identified asymptomatic gallstones?

a. Cholecystectomy

b. Low-cholesterol diet

c. Ursodeoxycholic acid

d. None of the above

55–32. A 31-year-old G2P1 20 weeks' gestation complains of vomiting, fever, and right upper quadrant pain. Examination reveals right upper quadrant tenderness. One diagnostic sonographic image is shown here. What is the most appropriate next step in her management?

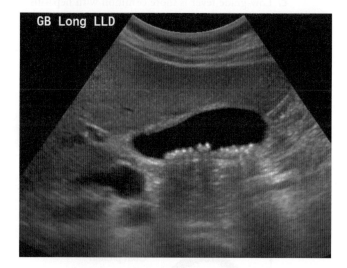

a. Cholecystectomy

b. Discharge home with oral antibiotics

c. Endoscopic retrograde cholangiopancreatography

d. Admission for serial abdominal examinations and intravenous antibiotics

CHAPTER 55 ANSWER KEY

Question number	Letter answer	Page cited	Header cited
55–1	a	p. 1084	Hepatic Disorders
55–2	b	p. 1085	Intrahepatic Cholestasis of Pregnancy—Pathogenesis
55–3	c	p. 1085	Intrahepatic Cholestasis of Pregnancy—Clinical Presentation
55–4	a	p. 1085	Intrahepatic Cholestasis of Pregnancy—Clinical Presentation
55–5	b	p. 1085	Intrahepatic Cholestasis of Pregnancy—Clinical Presentation
55–6	d	p. 1085	Intrahepatic Cholestasis of Pregnancy—Management
55–7	a	p. 1086	Cholestasis and Pregnancy Outcomes
55–8	b	p. 1086	Acute Fatty Liver of Pregnancy
55–9	c	p. 1086	Acute Fatty Liver of Pregnancy—Etiopathogenesis
55–10	a	p. 1086	Acute Fatty Liver of Pregnancy—Etiopathogenesis
55–11	b	p. 1087	Acute Fatty Liver of Pregnancy—Clinical and Laboratory Findings
55–12	c	p. 1087	Acute Fatty Liver of Pregnancy—Clinical and Laboratory Findings
55–13	d	p. 1087	Acute Fatty Liver of Pregnancy—Clinical and Laboratory Findings
55–14	d	p. 1088	Acute Fatty Liver of Pregnancy—Management
55–15	d	p. 1088	Acute Fatty Liver of Pregnancy—Management
55–16	c	p. 1088	Viral Hepatitis
55–17	a	p. 1088	Acute Hepatitis
55–18	c	p. 1088	Acute Hepatitis
55–19	c	p. 1088	Acute Hepatitis
55–20	b	p. 1090	Hepatitis B
55–21	a	p. 1090	Hepatitis B
55–22	a	p. 1090	Hepatitis B
55–23	b	p. 1091	Hepatitis C
55–24	d	p. 1091	Hepatitis C
55–25	d	p. 1090	Hepatitis B and Hepatitis C
55–26	d	p. 1092	Hepatitis E
55–27	d	p. 1092	Autoimmune Hepatitis
55–28	b	p. 1092	Nonalcoholic Fatty Liver Disease
55–29	b	p. 1093	Cirrhosis
55–30	b	p. 1093	Cirrhosis
55–31	d	p. 1095	Cholelithiasis and Cholecystitis
55–32	a	p. 1096	Medical versus Surgical Management

CHAPTER 56

Hematological Disorders

56–1. A hemoglobin concentration below which of the following thresholds would indicate anemia in an iron-supplemented pregnant woman in any trimester?

a. 9.0 g/dL

b. 9.5 g/dL

c. 10.0 g/dL

d. 10.5 g/dL

56–2. What is the most common cause of antepartum anemia in pregnant women?

a. Thalassemia

b. Iron deficiency

c. Folic acid deficiency

d. Anemia of chronic disease

56–3. A 19-year-old primigravida at 29 weeks' gestation is noted to have anemia with a hemoglobin concentration of 8 g/dL. The peripheral blood smear below is obtained. Which of the following laboratory findings are likely to accompany this condition?

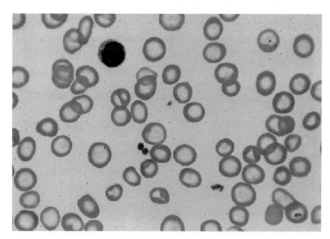

Reproduced with permission from Beutler E: Disorders of iron metabolism. In Lichtman MA, Kipps TJ, Seligsohn U (eds): Williams Hematology, 8th ed. New York, McGraw-Hill, 2010, Figure 42-10C.

a. Decreased serum ferritin level

b. Elevated mean corpuscular volume

c. Decreased total iron binding capacity

d. Positive sickle-cell screen (Sickledex) result

56–4. For the patient described in Question 56–3, what is the most appropriate initial treatment?

a. Red cell transfusion

b. Folic acid, 4 mg orally daily

c. Hydroxyurea, 1 g orally daily

d. Elemental iron, 200 mg orally daily

56–5. Of medical conditions associated with anemia of chronic disease, which is most frequently encountered in pregnancy?

a. Crohn disease

b. Hodgkin lymphoma

c. Chronic renal insufficiency

d. Systemic lupus erythematosus

56–6. A 36-year-old G3P2 at 18 weeks' gestation reports extreme fatigue and is found to be have a hemoglobin concentration of 7.5 g/dL. The erythrocyte mean corpuscular volume is markedly elevated and measures 124 fL. A peripheral blood smear is obtained and is shown here. What is the most likely etiology?

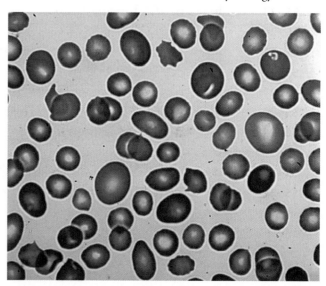

Reproduced with permission from Green R: Folate, cobalamin, and megaloblastic anemia. In Lichtman MA, Kipps TJ, Seligsohn U (eds): Williams Hematology, 8th ed. New York, McGraw-Hill, 2010, Figure 41-12A.

a. Iron deficiency

b. Vitamin B_6 deficiency

c. Folic acid deficiency

d. Vitamin B_{12} deficiency

56–7. All **EXCEPT** which of the following statements regarding autoimmune hemolytic anemia in pregnancy are true?

a. Pregnancy can accelerate hemolysis.

b. The direct Coombs test is usually positive.

c. The indirect Coombs test is usually positive.

d. The cause of aberrant antibody production originates from fetal microchimerism.

56–8. Pregnant women with paroxysmal nocturnal hemoglobinuria are at increased risk for which of the following?

a. Renal failure

b. Venous thrombosis

c. Maternal mortality

d. All of the above

56–9. What is the typical inheritance pattern of the mutation in the *spectrin* gene that results in hereditary spherocytosis?

a. Mitochondrial

b. X-linked dominant

c. Autosomal dominant

d. Autosomal recessive

56–10. The following image demonstrates the appearance of spherocytes using scanning electron microscopy. In addition to identifying erythrocytes with this appearance, what other laboratory finding helps confirm the diagnosis of hereditary spherocytosis?

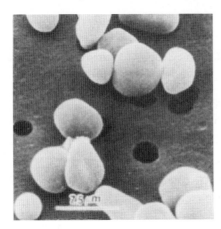

Reproduced with permission from Cunningham FG, Leveno KJ, Bloom SL, et al (eds): Hematological disorders. In Williams Obstetrics, 24th ed. New York, McGraw-Hill, 2014, Figure 56-2B.

a. Low serum haptoglobin level

b. Elevated serum bilirubin level

c. Increased erythrocyte osmotic fragility

d. Increased serum level of fibrin split products

56–11. Which of the following statements is true regarding women who are *heterozygous* for the glucose-6-phosphate dehydrogenase mutation?

a. Infections in pregnancy can precipitate hemolysis.

b. Some degree of protection against malaria is conferred.

c. Lyonization results in a variable degree of enzyme activity.

d. All of the above

56–12. Which of the following pregnancy complications has been associated with polycythemia vera?

a. Stillbirth

b. Coagulopathy

c. Placenta previa

d. Placental abruption

56–13. What is the prevalence of sickle-cell trait among African-American women in the United States?

a. 1%

b. 4%

c. 8%

d. 25%

56–14. In patients with sickle-cell disease, red cells may assume the following configuration under which of the following conditions?

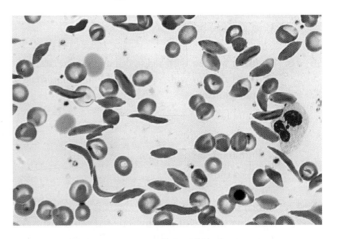

Reproduced with permission from Longo DL: Atlas of hematology and analysis of peripheral blood smears. In Longo DL, Fauci AS, Kasper DL, et al (eds): Harrison's Principles of Internal Medicine, 18th ed. New York, McGraw-Hill, 2012, Figure e17-12.

a. Hyperglycemia

b. Low oxygen tension

c. Dietary protein deficiency

d. Administration of certain antibiotics

56–15. A 22-year-old primigravida with sickle-cell disease presents with complaints of fever, cough, and increasing dyspnea. The following chest radiograph is obtained. All **EXCEPT** which of the following are precipitants of this condition?

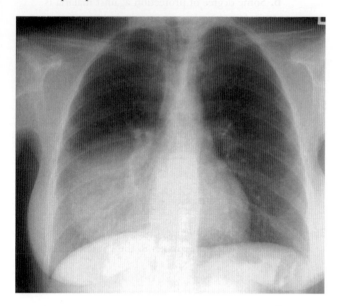

Reproduced with permission from Cunningham FG, Leveno KJ, Bloom SL, et al (eds): Pulmonary disorders. In Williams Obstetrics, 22nd ed. New York, McGraw-Hill, 2005, Figure 46-1.

    a. Infection

    b. Atelectasis

    c. Coagulopathy

    d. Marrow emboli

56–16. Pregnant women with sickle-cell anemia are at increased risk for which of the following maternal complications?

    a. Renal failure

    b. Cardiomyopathy

    c. Pulmonary hypertension

    d. All of the above

56–17. Which of the following statements is accurate regarding the use of prophylactic red cell transfusions for pregnant women with sickle-cell anemia?

    a. Gestation duration is increased.

    b. Perinatal mortality rate is decreased.

    c. Rate of fetal-growth restriction is decreased.

    d. Risk of red cell alloimmunization is increased.

56–18. Which of the following contraceptive choices may help prevent painful crises in women with sickle-cell disease?

    a. Intrauterine device

    b. Surgical sterilization

    c. Depot medroxyprogesterone acetate

    d. Combination oral contraceptive pills

56–19. Sickle-cell trait (hemoglobin AS) has been associated with an increased risk for which of the following?

    a. Preeclampsia

    b. Placental abruption

    c. Gestational diabetes

    d. Urinary tract infections

56–20. Women with which of the following α-globin genotypes are at risk to have offspring with homozygous α-thalassemia?

    a. $\alpha\alpha/--$

    b. $\alpha-/\alpha\alpha$

    c. $\alpha-/\alpha-$

    d. $\alpha\alpha/\alpha\alpha$

56–21. Which of the following findings on hemoglobin electrophoresis would be most consistent with a diagnosis of β-thalassemia minor?

    a. Hemoglobin A2 less than 1%; normal fetal hemoglobin level

    b. Hemoglobin A2 less than 1%; fetal hemoglobin greater than 2%

    c. Hemoglobin A2 greater than 3.5%; normal fetal hemoglobin level

    d. Hemoglobin A2 greater than 3.5%; fetal hemoglobin greater than 2%

56–22. What is the most common cause of thrombocytopenia in pregnancy?

    a. Severe preeclampsia

    b. Consumptive coagulopathy

    c. Gestational thrombocytopenia

    d. Immune thrombocytopenic purpura

56–23. When indicated in pregnancy, which of the following is the most appropriate initial treatment of immune thrombocytopenic purpura?

    a. Azathioprine

    b. Laparoscopic splenectomy

    c. Systemic corticosteroids

    d. Intravenous anti-D immunoglobulin G

56–24. Which of the following management strategies is recommended to detect fetal thrombocytopenia in women who have chronic immune thrombocytopenic purpura?

a. Cordocentesis

b. Scalp sampling

c. Cesarean delivery

d. None of the above

56–25. Most cases of thrombocytosis in which the platelet count exceeds 1 million/μL are caused by which of the following conditions?

a. Malignancy

b. Iron deficiency

c. Autoimmune conditions

d. Essential thrombocytosis

56–26. Although there is considerable clinical overlap between thrombotic thrombocytopenic purpura (TTP) and hemolytic uremic syndrome (HUS), these entities can be distinguished by all **EXCEPT** which of the following?

a. HUS has more renal dysfunction.

b. HUS is seen primarily in adults.

c. TTP more frequently has associated neurologic aberrations.

d. All statements are true.

56–27. What is the cornerstone of treatment for thrombotic thrombocytopenic purpura?

a. Anticoagulation

b. Plasmapheresis

c. Platelet transfusion

d. Intravenous immunoglobulin (IVIG)

56–28. Because the treatment of the two conditions is very different, differentiating severe preeclampsia from thrombotic thrombocytopenic purpura (TTP) is important. Which of the following clinical findings favors TTP?

a. Moderate thrombocytopenia

b. Severe hemolysis

c. Mild disseminated intravascular coagulation

d. Marked transaminase elevation

56–29. Hemophilia A, characterized by a severe deficiency in factor VIII, is inherited in what fashion?

a. X-linked dominant

b. X-linked recessive

c. Autosomal dominant

d. Autosomal recessive

56–30. In women affected by hemophilia A, the risk for excessive hemorrhage at delivery can be reduced by all **EXCEPT** which of the following?

a. Uterotonics

b. Desmopressin

c. Avoiding episiotomy

d. Operative vaginal delivery

56–31. Pregnancy physiology results in which of the following changes to factor VIII and von Willebrand factor (vWF) levels?

a. Increased factor VIII and vWF levels

b. Decreased factor VIII and vWF levels

c. Increased factor VIII levels; decreased vWF factor levels

d. Decreased factor VIII levels; increased vWF factor levels

56–32. Although pregnancy outcomes are generally good in women who have von Willebrand disease, which of the following pregnancy-related complications may be encountered in up to 50 percent of such cases?

a. Preterm birth

b. Placental abruption

c. Postpartum hemorrhage

d. Fetal-growth restriction

CHAPTER 56 ANSWER KEY

Question number	Letter answer	Page cited	Header cited
56–1	d	p. 1101	Anemias
56–2	b	p. 1102	Iron Deficiency Anemia
56–3	a	p. 1103	Iron Deficiency Anemia—Diagnosis
56–4	d	p. 1103	Iron Deficiency Anemia—Treatment
56–5	c	p. 1103	Anemia Associated with Chronic Disease—Pregnancy
56–6	c	p. 1104	Folic Acid Deficiency
56–7	b	p. 1104	Autoimmune Hemolysis
56–8	d	p. 1105	Paroxysmal Nocturnal Hemoglobinuria
56–9	c	p. 1106	Hereditary Spherocytosis
56–10	c	p. 1106	Hereditary Spherocytosis
56–11	d	p. 1106	Erythrocyte Enzyme Deficiency
56–12	a	p. 1107	Polycythemia Vera
56–13	c	p. 1108	Sickle-Cell Hemoglobinopathies—Inheritance
56–14	b	p. 1108	Sickle-Cell Hemoglobinopathies—Pathophysiology
56–15	c	p. 1108	Pregnancy and Sickle-Cell Syndromes
56–16	d	p. 1108	Pregnancy and Sickle-Cell Syndromes, Table 56-2
56–17	d	p. 1110	Prophylactic Red Cell Transfusions
56–18	c	p. 1111	Contraception and Sterilization
56–19	d	p. 1111	Sickle-Cell Trait
56–20	a	p. 1112	Alpha Thalassemias
56–21	d	p. 1113	Beta Thalassemias
56–22	c	p. 1114	Thrombocytopenia
56–23	c	p. 1114	Immune Thrombocytopenia—Diagnosis and Management
56–24	d	p. 1115	Detection of Fetal Thrombocytopenia
56–25	d	p. 1115	Thrombocytosis
56–26	b	p. 1116	Thrombotic Microangiopathies—Etiopathogenesis
56–27	b	p. 1116	Thrombotic Microangiopathies—Treatment
56–28	b	p. 1116	Thrombotic Microangiopathies—Pregnancy
56–29	b	p. 1117	Hemophilia A and B
56–30	d	p. 1117	Hemophilia A and B—Pregnancy
56–31	a	p. 1118	Von Willebrand Disease—Pregnancy
56–32	c	p. 1118	Von Willebrand Disease—Pregnancy

CHAPTER 57

Diabetes Mellitus

57–1. The number of Americans with diabetes is increasing, in part, because of which of the following?

    a. An obesity prevalence that has plateaued

    b. An aging population that is more likely to develop type 2 diabetes

    c. Decreased populations within minority groups, who are more likely to develop type 1 diabetes

    d. All of the above

57–2. In 2006 in the United States, the rate of diabetes during pregnancy approximated which of the following?

    a. 0.5%

    b. 4%

    c. 9%

    d. 14%

57–3. The graphic below concerning the age-specific incidence of gestational diabetes suggests which of the following?

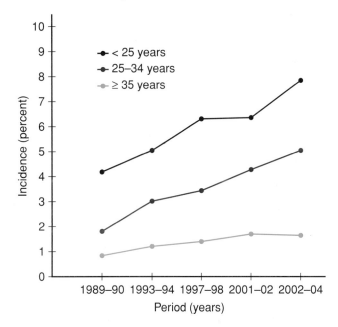

Reproduced with permission from Cunningham FG, Leveno KJ, Bloom SL, et al (eds): Diabetes mellitus. In Williams Obstetrics, 24th ed. New York, McGraw-Hill, 2014, Figure 57-1.

    a. The greatest increase in incidence was in the group of women ≥ 35 years.

    b. For all maternal age groups, the incidence of gestational diabetes has increased since 1989.

    c. The decreases seen in the group of women younger than 25 years may be explained by improved dietary intake.

    d. None of the above

57–4. A 27-year-old woman with proliferative retinopathy would have what diagnosis by the White classification?

    a. R diabetes

    b. H diabetes

    c. RF diabetes

    d. A2 gestational diabetes

57–5. What fasting plasma glucose level is used as the threshold to diagnose overt diabetes?

   a. 105 mg/dL

   b. 116 mg/dL

   c. 126 mg/dL

   d. 140 mg/dL

57–6. Which of the following is a risk factor in pregnant women for impaired carbohydrate metabolism?

   a. Family history of diabetes

   b. Previous infant with polycystic kidney disease

   c. High serum levels of antiphospholipid antibodies

   d. All of the above

57–7. Fetuses of overtly diabetic mothers have an increased risk for which of the following?

   a. Preterm delivery

   b. Spontaneous abortion

   c. Congenital malformation

   d. All of the above

57–8. This figure illustrates the frequency of congenital malformations at given maternal glycohemoglobin levels early in pregnancy. What can be said regarding this relationship?

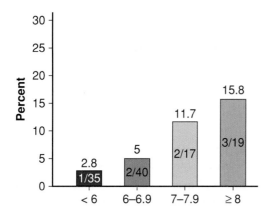

Reproduced with permission from Cunningham FG, Leveno KJ, Bloom SL, et al (eds): Diabetes mellitus. In Williams Obstetrics, 24th ed. New York, McGraw-Hill, 2014, Figure 57-2.

   a. Gestational diabetes confers an increased risk of congenital malformation.

   b. If the glycohemoglobin A_{1C} is < 6, there is no risk of congenital malformation.

   c. As preconceptional glucose control worsens, the incidence of congenital malformation increases.

   d. The highest risk for congenital malformation is seen with a glycohemoglobin A_{1C} level between 7 and 8.

57–9. Fetal hyperinsulinemia in the second half of pregnancy is associated with which of the following?

   a. Altered fetal growth

   b. Neonatal hypoglycemia

   c. Maternal hyperglycemia

   d. All of the above

57–10. What might be said of the pregnancy yielding this 6050 g newborn?

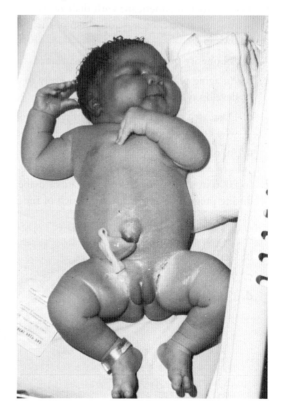

Reproduced with permission from Cunningham FG, Leveno KJ, Bloom SL, et al (eds): Diabetes mellitus. In Williams Obstetrics, 24th ed. New York, McGraw-Hill, 2014, Figure 57-3.

   a. The baby was at risk for neonatal hyperglycemia.

   b. The mother probably had excellent glycemic control.

   c. The mother had an increased risk for shoulder dystocia.

   d. All of the above

57–11. This graphic comparing birthweight distributions of neonates born to diabetic and nondiabetic mothers illustrates which of the following?

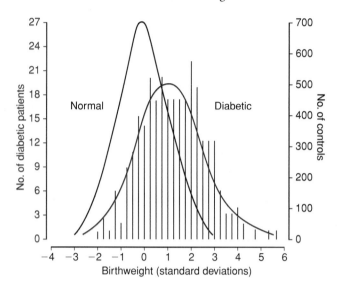

Reproduced with permission from Cunningham FG, Leveno KJ, Bloom SL, et al (eds): Diabetes mellitus. In Williams Obstetrics, 24th ed. New York, McGraw-Hill, 2014, Figure 57-4.

a. Newborns of diabetic mothers are "growth promoted."

b. The birthweight distribution of newborns of diabetic mothers is skewed toward consistently heavier birthweights.

c. Growth promotion from maternal hyperglycemia does not precluded fetal-growth restriction, which is defined as 2 standard deviations below the mean.

d. All of the above

57–12. The incidence of stillbirth is highest in pregnancies complicated by which of the following?

a. Overt diabetes

b. Gestational diabetes

c. Overt diabetes and hypertension

d. Gestational diabetes and hypertension

57–13. Which of the following is a reasonable explanation for hydramnios in diabetic pregnancy?

a. Maternal endothelial leak caused by hyperglycemia

b. Glucose reabsorption by the fetal glomerular collecting system

c. Osmotic gradient created by high glucose concentrations in the amnionic fluid

d. All of the above

57–14. What is the most likely cause for the increased incidence of respiratory distress syndrome in the neonates of diabetic mothers?

a. Indicated preterm delivery

b. Delayed maturation of type II pneumocytes

c. Decreased production of surfactant in a hyperglycemic environment

d. All of the above

57–15. Hyperbilirubinemia in the newborns of diabetic mothers is related to which of the following?

a. Newborn polycythemia

b. Relative fetal hypoxia

c. Hyperglycemia-mediated increases in maternal affinity for oxygen and fetal oxygen consumption

d. All of the above

57–16. What can be said regarding the inheritance of diabetes?

a. Breast feeding increases the inheritance risk.

b. There is a genetic component to the inheritance of type I diabetes.

c. If both parents have type 2 diabetes, the risk of inheritance approximates 20%.

d. None of the above

57–17. What is the maternal mortality rate associated with class H diabetes?

a. 10%

b. 25%

c. 50%

d. 75%

57–18. For women with chronic hypertension and diabetic nephropathy, what is the associated risk of developing preeclampsia?

a. 20%

b. 40%

c. 60%

d. 80%

57–19. The adverse effects of pregnancy on diabetic retinopathy may be reduced by which of the following during pregnancy?

a. Good glycemic control

b. Laser retina photocoagulation in pregnancy

c. Folate, 4 mg orally daily throughout pregnancy

d. A and B

57–20. What is the most important component of diabetic ketoacidosis treatment in pregnancy?

a. Restore euglycemia

b. Provide intravenous hydration

c. Provide intravenous potassium repletion

d. Provide intravenous bicarbonate to correct acidosis

57–21. Which of the following infections is increased in gravidas with overt diabetes?

a. Pyelonephritis

b. Respiratory infections

c. Wound infection after cesarean delivery

d. All of the above

57–22. Concerning the preconceptional period, what can be said of care for the diabetic woman?

a. Should achieve euglycemia

b. Should begin daily folate

c. Should have an ophthalmological appointment to screen for retinopathy

d. All of the above

57–23. Women with type 1 diabetes should achieve glycemic control with which of the following during pregnancy?

a. Insulin

b. Diet alone

c. Insulin and diet

d. Oral hypoglycemic agents

57–24. During which of the following epochs in pregnancy is the peak incidence of maternal hypoglycemia noted?

a. 10–14 weeks

b. 20–24 weeks

c. 28–32 weeks

d. 34–38 weeks

57–25. In pregnant women with overt diabetes, which of the following statements is true regarding detection of fetal anomalies?

a. Sonographic anatomical evaluation is best performed at 18–22 weeks' gestation.

b. The accuracy of sonographic fetal anatomical evaluation is not diminished by concurrent maternal obesity.

c. Maternal serum alpha-fetoprotein determination should be completed early, between 12 and 16 weeks, in mothers with overt diabetes.

d. None of the above

57–26. Concerning labor and delivery in insulin-requiring diabetics, which of the following is true?

a. The patient should receive insulin as usual and have breakfast prior to induction.

b. The mother should be adequately hydrated, and euglycemia is maintained by a continuous insulin infusion.

c. Primary cesarean is preferred for any insulin-requiring diabetic mother whose baby has an estimated fetal weight ≥ 4000 g.

d. Euglycemia is best achieved by administering dextrose-containing intravenous fluids and regularly scheduled insulin injections.

57–27. Which of the following defines gestational diabetes?

a. Any diabetes that is first detected in pregnancy.

b. Diabetes that does not require insulin during pregnancy.

c. A glycohemoglobin A_{1C} level < 7 found early in pregnancy.

d. None of the above

57–28. Concerning the screening of gravidas for gestational diabetes, which of the following is true?

a. Approximately 80% of institutions in the United States use universal screening.

b. Universal screening is endorsed by the International Workshop Conference on Gestational Diabetes.

c. The American College of Obstetricians and Gynecologists (ACOG) endorses one-step glucose screening that uses a 75-g glucose tolerance test.

d. The American College of Obstetricians and Gynecologists (ACOG) endorses a two-step screening process that begins with a 50-g oral glucose screen.

57–29. Reported by Landon (2009), the Maternal-Fetal Medicine Units Network evaluated women with mild gestational diabetes, defined as a fasting blood glucose level > 95 mg/dL. Compared with women receiving only standard obstetrical care, those receiving dietary counseling and glucose monitoring had decreased rates of which of the following morbidities?

a. Fetal macrosomia

b. Cesarean delivery

c. Shoulder dystocia

d. All of the above

57–30. In women with gestational diabetes, early fasting hyperglycemia is associated with increased rates of which of the following?

   a. Fetal macrosomia

   b. Cesarean delivery

   c. Maternal hypertension

   d. All of the above

57–31. Which of the following factors have been implicated in fetal macrosomia?

   a. Leptin

   b. C-peptide

   c. Insulin-like growth factor

   d. All of the above

57–32. As reported by Metzger (2007), the Fifth International Working Conference on Gestational Diabetes recommended fasting blood glucose levels be kept below what value?

   a. 95 mg/dL

   b. 100 mg/dL

   c. 110 mg/dL

   d. 120 mg/dL

57–33. Concerning nutritional instructions for women with gestational diabetes, which of the following is true?

   a. Daily caloric intake should range between 30 and 35 kcal/kg.

   b. A carbohydrate-controlled diet should maintain mild hyperglycemia and avoid ketosis.

   c. The American College of Obstetricians and Gynecologists (ACOG) recommends that carbohydrate intake should comprise no more than 20% of the total daily calories.

   d. All of the above

57–34. Which of the following reflects the American College of Obstetricians and Gynecologists (ACOG) recommendations concerning activity in gravidas with gestational diabetes?

   a. Modified bed rest near term

   b. Moderate exercise for those without contraindications

   c. Maintenance of the same exercise routine established before conception

   d. None of the above

57–35. Concerning glucose monitoring in pregnancy, which of the following is true?

   a. Fasting blood glucose levels < 100 mg/dL should be the goal.

   b. Preprandial surveillance is superior to postprandial testing.

   c. Daily monitoring with reflectance meters may reduce fetal macrosomia rates.

   d. Weekly monitoring to achieve fasting blood glucose levels < 110 mg/dL reduces cesarean delivery rates.

57–36. Which of the following is appropriate initial insulin dosing for pregnant women who meet criteria for therapy?

   a. 0.5 units/kg NPH, administered daily in two divided doses

   b. 20 units NPH and 10 units regular insulin, administered daily each morning

   c. 0.7–1.0 units/kg insulin, using a combination of NPH and regular insulin, administered daily in divided doses

   d. None of the above

57–37. Regarding metformin therapy for gestational diabetes, which of the following is true?

   a. It crosses the placenta.

   b. Compared with insulin therapy, rates of neonatal hypoglycemia are increased.

   c. Compared with insulin therapy, rates of adverse perinatal outcomes are increased.

   d. All of the above

57–38. Your patient is a 33-year-old G3P2 white female who presents for her first prenatal visit at 16 weeks' gestation. She had a newborn weighing 9 lb and gestational diabetes in her last pregnancy. At this visit, all **EXCEPT** which of the following are appropriate prenatal laboratory tests?

   a. Rapid plasma reagin test

   b. Serum total cholesterol level

   c. 50-g oral glucose tolerance test

   d. Quad screen to assess fetal risk of aneuploidy and neural-tube defect

57–39. Testing of the patient in Question 57–38 shows a negative quad screen result, a glucose level of 146 mg/dL, and a negative rapid plasma reagin test result. Which of the following should be ordered next?

    a. 3-hour oral glucose tolerance test

    b. Genetic counseling and offer genetic amniocentesis

    c. Microhemagglutination assay *Treponema pallidum* (MHA-TP)

    d. None of the above

57–40. Three-hour oral glucose tolerance testing of the patient in Question 57–38 yields normal results. Subsequently, she returns to her prenatal clinic at normal intervals. At 26 weeks' gestation, what test should be ordered?

    a. Rapid plasma reagin test

    b. Targeted fetal sonography

    c. 3-hour glucose tolerance test

    d. 50-g oral glucose tolerance screen

57–41. Ms. Smith is diagnosed with gestational diabetes that is controlled solely with diet. Which of the following are important for the management of her pregnancy at term?

    a. Induction at 38 weeks' gestation

    b. Weekly umbilical artery Doppler studies

    c. Cesarean delivery if the estimated fetal weight is 4250 g

    d. None of the above

References

HAPO Study Cooperative Research Group: Hyperglycemia and adverse pregnancy outcomes. N Engl J Med 358:2061, 2008

Landon MB, Spong CY, Thom E, et al: A multicenter, randomized treatment trial of mild gestational diabetes. N Engl J Med 361(14):1339, 2009

Metzger BE, Buchanan TA, Coustan DR, et al: Summary and recommendations of the Fifth International Workshop-Conference on Gestational Diabetes. Diabetes Care 30(Suppl 2):S251, 2007

CHAPTER 57 ANSWER KEY

Question number	Letter answer	Page cited	Header cited
57–1	b	p. 1125	Introduction
57–2	b	p. 1125	Classification During Pregnancy
57–3	b	p. 1125	Classification During Pregnancy
57–4	a	p. 1126	White Classification in Pregnancy
57–5	c	p. 1127	Diagnosis
57–6	a	p. 1127	Diagnosis
57–7	d	p. 1128	Fetal Effects
57–8	c	p. 1128	Malformations
57–9	d	p. 1129	Altered Fetal Growth
57–10	c	p. 1129	Altered Fetal Growth, Hypoglycemia
57–11	d	p. 1129	Altered Fetal Growth
57–12	c	p. 1129	Unexplained Fetal Demise
57–13	c	p. 1130	Hydramnios
57–14	a	p. 1130	Respiratory Distress Syndrome
57–15	d	p. 1130	Hyperbilirubinemia and Polycythemia
57–16	b	p. 1131	Inheritance of Diabetes
57–17	c	p. 1131	Maternal Effects
57–18	c	p. 1131	Diabetic Nephropathy
57–19	d	p. 1132	Diabetic Retinopathy
57–20	b	p. 1133	Diabetic Ketoacidosis
57–21	d	p. 1133	Infections
57–22	d	p. 1134	Preconceptional Care
57–23	c	p. 1134	Insulin Treatment
57–24	a	p. 1135	Hypoglycemia
57–25	a	p. 1135	Second Trimester
57–26	b	p. 1135	Third Trimester and Delivery
57–27	a	p. 1136	Gestational Diabetes
57–28	d	p. 1136	Gestational Diabetes
57–29	d	p. 1136	Screening and Diagnosis
57–30	d	p. 1139	Maternal and Fetal Effects
57–31	d	p. 1140	Fetal Macrosomia
57–32	a	p. 1140	Management
57–33	a	p. 1140	Diabetic Diet
57–34	b	p. 1141	Exercise
57–35	c	p. 1141	Glucose Monitoring
57–36	c	p. 1141	Insulin Treatment
57–37	a	p. 1141	Oral Hypoglycemic Agents
57–38	b	p. 1137	Table 57-12
57–39	a	p. 1136	Screening and Diagnosis
57–40	c	p. 1137	Table 57-12
57–41	d	p. 1142	Obstetrical Management

CHAPTER 58

Endocrine Disorders

58–1. Which of the following is true of thyroid-stimulating hormone (TSH) during pregnancy?

 a. Decreased levels are found in early pregnancy.

 b. TSH crosses the placenta and stimulates fetal thyroxine production.

 c. TSH levels are increased in early pregnancy because of the effects of human chorionic gonadotropin (hCG).

 d. None of the above

58–2. Maternal sources account for what percentage of fetal thyroxine at term?

 a. 10%

 b. 30%

 c. 50%

 d. 70%

58–3. In a study of more than 1000 women with thyroid peroxidase (TPO) antibodies, there was an associated increased risk of which of the following?

 a. Placenta previa

 b. Preterm delivery

 c. Placental abruption

 d. Preterm rupture of membranes

58–4. Which clinical symptom is not characteristic of mild thyrotoxicosis?

 a. Thyromegaly

 b. Tachycardia

 c. Cold intolerance

 d. Poor maternal weight

58–5. The condition shown here is commonly associated with which of the following maternal signs?

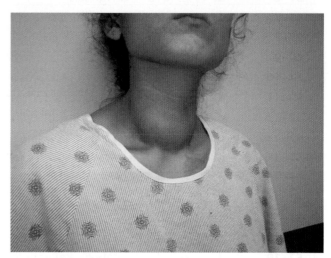

 a. Tachycardia

 b. Enophthalmos

 c. Maternal androgen insensitivity

 d. All of the above

58–6. The following fetal condition is associated with fetal thyrotoxicosis. If identified antenatally, the mother may be treated with which of the following agents, which is subsequently transported transplacentally to the fetus?

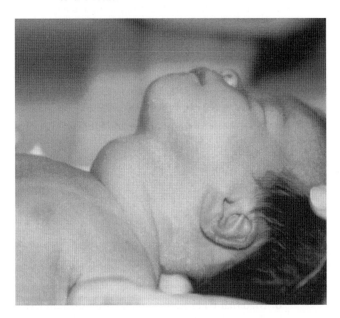

Reproduced with permission from Cunningham FG, Leveno KJ, Bloom SL, et al (eds): Endocrine disorders. In Williams Obstetrics, 24th ed. New York, McGraw-Hill, 2014, Figure 58-2.

    a. Iodine

    b. Prednisone

    c. Propylthiouracil (PTU)

    d. Intravenous immune globulin G (IVIG)

58–7. If a pregnant woman develops fever or sore throat while taking a thionamide, how should this be managed?

    a. Stop the medication immediately

    b. Increase her dose of propylthiouracil

    c. Change from propylthiouracil to methimazole

    d. None of the above

58–8. Which of the following is an appropriate initial thionamide dose for pregnant women with hyperthyroidism and is the one typically used at Parkland Hospital?

    a. 50 mg po tid

    b. 100 mg po tid

    c. 200 mg po tid

    d. 300 mg po bid

58–9. Which of the following is the initial treatment consideration for thyrotoxicosis in the pregnant woman?

    a. Administer sodium iodide

    b. Initiate corticosteroids

    c. Administer potassium iodide

    d. None of the above

58–10. Untreated maternal thyrotoxicosis may lead to which of the following fetal complications?

    a. Stillbirth

    b. Macrosomia

    c. Postterm gestation

    d. All of the above

58–11. Subclinical hyperthyroidism is characterized by which of the following changes in serum hormone levels?

    a. High total thyroxine level

    b. Low free thyroxine (FT_4) level

    c. Low thyroid-stimulating hormone and normal FT_4 levels

    d. High thyroid-stimulating hormone and normal FT_4 levels

58–12. Which of the following is true of routine thyroid-stimulating hormone screening in pregnancy?

    a. It is advocated by the American Association of Clinical Endocrinologists.

    b. It is not advocated by the American College of Obstetricians and Gynecologists (ACOG).

    c. It leads to improved outcome in neonates whose mothers have subclinical hypothyroidism.

    d. All of the above

58–13. Severe hypothyroidism is uncommon in later pregnancy for which of the following reasons?

    a. It is often associated with infertility.

    b. It is associated with increased abortion rates.

    c. Most women with severe hypothyroidism elect first-trimester termination.

    d. A and B

58–14. Concerning initial treatment of maternal hypothyroidism, which of the following is true?

    a. Approximately 400 µg thyroxine should be given orally daily.

    b. Thyroid-stimulating hormone (TSH) levels should be measured at 2-week intervals.

    c. The thyroxine dose should be adjusted in 25- to 50-µg increments to achieve TSH levels between 0.5 and 2.5 mU/L.

    d. All of the above

58–15. An increased incidence of which of the following pregnancy outcomes have been linked with maternal subclinical hypothyroidism?

   a. Stillbirth

   b. Preeclampsia

   c. Placenta previa

   d. None of the above

58–16. What condition is described by a low serum free thyroxine level and normal thyroid-stimulating hormone values?

   a. Isolated hypothyroxinemia

   b. Isolated hyperthyroxinemia

   c. Subclinical hypothyroidism

   d. Subclinical hyperthyroidism

58–17. Mild iodine deficiency during pregnancy typically may cause which of the following?

   a. Neonatal goiter

   b. Endemic cretinism

   c. Placental abruption

   d. Neurodevelopmental abnormalities in offspring

58–18. What is the incidence of congenital hypothyroidism?

   a. 1/500

   b. 1/1000

   c. 1/3000

   d. 1/9000

58–19. Which of the following is true of postpartum thyroiditis?

   a. It affects 5–10% of women during the first year postpartum.

   b. It develops at a higher rate in women with type 1 diabetes mellitus.

   c. It is related to increasing serum levels of thyroid autoantibodies.

   d. All of the above

58–20. In regard to postpartum thyroiditis, which of the following is true?

   a. Initially, there is a hypothyroid phase.

   b. Initial hyperthyroidism responds well to thionamides.

   c. Beta blockers may be of help in the initial phase of postpartum thyroiditis.

   d. All of the above

58–21. Which of the following is true of thyroid nodules during pregnancy.

   a. Are poorly assessed by fine-needle aspiration

   b. Can be safely removed before 24 weeks' gestation

   c. When smaller than 0.5 cm, can be reliably detected sonographically

   d. If cancerous, confer a worse prognosis than if found in nonpregnant controls

58–22. Which of the following is true regarding parathyroid hormone activity in pregnancy?

   a. It acts directly on the bone and kidney.

   b. It maintains intracellular calcium concentration.

   c. It acts indirectly on the small intestine through its effects on vitamin D synthesis and lowers serum calcium levels.

   d. None of the above

58–23. What is true concerning parathyroid hormone (PTH) during pregnancy?

   a. Maternal PTH levels are increased.

   b. Maternal PTH leads to total serum calcium levels that are higher than nonpregnant levels.

   c. PTH that provides the greatest clinical effects is probably of placental and decidual origin.

   d. All of the above

58–24. Which of the following is true of hyperparathyroidism?

   a. It is generally a disease of young females.

   b. It has a reported prevalence of 2–3 per 10,000 women.

   c. It is caused mainly by hyperfunctioning of all four parathyroid glands.

   d. It may be masked by pregnancy due to significant calcium shunting to the fetus.

58–25. Which management strategies are considered appropriate for the pregnant patient with hyperparathyroidism?

   a. With hypercalcemic crisis, intravenous saline infusion and diuresis should be implemented.

   b. If a gravida is symptomatic, then oral calcium, 1–1.5 g daily in divided doses, is implemented.

   c. If a gravida is asymptomatic, surgical removal should be performed early and before the end of the first trimester.

   d. Hyperkalemia and hypermagnesemia are complications of hypercalcemic crisis, and levels of these electrolytes should be monitored.

58–26. What is true concerning hypocalcemia in pregnancy?

  a. The most common cause is renal insufficiency.

  b. Maternal treatment consists of large oral doses of phosphate.

  c. Associated hypoparathyroidism follows 20% of thyroidectomy cases.

  d. Hypocalcemic gravidas may have neonates with bone demineralization.

58–27. Which of the following is true of a pheochromocytoma?

  a. It is called the *10-percent tumor.*

  b. It is found in 0.1% of hypertensive patients during pregnancy.

  c. It is detected by a 24-hour urine collection for free catecholamines, metanephrines, or vanillylmandelic acid (VMA).

  d. All of the above

58–28. The patient whose magnetic resonance (MR) imaging is shown here has a history of hypertension, palpitations, and frequent flushing episodes. The most likely diagnosis is which of the following?

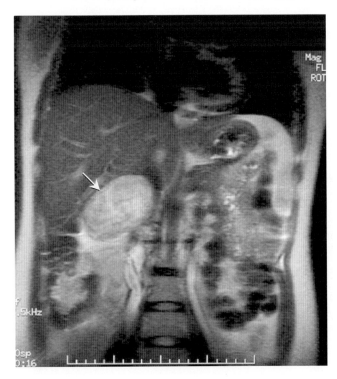

Reproduced with permission from Cunningham FG, Leveno KJ, Bloom SL, et al (eds): Endocrine disorders. In Williams Obstetrics, 24th ed. New York, McGraw-Hill, 2014, Figure 58-6.

  a. Wilms tumor

  b. Adrenal tumor

  c. Liver hepatoma

  d. Renal medulloblastoma

58–29. Which of the following is preferred medical therapy in pregnancy for hypertension with pheochromocytoma?

  a. Hydralazine

  b. Beta blockers

  c. Alpha blockers

  d. Calcium-channel blockers

58–30. Concerning Cushing syndrome in general, which of the following is true?

  a. Most cases arise from long-term corticosteroid treatment.

  b. This syndrome is rare, with an annual incidence of 1 in 3000.

  c. Occasionally, severe Cushing-associated estrogen excess may lead to severe feminization.

  d. All of the above

58–31. Complications of Cushing syndrome in pregnancy include which of the following?

  a. Greater than 50% of mothers will have hypertension.

  b. Greater than 50% of mothers will develop diabetes mellitus.

  c. Maternal Cushing syndrome carries a maternal mortality rate of 7%.

  d. All of the above

58–32. Concerning Addison disease, which of the following is true?

  a. The most frequent cause is tuberculosis.

  b. Cortisone therapy may be discontinued postpartum.

  c. Adrenal hypofunction does not usually affect fertility.

  d. Low serum cortisol levels in pregnancy should prompt adrenocorticotropic hormone (ACTH) stimulation testing.

58–33. Hyperaldosteronism is pregnancy is most likely caused by which of the following?

  a. Adrenal carcinoma

  b. Adrenal aldosteronoma

  c. Bilateral adrenal hyperplasia

  d. None of the above

58–34. Normal prolactin levels in pregnancy are considered those below what threshold?

  a. 12 pg/mL

  b. 18 pg/mL

  c. 25 pg/mL

  d. 30 pg/mL

CHAPTER 58 ANSWER KEY

Question number	Letter answer	Page cited	Header cited
58–1	a	p. 1147	Thyroid Physiology and Pregnancy
58–2	b	p. 1147	Thyroid Physiology and Pregnancy
58–3	c	p. 1148	Autoimmunity and Thyroid Disease
58–4	c	p. 1148	Hyperthyroidism
58–5	a	p. 1148	Hyperthyroidism
58–6	c	p. 1149	Treatment
58–7	a	p. 1149	Treatment
58–8	b	p. 1149	Treatment
58–9	d	p. 1151	Management
58–10	a	p. 1151	Thyroid Storm and Heart Failure
58–11	c	p. 1151	Subclinical Hyperthyroidism
58–12	b	p. 1155	TSH Level Screening in Pregnancy
58–13	d	p. 1152	Hypothyroidism
58–14	c	p. 1153	Treatment
58–15	b	p. 1154	Subclinical Hypothyroidism and Pregnancy
58–16	a	p. 1155	Isolated Maternal Hypothyroxinemia
58–17	a	p. 1155	Iodine Deficiency
58–18	c	p. 1156	Congenital Hypothyroidism
58–19	d	p. 1156	Postpartum Thyroiditis
58–20	c	p. 1156	Clinical Manifestations
58–21	b	p. 1157	Nodular Thyroid Disease
58–22	a	p. 1157	Parathyroid Diseases
58–23	c	p. 1157	Parathyroid Diseases
58–24	d	p. 1158	Hyperparathyroidism
58–25	a	p. 1158	Management in Pregnancy
58–26	d	p. 1158	Hypoparathyroidism
58–27	d	p. 1159	Pheochromocytoma
58–28	b	p. 1160	Pheochromocytoma Complicating Pregnancy
58–29	c	p. 1160	Management
58–30	a	p. 1160	Cushing Syndrome
58–31	a	p. 1161	Cushing Syndrome and Pregnancy
58–32	d	p. 1161	Adrenal Insufficiency—Addison Disease
58–33	b	p. 1162	Primary Aldosteronism
58–34	c	p. 1162	Prolactinomas

CHAPTER 59

Connective-Tissue Disorders

59–1. All **EXCEPT** which of the following disorders are acquired connective tissue disorders?

a. Rheumatoid arthritis

b. Osteogenesis imperfecta

c. Systemic lupus erythematosus

d. Antiphospholipid antibody syndrome

59–2. Which of the following statements is true regarding immune-mediated connective tissue disorders?

a. They typically have no renal involvement.

b. They have a clearly elucidated pathogenesis.

c. They are always associated with rheumatoid factor.

d. They may or may not have an association with autoantibody formation.

59–3. How should a patient with a connective-tissue disorder be counseled regarding disease activity during pregnancy?

a. It will worsen.

b. It will improve.

c. It will be unchanged.

d. It will be modulated by the effect of pregnancy hormones.

59–4. A patient presents with photosensitivity and the rash seen here. What is the best screening test for systemic lupus erythematosus?

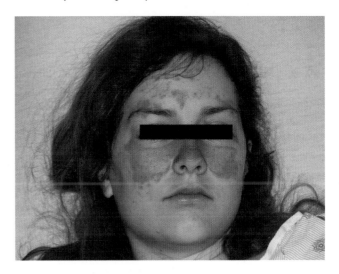

Used with permission from Dr. Martha Rac.

a. Anti-Smith antibody

b. Antinuclear antibody

c. Antiphospholipid antibody

d. Anti-double-stranded-DNA antibody

59–5. How early can fetal cells and free fetal DNA be detected in maternal blood?

a. 1st trimester

b. 2nd trimester

c. 3rd trimester

d. Puerperium

59–6. The "autoimmunity gene," which predisposes to lupus, rheumatoid arthritis, and Crohn disease, is located on what chromosome?

a. Chromosome 6

b. Chromosome 16

c. Chromosome 21

d. Chromosome 22

59–7. Which systemic lupus erythematosus-specific antibody correlates with nephritis and vasculitis activity when seen in high titers?

   a. Anti-Ro

   b. Anti-La

   c. Antinuclear

   d. Anti-double-stranded-DNA

59–8. Which autoantibody is associated with thrombosis, fetal loss, and thrombocytopenia?

   a. Anti-Ro

   b. Antinuclear

   c. Antiplatelet

   d. Antiphospholipid

59–9. Ninety-five percent of patients with systemic lupus erythematosus experience all **EXCEPT** which of the following clinical manifestations?

   a. Fever

   b. Arthralgias

   c. Proteinuria

   d. Weight loss

59–10. Which of the following autoantibodies are specific for lupus?

   a. Anti-double-stranded-DNA and anti-Ro

   b. Anti-double-stranded-DNA and anti-La

   c. Anti-Smith and anti-RNP

   d. Anti-Smith and Anti-double-stranded-DNA

59–11. In addition to systemic lupus erythematosus (SLE), what other conditions could present with low titers of antinuclear antibody?

   a. Chronic inflammation

   b. Acute viral infection

   c. Autoimmune disorder other than SLE

   d. All of the above

59–12. All **EXCEPT** which of the following laboratory findings may be consistent with a diagnosis of systemic lupus erythematosus?

   a. Anemia

   b. Leukopenia

   c. Decreased D-dimer levels

   d. False-positive Venereal Disease Research Laboratory (VDRL) test result

59–13. Based on the 1997 Revised Criteria of the American Rheumatism Association, a patient could be diagnosed with systemic lupus erythematosus if she had which of the following findings?

   a. Diarrhea, arthritis, anemia, weight loss

   b. Malar rash, anemia, oral ulcers, anti-Smith antibodies

   c. Discoid rash, renal failure, increased antinuclear antibody titers

   d. History of preeclampsia, antiphospholipid antibodies, fetal loss

59–14. What is the incidence of systemic lupus erythematosus in pregnancy?

   a. 1:1200

   b. 1:3300

   c. 1:6000

   d. 1:10,000

59–15. A patient presents for preconceptional counseling with a history of systemic lupus erythematosus (SLE). She was diagnosed as an adolescent but has done well during the past few years and is currently in remission. She wants to know what her chances are of having an uncomplicated pregnancy. Which of the following does not factor into the obstetrical outcome of a patient with SLE?

   a. Time since last flare

   b. Presence of antinuclear antibodies

   c. Presence of antiphospholipid antibodies

   d. Disease activity at the beginning of pregnancy

59–16. Following counseling, the patient in Question 59–15 would like to pursue pregnancy. What is the most common complication that she will likely encounter during her pregnancy?

   a. Anemia

   b. Preeclampsia

   c. Deep-vein thrombosis

   d. Fetal-growth restriction

59–17. A patient with systemic lupus erythematosus presents for prenatal care. She is currently asymptomatic on azathioprine. Her 24-hour urine collection shows 5 g of protein. What can be said regarding this patient's potential pregnancy outcome?

   a. Her fetus has an increased risk of fetal death.

   b. Her fetus has a perinatal mortality risk > 50%.

   c. Immunosuppressive treatment should be discontinued during pregnancy.

   d. She will have a poor outcome whether her disease remains in remission or not.

59–18. The patient in Question 59–17 would like to know how you will diagnose a pending lupus flare. She states that her rheumatologist follows her complement levels routinely. What can be said regarding lupus disease activity in pregnancy and serial evaluation of complement levels?

a. Disease activity does not correlate well with complement levels.

b. Disease activity correlates best with decreasing levels of C_3 complement.

c. Disease activity correlates best with decreasing levels of C_4 complement.

d. Disease activity correlates best with decreasing levels of CH_{50} complement.

59–19. Which of the following drugs should be avoided if at all possible during the treatment of obstetrical patients with systemic lupus erythematosus?

a. Aspirin

b. Azathioprine

c. Corticosteroids

d. Mycophenolate mofetil

59–20. Which drug is most helpful in managing dermatological manifestations of systemic lupus erythematosus?

a. Gold salts

b. Azathioprine

c. Cyclophosphamide

d. Hydroxychloroquine

59–21. The children of patients with systemic lupus erythematosus may have increased rates of which of the following complications?

a. Neonatal lupus

b. Learning disorders

c. Congenital heart block

d. All of the above

59–22. A postpartum patient with systemic lupus erythematosus (SLE) is concerned after her baby was born with a rash. Her pediatrician says it is related to lupus. What can you tell the patient regarding the cutaneous manifestations of neonatal lupus?

a. They are usually transient.

b. They never present beyond the first week of life.

c. The recurrence risk in a future pregnancy approximates 5%.

d. All of the above

59–23. A patient with systemic lupus erythematosus has anti-SS-A antibodies. She is worried about the risk of the condition seen in this M-mode image. What is the risk of this complication in her fetus or neonate?

a. < 1%

b. 2–3%

c. 6–7%

d. 10–15%

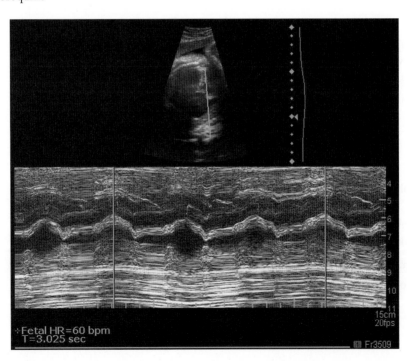

59–24. Which of the following are safe and effective contraceptive methods for patients with systemic lupus erythematosus who lack antiphospholipid antibodies?

  a. Progesterone only pills

  b. Progesterone intrauterine device

  c. Combination estrogen-progesterone pills

  d. All of the above

59–25. All **EXCEPT** which of the following are common features of antiphospholipid antibody syndrome?

  a. Thrombocytosis

  b. Central nervous system involvement

  c. Recurrent arterial or venous thrombosis

  d. Fetal loss in the second half of pregnancy

59–26. Which of the following might be associated with the presence of anti-β2 glycoprotein I antibodies?

  a. Neonatal lupus

  b. Intervillous space thrombosis

  c. Systemic lupus erythematosus flare

  d. All of the above

59–27. Nonspecific antiphospholipid antibodies are present in low titers in what percentage of the normal *nonpregnant* population?

  a. 1%

  b. 5%

  c. 10%

  d. 15%

59–28. Nonspecific antiphospholipid antibodies are present in low titers in what percentage of the normal *pregnant* population?

  a. 1%

  b. 5%

  c. 10%

  d. 15%

59–29. Which of the following tests is least specific for lupus anticoagulant?

  a. Partial thromboplastin time

  b. Dilute Russell viper venom time

  c. Platelet neutralization procedure

  d. All of the above are highly specific

59–30. Once clinical criteria are present, all **EXCEPT** which of the following tests are useful in diagnosing antiphospholipid antibody syndrome?

  a. Lupus anticoagulant

  b. Antiplatelet antibodies

  c. Anticardiolipin antibodies

  d. Anti-β2 glycoprotein I antibodies

59–31. Which is the main mechanism by which antiphospholipid antibodies cause damage?

  a. Deactivation of the tissue factor pathway

  b. Increased protein C and protein S activity

  c. Increased decidual production of prostaglandin E_2

  d. Exposure of the basement membrane of endothelium and syncytiotrophoblast

59–32. A pregnant patient has known antiphospholipid antibodies. Last year, she was hospitalized for pulmonary embolism. Which of the following therapies is most effective during her current pregnancy?

  a. Glucocorticoids

  b. Low-dose aspirin

  c. Low-molecular-weight heparin

  d. Low-dose aspirin and unfractionated heparin

59–33. Which statement is false regarding the connective-tissue disorder in which these joint findings are most classically seen?

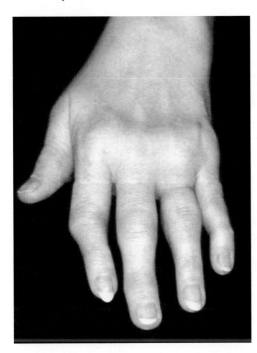

Reproduced with permission from Shah A, St. Clair W: Rheumatoid arthritis. In Longo DL, Fauci AS, Kasper DL, et al (eds): Harrison's Principles of Internal Medicine, 18th ed. New York, McGraw-Hill, 2012, Figure 321-1.

   a. It is more common in women than in men.

   b. It is characterized by chronic polyarthritis.

   c. It is more likely to develop in women who have been pregnant.

   d. Cigarette smoking increases the risk of this disorder.

59–34. Which of the following factors contributes the highest score when determining whether a patient meets criteria for a diagnosis of rheumatoid arthritis?

   a. Symptom duration > 6 weeks

   b. Involvement of two large joints

   c. Abnormal C-reactive protein levels

   d. High-positive rheumatoid factor level

59–35. All **EXCEPT** which of the following drugs may be used safely in early pregnancy to treat rheumatoid arthritis?

   a. Adalimumab

   b. Leflunomide

   c. Sulfasalazine

   d. Cyclooxygenase-2 (COX-2) inhibitors

59–36. Which connective-tissue disorder is characterized by a necrotizing granulomatous vasculitis affecting the respiratory tract and kidneys?

   a. Systemic sclerosis

   b. Takayasu arteritis

   c. Ehlers-Danlos syndrome

   d. Wegener granulomatosis

59–37. Which disorder is characterized by chronic inflammatory arteritis of the great vessels?

   a. Systemic sclerosis

   b. Takayasu arteritis

   c. Ehlers-Danlos syndrome

   d. Wegener granulomatosis

59–38. A pregnant patient presents with a characteristic rash, shown here, and asymmetrical muscle weakness. A muscle biopsy reveals inflammation and muscle fiber degeneration. Which of the following is false?

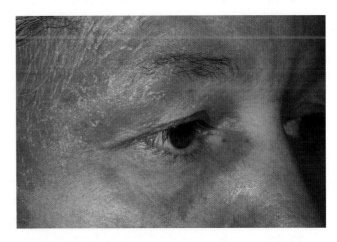

Reproduced with permission from Allred A, Usatine RP: Dermatomyositis. In Usatine RP, Smith MA, Chumley H, et al (eds): The Color Atlas of Family Medicine. New York, McGraw-Hill, 2009, Figure 174-2.

   a. She most likely has polymyositis.

   b. An abnormal electromyogram is expected.

   c. She may have an associated malignant tumor.

   d. The disease typically responds to intravenous immune globulin (IVIG) and corticosteroids.

59–39. Which of the following inherited disorders has been associated with spontaneous uterine rupture?

   a. Chondrodysplasia

   b. Huntington disease

   c. Epidermolysis bulla

   d. Ehlers-Danlos syndrome

CHAPTER 59 ANSWER KEY

Question number	Letter answer	Page cited	Header cited
59–1	b	p. 1168	Introduction
59–2	d	p. 1168	Immune-Mediated Connective-Tissue Diseases
59–3	d	p. 1168	Immune-Mediated Connective-Tissue Diseases
59–4	b	p. 1169	Clinical Manifestations and Diagnosis
59–5	a	p. 1168	Immune-Mediated Connective-Tissue Diseases
59–6	b	p. 1169	Systemic Lupus Erythematosus
59–7	d	p. 1169	Table 59-1
59–8	d	p. 1169	Table 59-1
59–9	c	p. 1169	Table 59-2
59–10	d	p. 1169	Table 59-1; Clinical Manifestations and Diagnosis
59–11	d	p. 1169	Clinical Manifestations and Diagnosis
59–12	c	p. 1170	Table 59-3; Clinical Manifestations and Diagnosis
59–13	b	p. 1170	Table 59-3
59–14	a	p. 1170	Lupus and Pregnancy
59–15	b	p. 1170	Lupus and Pregnancy
59–16	b	p. 1171	Table 59-4
59–17	a	p. 1170	Lupus Nephritis
59–18	a	p. 1171	Management During Pregnancy
59–19	d	p. 1172	Pharmacological Treatment
59–20	d	p. 1172	Pharmacological Treatment
59–21	d	p. 1172	Perinatal Mortality and Morbidity
59–22	a	p. 1172	Neonatal Lupus Syndrome
59–23	b	p. 1172	Congenital Heart Block
59–24	d	p. 1173	Long-Term Prognosis and Contraception
59–25	a	p. 1173	Table 59-5; Antiphospholipid Antibody Syndrome
59–26	b	p. 1173	Specific Antiphospholipid Antibodies
59–27	b	p. 1174	Pregnancy and Antiphospholipid Antibodies
59–28	b	p. 1174	Pregnancy and Antiphospholipid Antibodies
59–29	a	p. 1174	Antiphospholipid Antibody Syndrome Diagnosis
59–30	b	p. 1174	Antiphospholipid Antibody Syndrome Diagnosis
59–31	d	p. 1174	Pregnancy Pathophysiology
59–32	d	p. 1175	Treatment in Pregnancy
59–33	c	p. 1176	Rheumatoid Arthritis
59–34	d	p. 1177	Table 59-6
59–35	b	p. 1176	Management
59–36	d	p. 1180	Wegener Granulomatosis
59–37	b	p. 1180	Takayasu Arteritis
59–38	a	p. 1180	Inflammatory Myopathies
59–39	d	p. 1181	Ehlers Danlos Syndrome

Neurological Disorders

60–1. Neurovascular disorders account for what percent of maternal deaths in the United States?

    a. 1%

    b. 5%

    c. 10%

    d. 20%

60–2. Why is magnetic resonance imaging a preferred modality in the diagnosis of neurovascular disorders in pregnancy?

    a. It is the most cost effective.

    b. It does not involve ionizing radiation.

    c. It is excellent for detecting recent hemorrhage.

    d. None of the above

60–3. What is the most common neurologic complaint during pregnancy?

    a. Seizure

    b. Headache

    c. Leg numbness

    d. Hand weakness

60–4. Which type of headache is most likely to be affected by pregnancy-induced hormonal changes?

    a. Cluster

    b. Tension

    c. Migraine

    d. Intracranial nonvascular

60–5. Which of the following obstetrical complications is increased in women who experience migraine headaches?

    a. Preeclampsia

    b. Preterm labor

    c. Premature rupture of membranes

    d. None of the above

60–6. A 28-year-old woman who is 8 weeks pregnant presents with symptoms that are consistent with a migraine headache. Which of the following medications used to treat migraine headaches should be avoided?

    a. Ibuprofen

    b. Metoprolol

    c. Sumatriptan

    d. Ergotamine derivatives

60–7. A young woman presents for preconceptional counseling because of her history of seizure disorder. She currently takes phenytoin and phenobarbital, and her last seizure was 1 year ago. What should she be told about her medication use and imminent attempt at conception?

    a. An attempt should be made to reduce her medications to a single drug.

    b. She should change to valproate to reduce the risk of fetal teratogenicity.

    c. No change in her medication regimen is indicated if her seizure disorder is stable.

    d. Since she has been seizure free for 1 year, she should withdraw from all medication use.

60–8. Which of the following is not a reason for subtherapeutic anticonvulsant levels during pregnancy?

    a. Increased gastric motility

    b. Increased nausea and vomiting

    c. Increased glomerular filtration

    d. Induction of hepatic enzymes during pregnancy

60–9. Which of the following medications is not associated with an increased risk of this congenital anomaly when taken in early pregnancy?

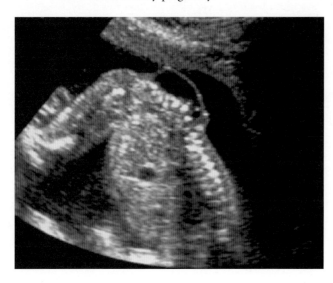

Reproduced with permission from Cunningham FG, Leveno KJ, Bloom SL, et al (eds): Fetal imaging. In Williams Obstetrics, 23rd ed. New York, McGraw-Hill, 2010, Figure 16-9A.

   a. Valproate

   b. Phenytoin

   c. Carbamazepine

   d. None of the above

60–10. Serum levels of antiepileptic medications are unreliable in pregnancy for which of the following reasons?

   a. Altered protein binding

   b. Increased glomerular filtration

   c. Levels are not available for new medications

   d. None of the above

60–11. Increased rates of which of the following have not contributed to the increase in stroke prevalence?

   a. Obesity

   b. Heart disease

   c. Smoking in women

   d. Diabetes mellitus

60–12. When do pregnancy-related strokes most commonly occur?

   a. Postpartum

   b. Intrapartum

   c. First trimester

   d. Second trimester

60–13. What is the most common etiology for ischemic stroke in pregnancy?

   a. Cocaine use

   b. Hypertension

   c. Saccular aneurysm

   d. Arteriovenous malformation

60–14. A 36-year-old African American primigravida who is 30 weeks pregnant had a headache earlier in the day. Her husband brings her to the emergency department after noticing she is unable to use her right hand and arm normally. Which of the following laboratory studies is not appropriate in her evaluation?

   a. Serum lipids

   b. Alkaline phosphatase

   c. Antiphospholipid antibody

   d. Hemoglobin electrophoresis

60–15. The patient in Question 60–14 presents for her postpartum visit and wants to discuss risks and management during a future pregnancy. Which of the following statements is most accurate?

   a. Prophylactic β-blocker therapy during pregnancy is indicated.

   b. There are no firm guidelines for prophylaxis during a future pregnancy.

   c. The recurrence risk is high, and she should not pursue another pregnancy.

   d. All women with prior stroke should be given prophylactic anticoagulation.

60–16. Which of the following is not an accurate statement regarding maternal middle cerebral artery embolism during pregnancy?

   a. May be caused by paradoxical embolism

   b. Occurs more commonly in the first trimester

   c. Must exclude thrombosis and hemorrhage prior to diagnosis

   d. Treatment includes antiplatelet therapy during pregnancy

60–17. How do the morbidity and mortality rates with the following lesion compare with those of subarachnoid hemorrhage?

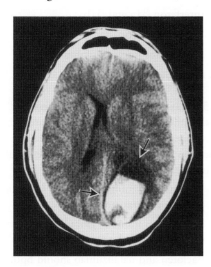

Reproduced with permission from Roberts HR, Key NS, Escobar MA: Hemophilia A and hemophilia B. In Lichtman MA, Kipps TJ, Seligsohn U (eds): Williams Hematology, 8th ed. New York, McGraw-Hill, 2010, Figure 124-14.

    a. Increased

    b. Decreased

    c. No difference

    d. No information available

60–18. What is the most important management strategy used to reduce complications associated with Charcot-Bouchard aneurysms?

    a. Control of systolic hypertension

    b. Appropriate prophylactic anticoagulation

    c. Prepregnancy closure of a patent foramen ovale

    d. None of the above

60–19. What is the most common cause of subarachnoid hemorrhage?

    a. Trauma

    b. Cerebral venous thrombosis

    c. Ruptured saccular aneurysm

    d. Ruptured arteriovenous malformation

60–20. During computed tomographic (CT) angiography performed as part of an evaluation for headache, the following was found in your patient. What is the risk of lesion rupture?

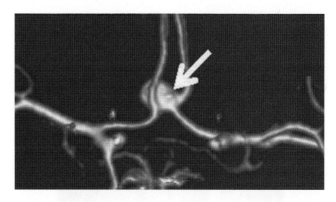

Reproduced with permission from Cowan JA Jr, Thompson BG: Neurosurgery. In Doherty GM (ed): Current Diagnosis & Treatment: Surgery, 13th ed. New York, McGraw-Hill, 2010, Figure 36-6B.

    a. 0.1%

    b. 0.5%

    c. 1%

    d. 5%

60–21. For a pregnant patient, which of the following statements regarding the lesion seen in Question 60–20 is most accurate?

    a. The cardinal symptom of rupture is hemiparesis.

    b. Aneurysms are most likely to bleed in the first trimester.

    c. Surgical repair is the preferred treatment for women remote from term.

    d. Cranial computed tomography with contrast is the preferred imaging modality.

60–22. Which of the following statements regarding arteriovenous malformations and pregnancy is true?

    a. The mortality rate associated with hemorrhage is 25–50%.

    b. Bleeding from this lesion is more frequent during pregnancy.

    c. They are the most common abnormality of the cerebrovascular system encountered during pregnancy.

    d. None of the above

60–23. Which of the following organisms is suggested to act as an environmental trigger in the development of multiple sclerosis?

    a. Influenza B

    b. Herpesvirus 6

    c. *Chlamydia trachomatis*

    d. None of the above

60–24. What percent of women will develop multiple sclerosis following an episode of isolated optic neuritis?

    a. 10%

    b. 25%

    c. 50%

    d. 75%

60–25. Identification of the lesions shown in this imaging study is most useful in what capacity?

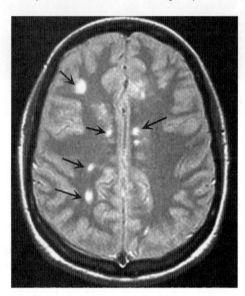

Reproduced with permission from Hauser SL, Goodin DS: Multiple sclerosis. In Longo DL, Fauci AS, Kasper DL, et al (eds): Harrison's Principles of Internal Medicine, 18th ed. New York, McGraw-Hill, 2012, Figure 380-3A.

    a. To determine the likelihood of a relapse

    b. To estimate the risk of obstetric complications

    c. To confirm the initial diagnosis of multiple sclerosis

    d. To evaluate response following treatment with interferon β1a

60–26. For patients with multiple sclerosis, which of the following is not associated with an increased risk of relapse in the puerperium?

    a. Breast feeding

    b. Relapses during pregnancy

    c. High relapse rate prior to pregnancy

    d. High multiple sclerosis disability score

60–27. Acute exacerbations of multiple sclerosis during pregnancy can safely be treated with which of the following therapies?

    a. Interferon β1a and β1b

    b. High-dose corticosteroids

    c. Intravenous immune globulin

    d. All of the above

60–28. A 34-year-old woman who was diagnosed with multiple sclerosis 2 years ago presents for preconceptional counseling. She currently takes baclofen and natalizumab. What she should be told about her condition?

    a. Patients with multiple sclerosis have slightly poorer perinatal outcomes.

    b. Intravenous immune globulin may prevent relapses during the puerperium.

    c. Baclofen and natalizumab should both be stopped before attempting to conceive.

    d. Breast feeding has a protective effect on the postpartum relapse rate.

60–29. Antibodies to which of the following structures are commonly found in patients with myasthenia gravis?

    a. Nonself antigens

    b. Acetylcholine receptor

    c. Oligodendrocyte glycoprotein

    d. Muscle-specific tyrosine kinase

60–30. A 30-year-old white woman with myasthenia gravis who is currently taking corticosteroids and azathioprine presents for prenatal care at 12 weeks' gestation. What is the most appropriate treatment to manage her disease?

    a. Stop azathioprine

    b. Continue her current medications

    c. Recommend prophylactic thymectomy

    d. Start plasmapheresis in the third trimester to reduce neonatal effects

60–31. The patient in Question 60–30 has a prenatal sonographic examination in the third trimester. What is the best explanation for the findings shown here?

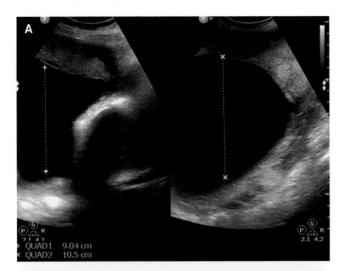

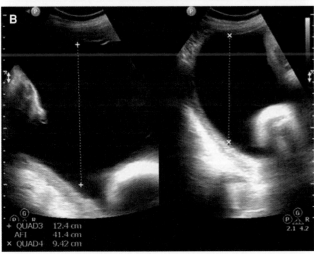

a. Her fetus also has a diagnosis of myasthenia gravis.

b. The finding is unrelated to her diagnosis of myasthenia gravis.

c. She has a higher likelihood of having developed gestational diabetes.

d. This is a transient side effect of transplacental passage of maternal antibodies.

60–32. Which of the following medications should be avoided during labor and delivery in a woman with a diagnosis of myasthenia gravis?

a. Gentamicin

b. Succinylcholine

c. Magnesium sulfate

d. All of the above

60–33. In which trimester do exacerbations of myasthenia gravis most commonly occur?

a. First

b. Second

c. Third

d. Equal rates across all trimesters

60–34. During pregnancy, what is the most appropriate treatment of acute Guillain-Barré syndrome?

a. Cyclosporine

b. Interferon 1β2

c. Intravenous dexamethasone

d. High-dose intravenous immune globulin

60–35. How is the frequency of the lesion shown here altered during pregnancy?

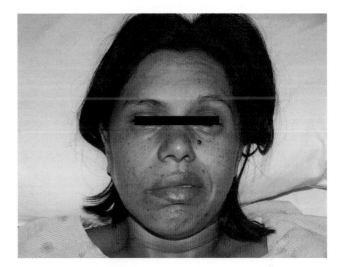

a. Doubled

b. No change

c. Quadrupled

d. Decreased by half

60–36. Which of the following is not a recommended therapy for the condition shown in Question 60–35?

a. Massage

b. Prednisone

c. Valacyclovir

d. Artificial tears

60–37. Which of the following complications is increased in women who experience Bell palsy during pregnancy?

a. Preeclampsia

b. Preterm labor

c. Premature rupture of membranes

d. None of the above

60–38. Which of the following complications is not increased in women with spinal cord injuries?

a. Preterm labor

b. Low birthweight

c. Gestational diabetes

d. Asymptomatic bacteriuria

60–39. Which of the following activities does not precipitate autonomic dysreflexia in parturients with spinal cord injuries?

a. Amniotomy

b. Foley catheter insertion

c. Epidural catheter placement

d. Uterine tocodynamometer transducer positioning

60–40. Which of the following is not a criteria for the diagnosis of idiopathic intracranial hypertension?

a. Recent weight gain > 20 lb

b. Intracranial pressure > 250 mm H_2O

c. Normal cerebral spinal fluid chemistries

d. Normal cerebral magnetic resonance imaging

60–41. Which of the following is not a common therapy used to treat the development of visual field defects associated with idiopathic intracranial hypertension in pregnancy?

a. Furosemide

b. Prednisone

c. Acetazolamide

d. Therapeutic lumbar puncture

CHAPTER 60 ANSWER KEY

Question number	Letter answer	Page cited	Header cited
60–1	c	p. 1187	Introduction
60–2	b	p. 1187	Central Nervous System Imaging
60–3	b	p. 1187	Headache
60–4	c	p. 1187	Headache
60–5	a	p. 1188	Migraine in Pregnancy
60–6	d	p. 1188	Management
60–7	a	p. 1189	Preconceptional Counseling
60–8	a	p. 1190	Epilepsy During Pregnancy
60–9	b	p. 1190	Table 60-2
60–10	a	p. 1191	Management in Pregnancy
60–11	c	p. 1191	Cerebrovascular Disease
60–12	a	p. 1191	Risk Factors
60–13	b	p. 1191	Risk Factors
60–14	b	p. 1191	Ischemic Stroke
60–15	b	p. 1193	Recurrence Risk of Ischemic Stroke
60–16	b	p. 1192	Cerebral Embolism
60–17	a	p. 1193	Intracerebral Hemorrhage
60–18	a	p. 1193	Intracerebral Hemorrhage
60–19	c	p. 1193	Subarachnoid Hemorrhage
60–20	c	p. 1194	Intracranial Aneurysm
60–21	c	p. 1194	Intracranial Aneurysm
60–22	d	p. 1194	Arteriovenous Malformations
60–23	b	p. 1194	Multiple Sclerosis
60–24	d	p. 1194	Multiple Sclerosis
60–25	c	p. 1194	Multiple Sclerosis
60–26	a	p. 1195	Effects of Pregnancy on MS
60–27	d	p. 1195	Management During Pregnancy and the Puerperium
60–28	b	p. 1195	Management During Pregnancy and the Puerperium
60–29	b	p. 1196	Myasthenia Gravis
60–30	b	p. 1196	Myasthenia and Pregnancy
60–31	d	p. 1197	Neonatal Effects
60–32	d	p. 1196	Myasthenia and Pregnancy
60–33	d	p. 1196	Myasthenia and Pregnancy
60–34	d	p. 1197	Pregnancy
60–35	c	p. 1197	Bell Palsy
60–36	c	p. 1198	Pregnancy
60–37	a	p. 1198	Pregnancy
60–38	c	p. 1198	Spinal-Cord Injury
60–39	d	p. 1198	Spinal-Cord Injury
60–40	a	p. 1199	Idiopathic Intracranial Hypertension
60–41	b	p. 1199	Effects of Pregnancy

Psychiatric Disorders

61–1. Which of the following has been associated with psychiatric disorders in pregnancy?

   a. Substance abuse

   b. Poor infant outcomes

   c. Poor obstetrical outcomes

   d. All of the above

61–2. A 20-year-old primipara presents for her 2-week postpartum appointment. During your conversation, she reports that she experienced some sadness with crying and insomnia when she came home from the hospital. Overall, she considers herself a fairly happy person, and those symptoms have since resolved. She mentions it only because it has never happened to her before. What is the most likely diagnosis?

   a. Postpartum blues

   b. Domestic violence

   c. Postpartum psychosis

   d. Postpartum depression

61–3. What is the best management plan for the patient in Question 61–2?

   a. Emotional support

   b. Initiate bupropion

   c. Brief course of fluoxetine

   d. Weekly therapy sessions for 4–6 months

61–4. Risk factors for depression include which of the following?

   a. History of abuse

   b. Nicotine dependence

   c. Family history of depression

   d. All of the above

61–5. What is the most common mood disorder?

   a. Schizophrenia

   b. Bipolar disorder

   c. Major depression

   d. Anorexia nervosa

61–6. A 35-year-old primipara presents to your office for routine follow-up. The patient reports feeling very sad, anxious, and exhausted. In addition, she has a great sense of hopelessness. Even when the baby sleeps, she finds that she cannot get to sleep. This has been going on for at least a month. The patient has a history of depression for which she took medication prior to pregnancy. She denies thoughts of suicide or infanticide. Which of the following statements is true?

   a. For women who discontinue treatment for depression, 70% relapse.

   b. If this patient goes untreated, there is a 25% chance that she will be depressed 1 year from now.

   c. Her condition could lead to insecure attachment and later behavioral problems in the child.

   d. All of the above

61–7. You diagnose the patient in Question 61–6 with a major depressive disorder. You think it is severe. Your best plan of management is which of the following?

   a. Psychotherapy

   b. Antidepressant treatment and psychotherapy

   c. Treatment with a mood stabilizer such as lithium

   d. Hospitalization under the care of a psychiatrist

61–8. In a woman with severe depression, which of the following medications might best be tried initially?

   a. Lithium

   b. Citalopram

   c. Amitriptyline

   d. Tranylcypromine

61–9. Which of the following selective serotonin-reuptake inhibitors has been most closely associated with fetal heart defects?

   a. Citalopram

   b. Fluoxetine

   c. Paroxetine

   d. Sertraline

61–10. A 25-year-old G1P0 at 12 weeks' gestation with a history of major depression presents for prenatal care. She reports that she was taking paroxetine up until 2 weeks ago when she found out she was pregnant. Her psychiatrist has changed her medication, and she is doing well. Based on her history, you should consider offering her which of the following?

    a. Amniocentesis

    b. Pregnancy termination

    c. Fetal echocardiography

    d. Maternal brain magnetic resonance imaging

61–11. A postpartum patient who is exclusively breast feeding is diagnosed with major depression. The decision is made to start a selective serotonin-reuptake inhibitor. Which of the following has the highest detectable concentrations in breast milk?

    a. Citalopram

    b. Fluoxetine

    c. Paroxetine

    d. Sertraline

61–12. Pregnant women not adequately prepared for electroconvulsive therapy are at increased for all **EXCEPT** which of the following?

    a. Aspiration

    b. Hypotension

    c. Respiratory acidosis

    d. Aortocaval compression

61–13. Which of the following statements regarding bipolar disorder is true?

    a. Periods of depression last at least 2 months.

    b. There is no genetic component to the illness.

    c. Up to 20% of patients with this illness commit suicide.

    d. It is more common among pregnant women compared with nonpregnant women.

61–14. A 25-year-old G1P0 at 18 weeks' gestation presents for prenatal care. The patient has a long history of debilitating bipolar disorder. She had been prescribed lithium and was taking this during the early weeks of her current pregnancy. Based on her history, you should offer her which of the following?

    a. Amniocentesis

    b. Pregnancy termination

    c. Fetal echocardiography

    d. Maternal brain magnetic resonance imaging

61–15. Lithium has been linked to which of the following fetal anomalies?

    a. Club foot

    b. Omphalocele

    c. Ebstein anomaly

    d. Pulmonary sequestration

61–16. Which of the following statements regarding postpartum psychosis is true?

    a. It is more common in multiparas.

    b. Its incidence is 1/10,000 deliveries.

    c. It usually manifests 6–8 weeks after delivery.

    d. It is more common in patients with obstetrical complications.

61–17. What is the most important risk factor for postpartum psychosis?

    a. Drug abuse

    b. Bipolar disorder

    c. Major depression

    d. Multifetal gestation

61–18. What is the recurrence risk of postpartum psychosis?

    a. 5%

    b. 10%

    c. 25%

    d. 50%

61–19. A 32-year-old G4P3 at 39 weeks' gestation presents in active labor. The patient had postpartum psychosis in her last pregnancy. In addition to close monitoring for recurrence and involvement of the family, you plan for her to initiate which of the following agents in the puerperium?

    a. Lithium

    b. Fluoxetine

    c. Citalopram

    d. No pharmacologic agent

61–20. Which of the following statements regarding anxiety disorders is true?

    a. They are more common in pregnant women than nonpregnant women.

    b. The prevalence of these disorders in adults in the United States is 1.8%.

    c. With generalized anxiety disorder, symptoms and severity increase across pregnancy.

    d. They are often characterized by irrational fear, nausea, insomnia, dizziness, and frequent urination.

61–21. A 21-year-old G1P0 at 15 weeks' gestation presents for prenatal care. She has a history of anxiety and is concerned for her baby. Which of the following counseling points are true?

    a. No pharmacotherapy agents can be used safely in pregnancy.

    b. Pharmacotherapy for anxiety has been strongly linked to cleft lip and palate.

    c. Benzodiazepines taken during the third trimester can cause neonatal withdrawal syndrome.

    d. All studies have shown that her child is at increased risk for various neuropsychiatric conditions.

61–22. Which of the following is not a prominent feature of schizophrenia spectrum disorders?

    a. Somnolence

    b. Hallucinations

    c. Disorganized thinking

    d. Abnormal motor behavior

61–23. If one parent has schizophrenia, what is the risk of this condition developing in offspring?

    a. <1%

    b. 5–10%

    c. 15–20%

    d. 50–60%

61–24. Within 5 years from the first signs of schizophrenia, what percent of patients are employed?

    a. 10%

    b. 30%

    c. 50%

    d. 70%

61–25. A 30-year-old G2P1 at 8 weeks' gestation with a history of schizophrenia controlled with haloperidol presents for prenatal care. Which medication regimen do you have planned for her during pregnancy?

    a. Continue her current medication regimen

    b. Stop haloperidol until the second trimester

    c. Change haloperidol to an atypical antipsychotic

    d. Stop haloperidol for the remainder of pregnancy and manage her with psychotherapy

61–26. Obstetrical complications of eating disorders include which of the following?

    a. Spontaneous abortion

    b. Low neonatal birthweight

    c. Poor maternal wound healing

    d. All of the above

61–27. Which of the following statements regarding eating disorders is true?

    a. Lifetime prevalence is 10–20%.

    b. Eating disorder symptoms worsen with pregnancy.

    c. Binge-eating disorder is associated with low neonatal birthweight.

    d. Pregnant women with a history of an eating disorder should be closely monitored for weight gain.

61–28. Which of the following is not a personality disorder?

    a. Paranoid

    b. Schizoid

    c. Schizotypal

    d. Schizoaffective

CHAPTER 61 ANSWER KEY

Question number	Letter answer	Page cited	Header cited
61–1	d	p. 1204	Psychiatric Disorders
61–2	a	p. 1205	Maternity Blues
61–3	a	p. 1205	Maternity Blues
61–4	d	p. 1205	Prenatal Evaluation
61–5	c	p. 1206	Major Depression
61–6	d	p. 1206	Major Depression
61–7	b	p. 1207	Fig 61-1 Treatment
61–8	b	p. 1207	Treatment
61–9	c	p. 1207	Fetal Effects of Therapy
61–10	c	p. 1207	Fetal Effects of Therapy
61–11	b	p. 1207	Fetal Effects of Therapy
61–12	c	p. 1209	Electroconvulsive Therapy
61–13	c	p. 1209	Bipolar and Related Disorders
61–14	c	p. 1209	Bipolar and Related Disorders
61–15	c	p. 1209	Bipolar and Related Disorders
61–16	d	p. 1210	Postpartum Psychosis
61–17	b	p. 1210	Postpartum Psychosis
61–18	d	p. 1210	Postpartum Psychosis
61–19	a	p. 1210	Postpartum Psychosis
61–20	d	p. 1210	Anxiety Disorders
61–21	c	p. 1210	Treatment
61–22	a	p. 1210	Schizophrenia Spectrum Disorders
61–23	b	p. 1210	Schizophrenia Spectrum Disorders
61–24	c	p. 1210	Schizophrenia Spectrum Disorders
61–25	a	p. 1211	Treatment
61–26	d	p. 1211	Feeding and Eating Disorders—Pregnancy
61–27	d	p. 1211	Feeding and Eating Disorders
61–28	d	p. 1211	Personality Disorders

CHAPTER 62

Dermatological Disorders

62–1. Which of the following is the most common, occurring in 1 percent of pregnancies?

 a. Pemphigoid

 b. Atopic eruptions

 c. Intrahepatic cholestasis of pregnancy

 d. Pruritic urticarial papules and plaques of pregnancy (PUPPP)

62–2. Which of the following statements regarding intrahepatic cholestasis of pregnancy is true?

 a. It has not been linked to adverse fetal outcome.

 b. Hepatic transaminase levels are commonly in the thousands.

 c. It is associated with abnormally elevated serum bile acid levels.

 d. An erythematous maculopapular rash precedes development of pruritus.

62–3. A 25-year-old G1P0 at 35 weeks' gestation presents to your office complaining of intense pruritus for one week. On examination, the patient has no lesions except for impressive excoriations covering a large portion of her body. She denies rash, fever, or sick contacts. The most likely diagnosis is which of the following?

 a. Eczema of pregnancy

 b. Pemphigoid gestationis

 c. Intrahepatic cholestasis of pregnancy

 d. Pruritic urticarial papules and plaques of pregnancy (PUPPP)

62–4. Which of the following statements about pemphigoid gestationis is true?

 a. It is most commonly seen on the face.

 b. It results from an infection with herpesvirus.

 c. It typically starts in the first trimester of pregnancy.

 d. It has been associated with preterm birth and fetal-growth restriction.

62–5. In pemphigoid gestationis, there is a reaction between maternal immunoglobulin G (IgG) and which of the following?

 a. Collagen V

 b. Collagen X

 c. Collagen XV

 d. Collagen XVII

62–6. A 22-year-old G1P0 at 26 weeks' gestation presents for her prenatal appointment. She complains of an itchy rash that started 2 to 3 days prior. She denies taking any medications. A photograph is provided below. What is your treatment plan?

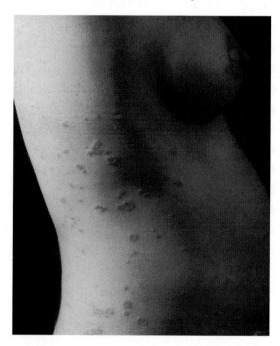

Reproduced with permission from Wolff K, Johnson RA (eds): Bullous diseases. In Fitzpatrick's Color Atlas and Synopsis of Clinical Dermatology, 6th ed. New York, McGraw-Hill, 2009, Figure 6-15.

 a. 7-day course of cephalexin

 b. 5-day course of oral acyclovir

 c. Over-the-counter clotrimazole cream

 d. Oral corticosteroids and oral antihistamine

62–7. You recommend that the patient in Question 62–6 take oral diphenhydramine and return in 1 week. One week later, she complains of vesicular lesions. A photograph is provided below. What should be included in your counseling?

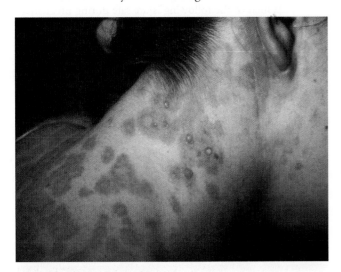

Reproduced with permission from Cunningham FG, Leveno KJ, Bloom SL, et al (eds): Dermatological disorders. In Williams Obstetrics, 23rd ed. New York, McGraw-Hill, 2010, Figure 56-5.

a. There is a 50-percent chance that the baby will have similar lesions.

b. This has never been associated with preterm birth or growth restriction.

c. Although the lesions may heal, there will likely be significant scarring.

d. If this does not respond to oral corticosteroids, other treatment modalities including intravenous immunoglobulin or plasmapheresis may be needed.

62–8. Which of the following has been used in the treatment of pemphigoid gestationis?

a. Oral prednisone

b. Oral antihistamines

c. High-dose intravenous immunoglobulin therapy

d. All of the above

62–9. An 18-year-old G1P0 at 37 weeks' gestation presents to your office complaining of rash and itching. A photograph is provided. On examination, you note striae and erythematous papules on her gravid abdomen. The papules extend to her thighs but spare the umbilicus. She otherwise feels well, and she denies fever or sick contacts. The most likely diagnosis is which of the following?

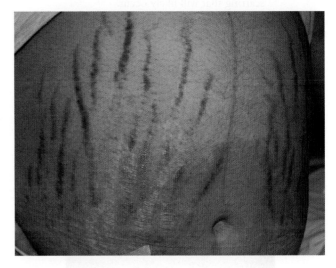

Used with permission from Dr. Kathryn Grande.

a. Scabies

b. Discomforts of pregnancy

c. Intrahepatic cholestasis of pregnancy

d. Pruritic urticarial papules and plaques of pregnancy (PUPPP)

62–10. Treatment for the patient in Question 62–9 is which of the following?

a. Antipruritics, acyclovir, topical corticosteroids

b. Antipruritics, cholestyramine, ursodeoxycholic acid

c. Antipruritics, skin emollients, topical corticosteroids

d. Antipruritics and an antibiotic with good gram-positive coverage

62–11. Which of the following is a risk factor for PUPPP?

a. Multiparity

b. Female fetus

c. Multifetal gestation

d. African American ethnicity

62–12. Which of the following statements regarding PUPPP is true?

    a. It seldom recurs in subsequent pregnancies.

    b. Lesions originate in the periumbilical area.

    c. Symptoms frequently persist for 6 to 9 months postpartum.

    d. Patients should be counseled about the significant scarring that will likely occur.

62–13. A 24-year-old G2P0 presents at 28 weeks' gestation complaining of a 4-week history of pruritic, erythematous arm papules. A photograph is provided. The patient otherwise feels well, and she denies sick contacts. Which of the following is the likely diagnosis?

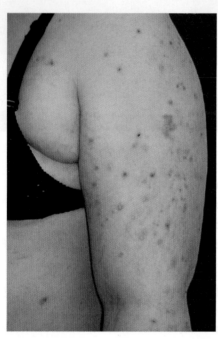

Reproduced with permission from Karen JK, Pomeranz MK: Skin changes and diseases in pregnancy. In Goldsmith LA, Katz SI, Gilcrest BA (eds): Fitzpatrick's Dermatology in General Medicine, 8th ed. New York, McGraw-Hill, 2012, Figure 108-6.

    a. Scabies

    b. Psoriasis

    c. Prurigo gestationis

    d. Eczema in pregnancy

62–14. Treatment for the patient in Question 62–13 would include which of the following?

    a. Oral fluconazole

    b. Permethrin 5-percent cream

    c. Oral trimethoprim-sulfamethoxazole

    d. Low- or moderate-potency topical corticosteroids

62–15. A 19-year-old G1P0 at 16 weeks' gestation presents for prenatal care. She has severe acne, and her dermatologist has resisted treating her because of the pregnancy. The patient would like to know what medications she can take for acne while pregnant. Which of the following is/are safe during pregnancy?

    a. Azelaic acid

    b. Benzoyl peroxide

    c. Topical erythromycin

    d. All of the above are acceptable

62–16. Which of the following is true about the condition represented in this photograph?

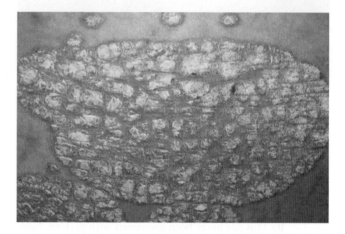

Reproduced with permission from Lawley TJ, Yancey KB: Approach to the patient with a skin disorder. In Longo DL, Fauci AS, Kasper DL, et al (eds): Harrison's Principles of Internal Medicine, 18th ed. New York, McGraw-Hill, 2012, Figure 51-7.

    a. Emollients should be avoided.

    b. Postpartum flares are uncommon.

    c. It has a variable course in pregnancy.

    d. It has been associated with postterm pregnancy.

62–17. Which of the following is the most common pregnancy-specific dermatosis?

    a. Cutaneous lupus

    b. Erythema nodosum

    c. Eczema in pregnancy

    d. Pruritic folliculitis of pregnancy

62–18. A 24-year-old G2P1 at 22 weeks' gestation complaining of a 2-day rash. It started in her axilla but has now spread to her torso. She reports having this rash before when she previously used oral contraceptives. She denies contact with new products or insect bites. A photograph is provided. What is the most likely diagnosis?

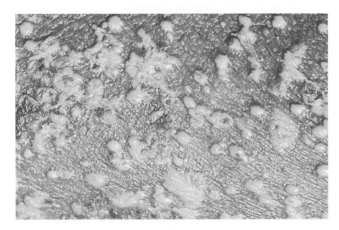

Reproduced with permission from Wolff K, Johnson RA (eds): Psoriasis. In Fitzpatrick's Color Atlas and Synopsis of Clinical Dermatology, 6th ed. New York, McGraw-Hill, 2009, Figure 3-13.

    a. Acne

    b. Pustular psoriasis

    c. Superinfected herpes

    d. Pemphigoid gestationis

62–19. Treatment for the patient in Question 62–18 should include which of the following?

    a. Acyclovir

    b. Acyclovir and antimicrobials for secondary infection

    c. Systemic corticosteroids and antimicrobials for secondary infection

    d. Systemic corticosteroids, acyclovir, and antimicrobials for secondary infection

62–20. A pregnant patient with a history of sarcoidosis reports having red, warm nodules of her legs that have since flattened and now look like bruises. She denies trauma. A photograph is provided. What is the most likely diagnosis?

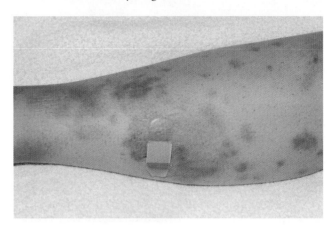

Used with permission from Dr. Stephan Shivvers.

    a. Erythema nodosum

    b. Pemphigoid gestationis

    c. Intrahepatic cholestasis of pregnancy

    d. Pruritic urticarial papules and plaques of pregnancy (PUPPP)

62–21. The condition in Question 62–20 is also associated with which of the following?

    a. Medications

    b. Malignancy

    c. Inflammatory bowel disease

    d. All of the above

62–22. A 35-year-old G4P3 at 30 weeks' gestation presents complaining of a "lump" on her tongue. It is not painful but does bleed easily. A photograph is provided. What is the most likely diagnosis?

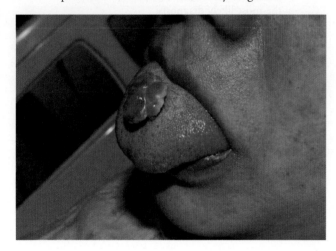

   a. Syphilis
   b. Condyloma
   c. Neurofibromatosis
   d. Pyogenic granuloma

62–23. Which of the following statements is true regarding the condition in Question 62–22?

   a. It is contagious.
   b. It is slow growing.
   c. It does not typically bleed.
   d. It occurs in response to low-grade local irritation or trauma.

62–24. Which of the following conditions is characterized by facial pustules and coalescing draining sinuses?

   a. Erythema nodosum
   b. Rosacea fulminans
   c. Neurofibromatosis
   d. Pyogenic granuloma

62–25. What is the initial choice of treatment for hidradenitis suppurativa?

   a. Coal tar
   b. Oral fluconazole
   c. Oral antimicrobials
   d. Oral corticosteroids

62–26. Which of the following is true regarding the effect of pregnancy on the size and number of neurofibromatosis lesions?

   a. Pregnancy has no effect.
   b. Lesions may increase in size and number.
   c. Lesions become smaller but more numerous.
   d. Lesions become smaller and less numerous.

62–27. Second-generation antihistamines are considered better than first-generation antihistamines for which of the following reasons?

   a. They are less sedating.
   b. They are much less expensive.
   c. They are pregnancy category A.
   d. They are pregnancy category C.

62–28. Which of the following is a second-generation antihistamine?

   a. Loratadine
   b. Diphenhydramine
   c. Chlorpheniramine
   d. None of the above

62–29. Regarding the use of high-potency topical corticosteroids, which of the following statements is true?

   a. They should only be used for 2 to 4 days.
   b. They are best reserved for refractory disorders.
   c. They should be used over extensive areas for best efficacy.
   d. They are the preferred agent for initial treatment of dermatological disorders.

62–30. Which of the following increases systemic absorption of topical corticosteroids?

   a. Occlusive dressings
   b. Prolonged treatment duration
   c. Compromised epidermal barrier
   d. All of the above

62–31. Coverage for which of the following is most important when treating skin disorders complicated by bacterial infections?

   a. Anaerobes
   b. Gram-positive organisms
   c. Gram-negative organisms
   d. All of the above

62–32. Which of the following therapeutic agents should be avoiding during pregnancy?

   a. Desonide
   b. Cetirizine
   c. Methotrexate
   d. Triamcinolone acetonide

CHAPTER 62 ANSWER KEY

Question number	Letter answer	Page cited	Header cited
62–1	c	p. 1214	Pregnancy-Specific Dermatoses
62–2	c	p. 1214	Intrahepatic Cholestasis of Pregnancy
62–3	c	p. 1215	Table 62-1
62–4	d	p. 1214	Pemphigoid Gestationis
62–5	d	p. 1214	Pemphigoid Gestationis
62–6	d	p. 1214	Pemphigoid Gestationis
62–7	d	p. 1214	Pemphigoid Gestationis
62–8	d	p. 1214	Pemphigoid Gestationis
62–9	d	p. 1216	Pruritic Urticarial Papules and Plaques of Pregnancy (PUPPP)
62–10	c	p. 1216	Pruritic Urticarial Papules and Plaques of Pregnancy (PUPPP)
62–11	c	p. 1216	Pruritic Urticarial Papules and Plaques of Pregnancy (PUPPP)
62–12	a	p. 1216	Pruritic Urticarial Papules and Plaques of Pregnancy (PUPPP)
62–13	c	p. 1216	Atopic Eruption of Pregnancy (AEP)
62–14	d	p. 1216	Atopic Eruption of Pregnancy (AEP)
62–15	d	p. 1216	Dermatological Conditions Not Specific to Pregnancy
62–16	c	p. 1216	Dermatological Conditions Not Specific to Pregnancy
62–17	c	p. 1216	Atopic Eruption of Pregnancy (AEP)
62–18	b	p. 1216	Dermatological Conditions Not Specific to Pregnancy
62–19	c	p. 1216	Dermatological Conditions Not Specific To Pregnancy
62–20	a	p. 1216	Dermatological Conditions Not Specific to Pregnancy
62–21	d	p. 1216	Dermatological Conditions Not Specific to Pregnancy
62–22	d	p. 1216	Dermatological Conditions Not Specific to Pregnancy
62–23	d	p. 1216	Dermatological Conditions Not Specific to Pregnancy
62–24	b	p. 1216	Dermatological Conditions Not Specific to Pregnancy
62–25	c	p. 1216	Dermatological Conditions Not Specific to Pregnancy
62–26	b	p. 1216	Dermatological Conditions Not Specific to Pregnancy
62–27	a	p. 1217	Dermatological Treatment
62–28	a	p. 1217	Dermatological Treatment
62–29	b	p. 1217	Dermatological Treatment
62–30	d	p. 1217	Dermatological Treatment
62–31	b	p. 1217	Dermatological Treatment
62–32	c	p. 1217	Dermatological Treatment

CHAPTER 63

Neoplastic Disorders

63–1. Which of the following is the most common benign neoplasm in pregnancy?

a. Ovarian cyst

b. Pyogenic granuloma

c. Endocervical polyp

d. Breast fibroadenoma

63–2. What are the most common cancers in pregnancy?

a. Breast, thyroid, cervix

b. Breast, cervix, lymphoma

c. Breast, thyroid, lymphoma

d. Thyroid, cervix, melanoma

63–3. Of the following imaging modalities, which is the safest during pregnancy?

a. Sonography

b. Computed tomography

c. Diagnostic radiography

d. Magnetic resonance imaging

63–4. When radiation therapy is needed during pregnancy, which of the following potential fetal risks should the patient be informed of?

a. Microcephaly

b. Mental retardation

c. Growth restriction

d. All of the above

63–5. Embryonic exposure to cytotoxic drugs may cause major congenital malformations in what percentage of cases?

a. 2%

b. 20%

c. 33%

d. 50%

63–6. Why is chemotherapy occasionally withheld in the last 3 weeks prior to delivery?

a. To allow the patient to breast feed

b. To decrease the likelihood of maternal neutropenia

c. To decrease the chance of fetal-growth restriction

d. To decrease the overall risk of late mutagenic effects

63–7. An ovarian cancer survivor presents for preconceptional counseling. She has had prior pelvic irradiation. With this history, she is at increased risk for all **EXCEPT** which of the following obstetrical complications?

a. Stillbirth

b. Preterm birth

c. Fetal birthweight < 2500 g

d. Fetal congenital malformations

63–8. Published case reports describe rare instances of maternal tumor metastasizing to the fetus. With which of the following cancer types does this most frequently occur?

a. Melanoma

b. Leukemia

c. Lymphoma

d. Breast cancer

63–9. An asymptomatic 19-year-old G1P0 presents for prenatal care. Her routine obstetrical care should include which of the following elements?

a. Pelvic examination alone

b. Pelvic examination and Pap smear

c. Pelvic examination, Pap smear, and human papillomavirus testing

d. Pelvic examination, Pap smear, and human papillomavirus vaccination

63–10. For at-risk women, cervical cytological screening is recommended more frequently than the routine screening guideline schedule. Which of the following patients should have more frequent cervical cancer screening?

a. 33-year-old with history of diabetes

b. 19-year-old with three lifetime sexual partners

c. 22-year-old with in utero diethylstilbestrol exposure

d. 26-year-old with prior human papillomavirus vaccination

63–11. Which of the following serovars are considered high-risk human papillomavirus serotypes?

　a. 6, 11

　b. 6, 16

　c. 11, 18

　d. 16, 18

63–12. A 40-year-old pregnant patient calls to discuss her Pap smear results. Her Pap smear shows atypical squamous cells of undetermined significance, and human papillomavirus testing is negative. Which of the following is your recommendation for subsequent evaluation?

　a. Colposcopy 6 weeks postpartum

　b. Colposcopy in the third trimester

　c. Repeat cytology 6 weeks postpartum

　d. Repeat cytology in the third trimester

63–13. For a cervical intraepithelial neoplasia (CIN) 1 lesion diagnosed in early pregnancy, what is the chance that repeat cytology at the end of the puerperium will be normal?

　a. 20–30%

　b. 40–50%

　c. 60–70%

　d. 80–90%

63–14. Cervical conization during pregnancy is associated with an increased risk of all **EXCEPT** which of the following?

　a. Preterm delivery

　b. Membrane rupture

　c. Residual neoplasia

　d. Inadequate diagnostic tissue sample

63–15. What is the incidence of invasive cervical cancer in the general obstetrical population?

　a. 1 in 2500

　b. 1 in 5500

　c. 1 in 8500

　d. 1 in 11,500

63–16. What percentage of cervical cancers are adenocarcinomas?

　a. 5%

　b. 20%

　c. 33%

　d. 50%

63–17. A 29-year-old G2P1 patient at 22 weeks' gestation is referred to your clinic for colposcopy due to a Pap smear report noting high-grade squamous intraepithelial lesion (HSIL). What can you tell her regarding colposcopy in pregnancy?

　a. It is best delayed to the puerperium.

　b. It is more likely to be unsatisfactory.

　c. She will need a repeat study at 26 weeks' gestation.

　d. It is indicated for the evaluation of HSIL lesions.

63–18. The cervical biopsy from the patient in Question 63–17 shows invasive squamous cell carcinoma. Which of the following is a part of formal cervical staging in pregnancy?

　a. Chest radiograph

　b. Renal sonography

　c. Abdominopelvic computed tomography

　d. None of the above

63–19. If microinvasive disease is diagnosed from a cervical conization specimen obtained in the early second trimester, which of the following statements is true regarding pregnancy management?

　a. She may deliver vaginally.

　b. She will need cesarean delivery.

　c. She will require adjuvant radiotherapy in the puerperium.

　d. She will need radical hysterectomy at the time of delivery.

63–20. All **EXCEPT** which of the following are reasons that surgical treatment is preferred to radiotherapy in the treatment of early-stage pregnancy-associated invasive cervical cancer?

　a. Radiation therapy destroys ovarian function.

　b. Radiation therapy can cause intestinal injury.

　c. Complication rates are higher with radiotherapy.

　d. Surgical treatment is more effective than radiotherapy.

63–21. A 32-year-old nulligravida requests fertility-sparing radical trachelectomy for her small Stage IB1 cervical cancer. How should you counsel her regarding this treatment option and future pregnancy outcomes?

　a. Her risk of premature delivery is decreased.

　b. She will need cesarean delivery in a future pregnancy.

　c. Her fertility remains the same as the general obstetrical population.

　d. Her chance of a live birth would be the same as the general obstetrical population.

63–22. You elect to perform transvaginal sonography for your patient with a uterus that is larger than expected based on her gestational age. Her sonogram is shown here. Regarding leiomyomas in pregnancy, which of the following statements is true?

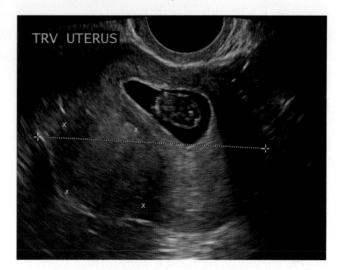

a. They require sonographic surveillance.

b. Their incidence in pregnancy approximates 2%.

c. They grow in pregnancy due to human chorionic gonadotropin stimulation.

d. The vaginal delivery rate is only 30% if leiomyomas are larger than 10 cm.

63–23. Prior to conception, uterine artery embolization (UAE) was recommended for your patient with symptomatic leiomyomas. Rates of which of the following are increased in pregnancies following UAE?

a. Miscarriage

b. Cesarean delivery

c. Postpartum hemorrhage

d. All of the above

63–24. What is the recommended standard of care for the treatment of endometrial carcinoma?

a. Curettage with progestational treatment

b. Curettage without progestational treatment

c. Total abdominal hysterectomy and bilateral salpingoophorectomy

d. All of the above

63–25. A 17-year-old gravida is referred for evaluation of an adnexal mass found at 9 weeks' gestation during sonography for first-trimester bleeding. A sonogram of her right ovary is shown, and dimensions of the mass are marked by calipers. Based on its appearance, what is the most likely diagnosis?

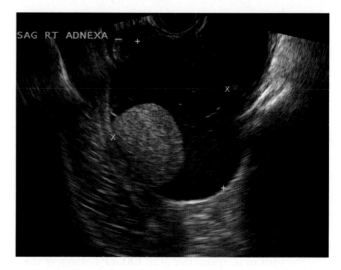

a. Serous cystadenoma

b. Corpus luteum cyst

c. Mature cystic teratoma

d. Ovarian hyperstimulation syndrome

63–26. A pregnant patient at 11 weeks' gestation complains of intermittent left lower quadrant pain and nausea and vomiting. She undergoes diagnostic exploratory laparotomy. Which of the following is true regarding management, in general, of patients with this diagnosis?

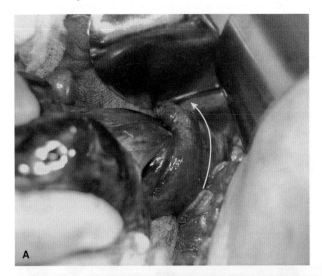

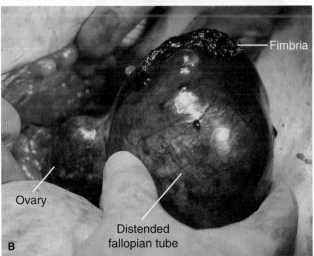

Reproduced with permission from Brooks Heinzman A, Hoffman BL: Pelvic mass. In Hoffman BL, Schorge JO, Schaffer JI, et al (eds): Williams Gynecology, 2nd ed. New York, McGraw-Hill, 2012, Figure 9-22.

    a. Excision of the adnexa is always required.

    b. All patients require progesterone replacement.

    c. Oophoropexy could prevent a recurrence of this complication.

    d. All of the above

63–27. A patient at 9 weeks' gestation is treated for a ruptured and excised corpus luteum cyst of pregnancy. Which of the following regimens is recommended?

    a. Micronized progesterone, 200 mg orally daily for 3 weeks

    b. 17-hydroxyprogesterone caproate, 150 mg intramuscularly × 1 dose

    c. 8% progesterone vaginal gel, one applicator vaginally daily for 1 week

    d. 17-hydroxyprogesterone caproate, 150 mg intramuscularly weekly for 3 weeks

63–28. Which of the following is a rare, solid benign ovarian tumor that can virilize a female fetus?

    a. Luteoma

    b. Brenner tumor

    c. Mature cystic teratoma

    d. Hyperreactio luteinalis

63–29. A pregnant patient presents with bilateral adnexal masses. She is pregnant with twins. Both masses are similar to the image shown below. What is the most likely diagnosis?

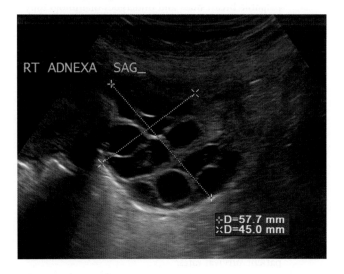

    a. Luteoma

    b. Granulosa cell tumor

    c. Mature cystic teratoma

    d. Hyperreactio luteinalis

63–30. Which of these pregnancy-associated adnexal masses can lead to hypovolemia with ascites, renal dysfunction, and adult respiratory distress syndrome?

   a. Luteoma

   b. Corpus luteum

   c. Granulosa cell tumor

   d. Hyperstimulated ovary

63–31. What percentage of ovarian cancer found in pregnancy is early-stage?

   a. 25%

   b. 50%

   c. 75%

   d. 90%

63–32. All **EXCEPT** which of the following are considered risk factors for breast cancer?

   a. Nulliparity

   b. Advancing age

   c. Breast feeding

   d. *BRCA1* and *BRCA2* gene mutation

63–33. A pregnant patient at 26 weeks' gestation has a palpable breast mass and undergoes mammography and needle biopsy of the identified lesion. Although clinical examination and biopsy results suggest a benign mass, mammogram findings suggest malignancy. What should be the next management step?

   a. Chemotherapy

   b. Mass excision

   c. Repeat mammography

   d. Repeat needle biopsy

63–34. Your evaluation of the patient in Question 63–33 confirms breast cancer in pregnancy. For women with this diagnosis, all **EXCEPT** which of the following treatments are associated with improved patient survival rates?

   a. Chemotherapy

   b. Total mastectomy

   c. Modified mastectomy

   d. Pregnancy termination

63–35. The patient in Question 63–33 is now 28 weeks pregnant. Her axillary nodes were positive for cancer, and chemotherapy is indicated. All **EXCEPT** which of the following agents are acceptable in pregnancy?

   a. Trastuzumab

   b. Doxorubicin

   c. 5-Fluorouracil

   d. Cyclophosphamide

63–36. All **EXCEPT** which of the following may be indicated in the management of thyroid cancer in pregnancy?

   a. Radioiodine

   b. Delay surgery until the second trimester

   c. Expectant management with thyroxine treatment

   d. Surgical treatment with thyroxine replacement

63–37. Reed-Sternberg cells, such as the one shown here, are consistent with which of the following lymphoid cell malignancies?

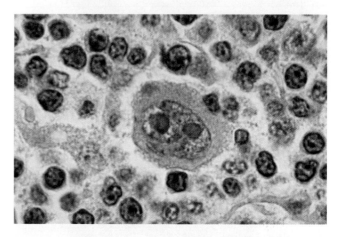

Reproduced with permission from Gascoyne RD, Skinnider BF: Pathology of malignant lymphomas. In Lichtman MA, Kipps TJ, Seligsohn U (eds): Williams Hematology, 8th ed. New York, McGraw-Hill, 2010, Figure 98-34.

   a. Hodgkin lymphoma

   b. Hairy cell leukemia

   c. Acute myeloid leukemia

   d. T cell derived lymphoma

63–38. What is the system used for staging Hodgkin and other lymphomas called?

   a. Clark

   b. Breslow

   c. Bethesda

   d. Ann Arbor

63–39. What standard single-agent chemotherapy regimen is recommended for treatment of Hodgkin disease during the first trimester?

   a. Bleomycin

   b. Vinblastine

   c. Dacarbadine

   d. Doxorubicin

63–40. Which virus is associated with Burkitt lymphoma?

    a. Hepatitis C

    b. Herpesvirus

    c. Epstein-Barr virus

    d. Human immunodeficiency virus

63–41. Which of the following statements regarding leukemia in pregnancy is false?

    a. Leukemias may arise from bone marrow.

    b. Remission is common during pregnancy.

    c. Termination of pregnancy will improve prognosis.

    d. Leukemias are more common in patients older than 40 years.

63–42. A patient presents at 14 weeks' gestation with the skin lesion shown below and palpable lymph nodes. Which of the following dermatological neoplasms is this is consistent with?

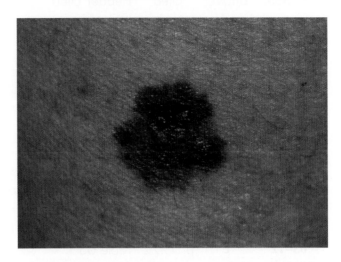

Reproduced with permission by Hardin MJ: Cutaneous conditions. In Knoop KJ, Stack LB, Storrow AB, et al (eds): The Atlas of Emergency Medicine, 3rd ed. New York, McGraw-Hill, 2010, Figure 13-80.

    a. Stage I melanoma

    b. Stage II melanoma

    c. Stage I basal cell carcinoma

    d. Stage II squamous cell carcinoma

CHAPTER 63 ANSWER KEY

Question number	Letter answer	Page cited	Header cited
63–1	a	p. 1219	Introduction
63–2	a	p. 1219	Introduction
63–3	a	p. 1219	Diagnostic Imaging
63–4	d	p. 1220	Radiation Therapy
63–5	b	p. 1220	Chemotherapy
63–6	b	p. 1220	Chemotherapy
63–7	d	p. 1220	Fertility and Pregnancy after Cancer Therapy
63–8	a	p. 1220	Placental Metastases
63–9	a	p. 1221	Cervix: Epithelial Neoplasia
63–10	c	p. 1221	Cervix: Epithelial Neoplasia
63–11	d	p. 1222	Oncogenic Human Papillomaviruses
63–12	c	p. 1222	Table 63-1
63–13	c	p. 1223	Cervical Intraepithelial Neoplasia
63–14	d	p. 1223	Cervical Conization
63–15	c	p. 1223	Invasive Cervical Cancer
63–16	b	p. 1223	Invasive Cervical Cancer
63–17	d	p. 1222	Table 63-1
63–18	d	p. 1223	Invasive Cervical Cancer
63–19	a	p. 1223	Management and Prognosis
63–20	d	p. 1223	Management and Prognosis
63–21	b	p. 1224	Pregnancy after Radical Trachelectomy
63–22	b	p. 1224	Leiomyomas
63–23	d	p. 1226	Fertility Considerations
63–24	c	p. 1226	Endometrial Carcinoma
63–25	c	p. 1227	Figure 63-6
63–26	c	p. 1227	Complications
63–27	b	p. 1227	Complications
63–28	a	p. 1228	Pregnancy Luteoma
63–29	d	p. 1228	Hyperreactio Luteinalis
63–30	d	p. 1228	Ovarian Hyperstimulation Syndrome
63–31	c	p. 1228	Ovarian Cancer
63–32	c	p. 1229	Risk Factors
63–33	b	p. 1229	Diagnosis
63–34	d	p. 1230	Management
63–35	a	p. 1230	Management
63–36	a	p. 1231	Thyroid Cancer
63–37	a	p. 1231	Hodgkin Disease
63–38	d	p. 1231	Staging and Treatment
63–39	b	p. 1231	Hodgkin Disease
63–40	c	p. 1232	Non-Hodgkin Lymphoma
63–41	c	p. 1232	Leukemias
63–42	b	p. 1233	Malignant Melanoma

CHAPTER 64

Infectious Diseases

64–1. Which of the following is the primary immunological fetal response to infection?

  a. IgA

  b. IgE

  c. IgG

  d. IgM

64–2. What percentage of women who have not previously had varicella will become infected after exposure?

  a. 1–2%

  b. 5–10%

  c. 20–30%

  d. 60–95%

64–3. Which of the following clinical intervals best describes the contagious period for varicella?

  a. From rash appearance until lesion crusting

  b. From varicella exposure until lesion appearance

  c. From 1 day before rash onset until lesion crusting

  d. From rash appearance until complete lesion resolution

64–4. A 26-year-old G1P0 at 32 weeks' gestation is seen in your office for fever, myalgias, and a rash of 2 days' duration. She has widely dispersed vesicular lesions that are pruritic. A picture of her face is provided here. Mortality from this infection is predominately due to which of the following?

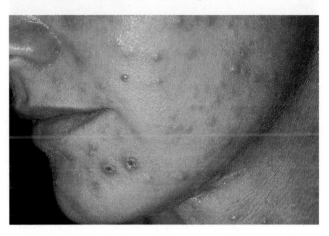

Reproduced with permission from Wolff K, Johnson RA (eds): Viral infections of skin and mucosa. In Fitzpatrick's Color Atlas and Synopsis of Clinical Dermatology, 6th ed. New York, McGraw-Hill, 2009, Figure 27-38.

  a. Pneumonia

  b. Meningitis

  c. Liver failure

  d. Renal failure

64–5. Which of the following statements regarding herpes zoster, shown here, is true?

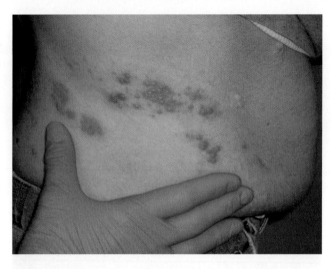

Used with permission from Dr. Mary Jane Pearson.

    a. It is painless.

    b. It is contagious if blisters are broken.

    c. It is responsible for many congenital malformations.

    d. It is more frequent and more severe in pregnant women.

64–6. One manifestation of congenital varicella syndrome is demonstrated in the photograph below. At which of the following gestational ages did infection most likely occur?

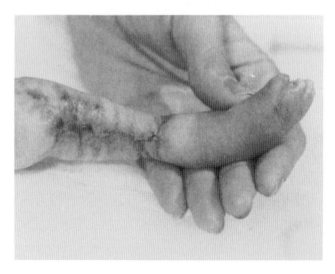

Reproduced with permission from Cunningham FG, Leveno KJ, Bloom SL, et al (eds): Infectious diseases. In Williams Obstetrics, 24th ed. New York, McGraw-Hill, 2014, Figure 64-1.

    a. < 6 weeks

    b. 6–10 weeks

    c. 13–20 weeks

    d. 28–32 weeks

64–7. An 18-year-old G1P0 at 36 weeks' gestation presents in active labor and appears to have active varicella. Despite all efforts, the infant delivers vaginally shortly thereafter. You are very concerned for which of the following reasons?

    a. Maternal antibody has not yet formed.

    b. Mortality rates for the newborn approach 30%.

    c. The infant may develop disseminated visceral and central nervous system disease.

    d. All of the above

64–8. A 19-year-old G2P0 at 37 weeks' gestation presents for her routine prenatal care appointment. While in the waiting room, she has a conversation with another patient who is coughing and scratching at a vesicular rash. The 19-year-old denies a prior history of chickenpox, and you are now concerned that she has been exposed to the varicella-zoster virus (VZV). What should be done for her now?

    a. Offer varicella vaccination with Varivax

    b. Defer VZV serology testing and proceed with varicella zoster immune globulin (VariZIG) administration

    c. Test for VZV serology and administer VariZIG if results are negative for antibodies to VZV

    d. Test for VZV serology and give VariZIG and Varivax if results are negative for antibodies to VZV

64–9. Which of the following statements regarding the varicella vaccine, Varivax, is false?

    a. Seroconversion is 98%.

    b. It is not secreted into breast milk.

    c. It is recommended in pregnancy to all women with no history of varicella.

    d. At 10 years postvaccination, the breakthrough infection rate approximates 5%.

64–10. During which of the following periods should influenza vaccination be avoided?

    a. First trimester

    b. Postpartum, if breastfeeding

    c. During pregnancy and for 1 month before becoming pregnant

    d. None of the above

64-11. A 22-year-old G1P0 at 32 weeks' gestation presents with fever, coryza, conjunctivitis, cough, and rash. The patient was raised in a separatist group that does not believe in immunizations. You suspect measles, and a photograph of her face is provided here. Which of the following counseling points is true?

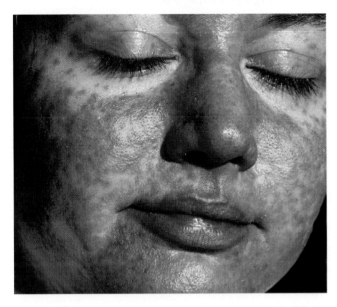

Reproduced with permission from Wolff K, Johnson RA (eds): Severe and life-threatening skin eruptions in the acutely ill patient. In Fitzpatrick's Color Atlas and Synopsis of Clinical Dermatology, 6th ed. New York, McGraw-Hill, 2009, Figure 8-5.

   a. Treatment is supportive.

   b. The virus is not teratogenic.

   c. There is an increased incidence of preterm delivery and low birthweight with maternal infection.

   d. All of the above

64-12. A 31-year-old G1P0 at 8 weeks' gestation presents complaining of a fever and rash of 5 day's duration. The rash started on her face and has spread to her trunk and extremities. A photograph of her chest is provided here. Given her gestational age, which of the following infections would be the most concerning for this patient and her fetus?

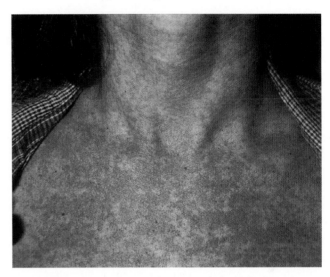

Reproduced with permission from Ryan KJ, Ray CG (eds): Mumps virus, measles, rubella, and other childhood exanthems. In Sherris Medical Microbiology, 5th ed. New York, McGraw-Hill, 2010, Figure 10-6.

   a. Rubeola

   b. Rubella

   c. Varicella

   d. Toxoplasmosis

64-13. If the patient in Question 64–12 has acute rubella, you would expect serologic testing to most likely show which of the following results?

   a. IgM positive, IgG negative

   b. IgM negative, IgG negative

   c. IgM negative; IgG positive, high affinity

   d. IgM positive; IgG positive, high affinity

64-14. With maternal rubella infection at 8 weeks' gestation, the risk of congenital infection most closely approximates which of the following?

   a. 1%

   b. 10%

   c. 25%

   d. up to 90%

64–15. The most common single defect associated with congenital rubella is which of the following?

    a. Glaucoma

    b. Microcephaly

    c. Sensorineural deafness

    d. Pulmonary artery stenosis

64–16. Hand foot and mouth disease is caused by which of the following viruses?

    a. Togavirus

    b. Parvovirus

    c. Coxsackievirus

    d. None of the above

64–17. A 20-year-old G1P0 at 18 weeks' gestation presents to your office for prenatal care. The patient just started working at a day-care center and is concerned about acquiring infections from the children. She reports several colds since starting the job. She wasn't feeling well last week and noted headache, nausea, and pharyngitis. Three weeks ago, one child in particular looked rather ill. She shows you a picture of the child on her cell phone, and the photograph is provided here. Your concern for this patient is infection with which of the following?

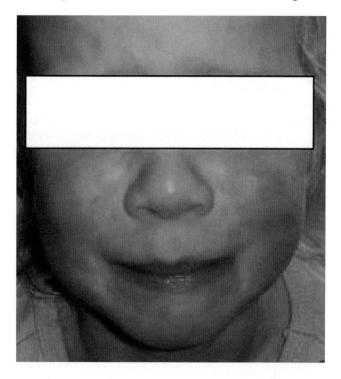

    a. Parvovirus

    b. Rubeola virus

    c. Rubella virus

    d. Coxsackievirus

64–18. For the patient in Question 64–17, you obtain and send serological testing for parvovirus B19. Which of the following testing outcomes would satisfy you that she is immune and needs no further evaluation?

    a. IgG positive, IgM negative

    b. IgG positive, IgM positive

    c. IgG negative, IgM negative

    d. IgG negative, IgM positive

64–19. The serological test results for the patient in Question 64–17 indicate that she has had a recent parvovirus B19 infection. Your management plan at this point should be which of the following?

    a. Offer pregnancy termination

    b. Begin serial measurement of maternal viral loads every 2 weeks for 10 weeks

    c. Begin serial fetal sonographic evaluation every 2 weeks for the first 10 weeks after infection

    d. Perform sonographic fetal evaluation now to identify hydrops and, if the scan results are normal, resume prenatal care with no further sonographic surveillance

64–20. Four weeks after first presenting for care, the fetus of the patient in Question 64–17 is now hydropic and shows elevated middle cerebral artery peak systolic velocities. You counsel her regarding fetal blood sampling and fetal transfusion. Which of the following is a true statement?

    a. Most fetuses require multiple transfusions.

    b. The mortality rate without transfusion is 90%.

    c. The overall mortality rate following transfusion is 50%.

    d. Reports of the neurodevelopmental outcomes of fetuses transfused for parvovirus-induced anemia are conflicting.

64–21. Which of the following statements regarding cytomegalovirus (CMV) is true?

    a. Pregnancy increases the severity of maternal CMV infection.

    b. It is the most common perinatal infection in the developed world.

    c. Most women who contract CMV will have symptoms that will alert the provider.

    d. Once a woman has been infected with CMV, she is immune and will never become ill again from CMV.

64–22. Which of the following is not a risk factor for intrapartum group B streptococcus (GBS) transmission?

  a. Membranes ruptured ≤ 18 hours

  b. Delivery at < 37 weeks' gestation

  c. Intrapartum temperature ≥ 38.0° Celsius

  d. Prior infant with invasive early-onset GBS disease

64–23. Which of the following antibiotics is never an appropriate choice for penicillin-allergic patients requiring group B streptococcus (GBS) chemoprophylaxis?

  a. Cefazolin

  b. Vancomycin

  c. Clindamycin

  d. Erythromycin

64–24. Which of the following is first-line inpatient therapy for methicillin-resistant *Staphylococcus aureus* infection?

  a. Rifampin

  b. Vancomycin

  c. Clindamycin

  d. Trimethoprim-sulfamethoxazole

64–25. A 25-year-old G3P2 at 34 weeks' gestation presents with decreased fetal movement, fever, myalgias, and headache for 4 days. Her fetus is dead. The patient's cervix is 3-cm dilated, and with rupture of membranes, dark-brown fluid is seen. Postpartum, the patient is diagnosed with listeriosis. Which of the following is preferred treatment for her?

  a. Vancomycin

  b. Ceftriaxone

  c. Erythromycin

  d. Ampicillin and gentamicin

64–26. Which of the following is not a typical sign or symptom of salmonellosis?

  a. Fever

  b. Abdominal pain

  c. Bloody diarrhea

  d. Nausea/vomiting

64–27. A 19-year-old G1P0 at 29 weeks' gestation presents to your office complaining of flulike symptoms and a target-shaped rash on her neck, which is shown in this photograph. She has just returned from a hiking trip in New Hampshire. Her history and rash are concerning for which of the following?

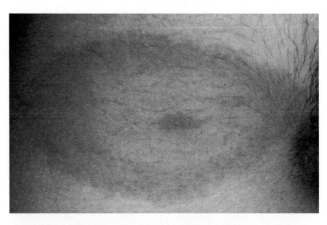

Reproduced with permission from Levinson W: Spirochetes. In Review of Medical Microbiology and Immunology, 12th ed. New York, McGraw-Hill, 2012, Figure 24-6.

  a. Lyme disease

  b. Toxoplasmosis

  c. West Nile virus infection

  d. Methicillin-resistant *Staphylococcus aureus* infection

64–28. Prompt treatment of the patient in Question 64–27 should prevent most adverse pregnancy outcomes. Assuming she has no allergies, which of the following is the preferred treatment?

  a. Spiramycin

  b. Vancomycin

  c. Amoxicillin

  d. Doxycycline

64–29. Which of the following statements regarding toxoplasmosis infection in pregnancy is true?

  a. The risk of fetal infection increases with gestational age.

  b. The risk of fetal infection decreases with gestational age.

  c. The severity of fetal infection is much greater in late pregnancy.

  d. The risk and severity of fetal infection are not dependent on gestational age.

64–30. Which of the following fetal outcomes is not associated with toxoplasmosis infection during pregnancy?

  a. Hydrocephalus

  b. Chorioretinitis

  c. Placental microabscesses

  d. Intracranial calcifications

64–31. A differential diagnosis for the findings seen in this fetal sonographic image would include all **EXCEPT** which of the following?

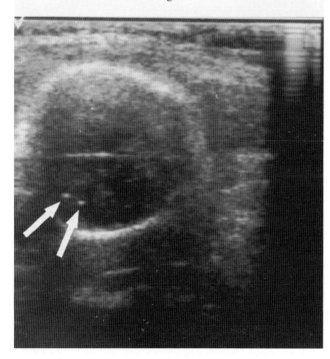

Reproduced with permission from Cunningham FG, Leveno KJ, Bloom SL, et al (eds): Infectious diseases. In Williams Obstetrics, 24th ed. New York, McGraw-Hill, 2014, Figure 64-1.

  a. Rubella

  b. Toxoplasmosis

  c. Parvovirus infection

  d. Cytomegalovirus infection

64–32. Which of the following statements regarding prenatal screening for toxoplasmosis is false?

  a. Screening is recommended in areas of low prevalence.

  b. The parasite is rarely detected in tissue or body fluids.

  c. IgM antibodies alone should not be used to detect acute toxoplasmosis.

  d. The presence of high-avidity IgG indicates that infection did not occur in the preceding 3 to 5 months.

64–33. For a pregnant woman with chloroquine-resistant malaria, the current recommended treatment is which of the following?

  a. Mefloquine

  b. Atovaquone

  c. Quinine and erythromycin

  d. Doxycycline and primaquine

64–34. Which of the following statements regarding West Nile virus is true?

  a. Treatment is with acyclovir.

  b. The incubation period is 3 to 4 weeks.

  c. Of those who are infected, 25% develop meningoencephalitis or acute flaccid paralysis.

  d. Diagnosis is by detection of viral IgG and IgM in serum and IgM in cerebrospinal fluid.

64–35. If a pregnant woman develops anthrax and has life-threatening allergies to both ciprofloxacin and penicillin, which of the following is a recommended alternative?

  a. Rifampin

  b. Vancomycin

  c. Doxycycline

  d. Trimethoprim-sulfamethoxazole

CHAPTER 64 ANSWER KEY

Question number	Letter answer	Page cited	Header cited
64–1	d	p. 1239	Fetal and Newborn Immunology
64–2	d	p. 1240	Varicella-Zoster Virus
64–3	c	p. 1240	Varicella-Zoster Virus
64–4	a	p. 1240	Maternal Infection
64–5	b	p. 1240	Maternal Infection
64–6	c	p. 1240	Fetal and Neonatal Infection
64–7	d	p. 1240	Fetal and Neonatal Infection
64–8	c	p. 1241	Maternal Viral Exposure
64–9	c	p. 1241	Vaccination
64–10	d	p. 1241	Vaccination
64–11	d	p. 1242	Rubeola (Measles)
64–12	b	p. 1243	Rubella—German Measles
64–13	a	p. 1243	Rubella—German Measles
64–14	d	p. 1243	Fetal Effects
64–15	c	p. 1243	Fetal Effects
64–16	c	p. 1244	Coxsackievirus
64–17	a	p. 1244	Parvovirus
64–18	a	p. 1245	Diagnosis and Management
64–19	c	p. 1245	Diagnosis and Management
64–20	d	p. 1245	Diagnosis and Management
64–21	b	p. 1245	Cytomegalovirus
64–22	a	p. 1249	Risk-Based Prevention
64–23	d	p. 1250	Intrapartum Antimicrobial Prophylaxis
64–24	b	p. 1252	Management
64–25	d	p. 1253	Maternal and Fetal Infection
64–26	c	p. 1253	Salmonellosis
64–27	a	p. 1254	Lyme Disease
64–28	c	p. 1254	Treatment and Prevention
64–29	a	p. 1255	Maternal and Fetal Infection
64–30	c	p. 1255	Maternal and Fetal Infection
64–31	c	p. 1255	Maternal and Fetal Infection
64–32	a	p. 1255	Screening and Diagnosis
64–33	a	p. 1256	Management
64–34	d	p. 1257	West Nile Virus
64–35	c	p. 1258	Anthrax

Sexually Transmitted Infections

65–1. Which of the following does not increase the risk of transmission of syphilis?

  a. Cervical inversion

  b. Cervical hyperemia

  c. Cervical friability

  d. Abrasions of the vaginal mucosa

65–2. The incubation period of syphilis is which of the following?

  a. 1–7 days

  b. 10 days

  c. 3–90 days

  d. 120–180 days

65–3. A 21-year-old G4P2 at 17 weeks' gestation presents for her first prenatal care visit. She has a history of prostitution, but she denies engaging in such activities for the past month. During examination, a painless lesion is noted on the right labia. A picture of the lesion is provided below. The most likely diagnosis is which of the following?

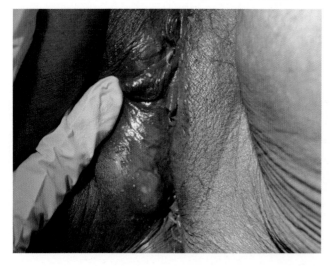

Reproduced with permission from Cunningham FG, Leveno KJ, Bloom SL, et al (eds): Sexually transmitted infections. In Williams Obstetrics, 24th ed. New York, McGraw-Hill, 2014, Figure 65-1.

  a. Chancroid

  b. Primary syphilis

  c. Bartholin gland duct abscess

  d. Herpes simplex virus infection

65–4. The best test to perform for the patient in Question 65–3 to ascertain a definitive diagnosis is which of the following?

  a. Rapid plasma reagin (RPR)

  b. Bacterial culture of lesion exudate

  c. Dark-field examination of lesion exudate

  d. Serum assay for herpes simplex virus 1 and 2 antibodies

65–5. The lesions in this photograph are most indicative of which stage of syphilis?

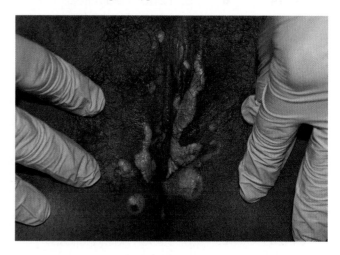

Used with permission from Dr. Jonathan Willms.

  a. Primary

  b. Secondary

  c. Late latent

  d. Early latent

65–6. Findings of secondary syphilis include all **EXCEPT** which of the following?

  a. Fever

  b. Macular rash

  c. Condylomata lata

  d. Strawberry cervix

65–7. A 40-year-old G9P8 at 10 weeks' gestation is found to have a rapid plasma reagin (RPR) of 1:4. Confirmatory testing is positive. She has no signs or symptoms of syphilis. The patient's RPR was nonreactive in all of her prior pregnancies, and she had a nonreactive RPR 6 months ago. Her stage is which of the following?

a. Primary

b. Secondary

c. Late latent

d. Early latent

65–8. A 20-year-old G1P0 at 10 weeks' gestation presents to your office for a rash of her palms and soles. She saw an informational poster on syphilis, and she is concerned that she has it. Her RPR titer is 1:64, and confirmatory testing is positive. The appropriate treatment is which of the following?

a. Benzathine penicillin G, 2.4 million units intramuscularly, weekly for two doses

b. Benzathine penicillin G, 2.4 million units intramuscularly, weekly for three doses

c. Benzathine penicillin G, 2.4 million units intramuscularly, weekly for four doses

d. Aqueous procaine penicillin, 2.4 million units intramuscularly, plus probenecid 500 mg orally four times daily, both for 10 days

65–9. The patient in Question 65–8 does not come to any of her subsequent appointments. Now at 36 weeks' gestation, she represents, you repeat her RPR, and it is 1:128. The most likely reason for this is which of the following?

a. Laboratory error

b. Successful treatment

c. Reinfection or treatment failure

d. Coexistent systemic lupus erythematosus

65–10. A pregnant woman with syphilis and a true penicillin allergy should be treated with which of the following?

a. Erythromycin

b. Azithromycin

c. Doxycycline, after delivery

d. Benzathine penicillin G, after desensitization

65–11. All **EXCEPT** which of the following are manifestations of a Jarisch-Herxheimer reaction in a pregnant woman treated for syphilis?

a. Contractions

b. Night sweats

c. Decreased fetal movement

d. Late fetal heart rate decelerations

65–12. In women with gonorrhea, what percent also have chlamydial infection?

a. 1%

b. 40%

c. 75%

d. 100%

65–13. Risk factors for gonorrhea that should prompt screening in pregnancy include all **EXCEPT** which of the following?

a. Drug use

b. Age > 25 years

c. New sexual partner

d. Prior gonococcal infection

65–14. The current recommendation for the treatment of uncomplicated gonococcal infection in pregnancy is which of the following?

a. Azithromycin 1 g orally as a single dose

b. Ceftriaxone 250 mg intramuscularly as a single dose

c. Erythromycin ethylsuccinate 400 mg orally four times daily for 14 days

d. Ceftriaxone 250 mg intramuscularly as a single dose plus azithromycin 1 g orally as a single dose

65–15. A 15-year-old G1P0 presents at 18 weeks' gestation complaining of pain of her wrists, the tops of her hands, ankles, and the tops of her feet. She has never experienced anything like this previously. She has no medical problems and eight lifetime sexual partners. A nucleic acid amplification test is positive for gonorrhea, and you suspect disseminated infection. The treatment for this is which of the following?

a. Azithromycin 1 g orally as a single dose

b. Ceftriaxone 250 mg intramuscularly as a single dose

c. Ceftriaxone 250 mg intramuscularly as a single dose plus azithromycin 1 g orally as a single dose

d. Ceftriaxone 1000 mg intravenously every 24 hours continued for 24 to 48 hours after improvement followed by oral therapy to complete a week of treatment

65–16. With 1.4 million cases reported in 2011, which of the following is the most commonly reported infectious disease in the United States?

a. Chancroid

b. Gonorrhea

c. Genital herpes

d. *Chlamydia trachomatis* infection

65–17. The most commonly identifiable infectious cause of ophthalmia neonatorum is which of the following?

a. *Haemophilus ducreyi*

b. *Chlamydia trachomatis*

c. *Trichomonas vaginalis*

d. *Neisseria gonorrhoeae*

65–18. First-line treatment for a chlamydial infection in pregnancy is which of the following?

a. Azithromycin 1000 mg orally as a single dose

b. Ofloxacin 300 mg orally twice a day for 7 days

c. Doxycycline 100 mg orally twice a day for 7 days

d. Erythromycin base 250 mg orally four times a day for 14 days

65–19. What percentage of pregnant women acquire herpes simplex virus-1 (HSV-1) or HSV-2 during pregnancy?

a. 0–0.1

b. 0.5–2

c. 5–7.5

d. 10–15

65–20. The most common route of neonatal HSV transmission is which of the following?

a. Postnatal

b. Peripartum

c. Intrauterine

d. Preconceptional

65–21. A patient who has HSV-2 isolated from genital secretions in the absence of HSV-1 or HSV-2 antibodies is classified as which of the following?

a. Transient infection

b. Reactivation disease

c. First episode primary infection

d. First episode nonprimary infection

65–22. A 19-year-old G2P0 at 18 weeks' gestation presents to the emergency room complaining of painful lesions of the perineum. She reports fever at home. A photograph of the patient's perineum is provided below. The best next step in the management of this patient is which of the following?

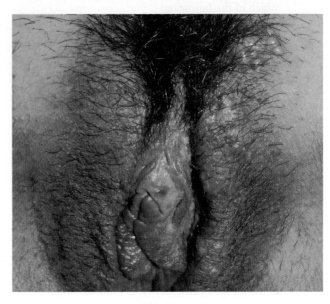

Reproduced with permission from Cunningham FG, Leveno KJ, Bloom SL, et al (eds): Sexually transmitted infections. In Williams Obstetrics, 24th ed. New York, McGraw-Hill, 2014, Figure 65-5.

a. Obtain lesion exudate for viral culture

b. Send human immunodeficiency virus (HIV) testing

c. Diagnose patient with HSV by clinical presentation alone

d. Send spinal fluid for HSV polymerase chain reaction (PCR) assay

65–23. At 36 weeks' gestation, you elect to provide the patient in Question 65–22 acyclovir suppression. You do this for all **EXCEPT** which of the following reasons?

a. It will decrease viral shedding.

b. It reduces the chances of the newborn acquiring herpes to zero.

c. It will decrease the chance of her having an outbreak at term.

d. It will decrease the chances of her requiring a cesarean delivery because of an outbreak.

65–24. A 27-year-old G2P1 at 39 weeks' gestation presents in active labor. The patient is known to have genital herpes, so a thorough exam is performed for lesions. No lesions are seen on the perineum or cervix, but a suspicious lesion is seen on her lower thigh. It is tender to the touch and suggestive of a herpetic lesion. Your plan of management is which of the following?

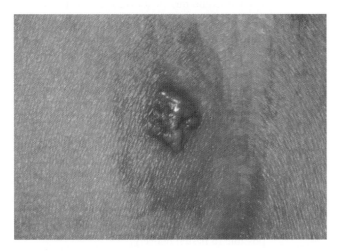

- **a.** Cesarean delivery
- **b.** Acyclovir and tocolysis
- **c.** Occlusive dressing over the lesion and vaginal delivery
- **d.** No change in management from any other patient in labor preparing for a vaginal delivery

65–25. After delivery of the patient in Question 65–24, she asks you if she can breast feed her infant given that she has active HSV. You counsel her which of the following?

- **a.** She should not breast feed.
- **b.** She can breast feed, but only if she is not taking acyclovir.
- **c.** She can breast feed while taking acyclovir but not valacyclovir.
- **d.** She can breast feed, provided she has no breast lesions and practices strict hand washing.

65–26. A 40-year-old G3P1 at 18 weeks' gestation comes to see you for a second opinion. A photograph of her perineum is provided below. She would like treatment, but her current doctor refuses because he feels the lesions will decrease in size after pregnancy. Which of the following treatments would be acceptable for use in pregnancy?

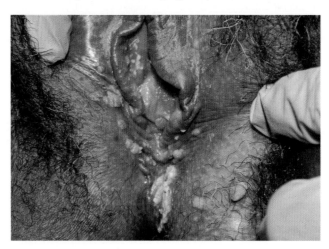

- **a.** Imiquimod
- **b.** Podophyllin resin
- **c.** Interferon therapy
- **d.** Trichloracetic acid

65–27. You see a 20-year-old G1P0 at 10 weeks' gestation in your office for Gardasil exposure. The patient reports that she received the first dose 1 month ago and before she knew she was pregnant. Your plan of care is which of the following?

- **a.** Continue the series as any damage has already been done
- **b.** Delay the remaining doses until the patient has delivered
- **c.** Delay the remaining doses until the patient has delivered and completed her breast feeding
- **d.** Recommend termination of pregnancy because of the strong likelihood of a significant fetal anomaly

65–28. Risk factors for bacterial vaginosis include all **EXCEPT** which of the following?

- **a.** Smoking
- **b.** Douching
- **c.** Vitamin D deficiency
- **d.** Advanced maternal age

65–29. A 15-year-old G1P0 at 15 weeks' presents to the emergency room complaining of foul-smelling, gray, watery discharge. She also has pruritus. The results of the wet mount are provided. The diagnosis is which of the following?

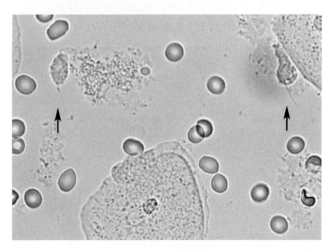

Used with permission from Dr. Lauri Campagna and Rebecca Winn, WHNP.

    a. Gonorrhea

    b. Candidiasis

    c. Trichomoniasis

    d. Bacterial vaginosis

65–30. When is transmission of human immunodeficiency virus (HIV) from a woman to her baby most likely to occur?

    a. Intrapartum

    b. Before 36 weeks' gestation

    c. In the days before delivery

    d. Transmission occurs equally throughout gestation

65–31. Which of the following statements about the treatment of HIV in pregnancy is true?

    a. Treatment is recommended for all HIV-infected pregnant women.

    b. All medications used for the treatment of HIV are safe in pregnancy.

    c. Treatment is only required if the HIV-infected woman would qualify for treatment when not pregnant.

    d. Zidovudine must be added to whatever regimen the woman is already taking, even if her viral load is adequately suppressed.

65–32. Which of the following statements regarding intrapartum management of HIV is true?

    a. If cesarean delivery is planned, it should be scheduled at 36 weeks' gestation.

    b. Cesarean delivery is recommended for women with a viral load > 1000 copies/mL.

    c. In labor, with a plan for vaginal delivery, amniotomy should be performed as soon as possible to hasten delivery.

    d. In labor, internal monitors should be placed because fetuses of HIV-infected women are at increased risk for distress.

CHAPTER 65 ANSWER KEY

Question number	Letter answer	Page cited	Header cited
65–1	a	p. 1265	Pathogenesis and Transmission
65–2	c	p. 1265	Pathogenesis and Transmission
65–3	b	p. 1266	Figure 65-1
65–4	c	p. 1267	Diagnosis
65–5	b	p. 1266	Clinical Manifestations
65–6	d	p. 1266	Clinical Manifestations
65–7	d	p. 1266	Clinical Manifestations
65–8	a	p. 1268	Treatment
65–9	c	p. 1268	Treatment
65–10	d	p. 1268	Penicillin Allergy
65–11	b	p. 1268	Penicillin Allergy
65–12	b	p. 1269	Gonorrhea
65–13	b	p. 1269	Gonorrhea
65–14	d	p. 1269	Screening and Treatment
65–15	d	p. 1270	Disseminated Gonococcal Infections
65–16	d	p. 1270	Chlamydial Infections
65–17	b	p. 1270	Chlamydial Infections
65–18	a	p. 1270	Screening and Treatment
65–19	b	p. 1271	Herpes Simplex Virus (HSV)
65–20	b	p. 1271	Pathogenesis and Transmission
65–21	c	p. 1271	Clinical Manifestations
65–22	a	p. 1273	Diagnosis
65–23	b	p. 1273	Peripartum Shedding Prophylaxis
65–24	c	p. 1273	Peripartum Shedding Prophylaxis
65–25	d	p. 1273	Peripartum Shedding Prophylaxis
65–26	d	p. 1275	Treatment
65–27	b	p. 1275	Immunization
65–28	d	p. 1276	Bacterial Vaginosis
65–29	c	p. 1276	Trichomoniasis
65–30	c	p. 1278	Maternal and Perinatal Transmission
65–31	a	p. 1279	Antiretroviral Therapy
65–32	b	p. 1281	Prenatal HIV Transmission

INDEX

Note: Page numbers followed by *f* represent figures.